T0227028

Functional Hand Reconstruction

Guest Editor

MICHAEL W. NEUMEISTER, MD, FRCSC, FACS

CLINICS IN PLASTIC SURGERY

www.plasticsurgery.theclinics.com

October 2011 • Volume 38 • Number 4

SAUNDERS an imprint of ELSEVIER, Inc.

W.B. SAUNDERS COMPANY
A Division of Elsevier Inc.

1600 John F. Kennedy Boulevard • Suite 1800 • Philadelphia, Pennsylvania 19103-2899

http://www.theclinics.com

CLINICS IN PLASTIC SURGERY Volume 38, Number 4
October 2011 ISSN 0094-1298, ISBN-13: 978-1-4557-0983-0

Editor: Joanne Husovski
Developmental Editor: Teia Stone

Clinics in Plastic Surgery (ISSN 0094-1298) is published quarterly by Elsevier Inc., 360 Park Avenue South, New York, NY 10010-1710. Months of issue are January, April, July, and October. Business and Editorial Offices: 1600 John F. Kennedy Blvd., Suite 1800, Philadelphia, PA 19103-2899. Periodicals postage paid at New York, NY and additional mailing offices. Subscription prices are $411.00 per year for US individuals, $617.00 per year for US institutions, $203.00 per year for US students and residents, $467.00 per year for Canadian individuals, $721.00 per year for Canadian institutions, $530.00 per year for international individuals, $721.00 per year for international institutions, and $256.00 per year for Canadian and foreign students/residents. To receive student/resident rate, orders must be accompanied by name of affiliated institution, date of term, and the *signature* of program/residency coordinator on institution letterhead. Orders will be billed at individual rate until proof of status is received. Foreign air speed delivery is included in all *Clinics* subscription prices. All prices are subject to change without notice. **POSTMASTER:** Send address changes to *Clinics in Plastic Surgery*, Elsevier Health Sciences Division, Subscription Customer Service, 3251 Riverport Lane, Maryland Heights, MO 63043. **Customer Service: 1-800-654-2452 (US and Canada). From outside of the United States and Canada, call 314-447-8871. Fax: 314-447-8029. E-mail: JournalsCustomerService-usa@elsevier.com (for print support); JournalsOnlineSupport-usa@ elsevier.com (for online support).**

Reprints. For copies of 100 or more of articles in this publication, please contact the Commercial Reprints Department, Elsevier Inc., 360 Park Avenue South, New York, New York 10010-1710. Tel.: (+1) 212-633-3812; Fax: (+1) 212-462-1935; E-mail: reprints@elsevier.com.

Clinics in Plastic Surgery is covered in *Current Contents, EMBASE/Excerpta Medica, Science Citation Index, MEDLINE/ PubMed (Index Medicus), ASCA,* and *ISI/BIOMED.*

Printed and bound by CPI Group (UK) Ltd, Croydon, CR0 4YY

Transferred to Digital Print 2011

Contributors

GUEST EDITOR

MICHAEL W. NEUMEISTER, MD, FRCSC, FACS
Professor and Division Chair, Department of Plastic Surgery, Division of Plastic Surgery, Southern Illinois University School of Medicine, Springfield, Illinois

AUTHORS

ASHLEY AMALFI, MD
PGY IV Resident, Department of Plastic Surgery, Division of Plastic Surgery, Southern Illinois University School of Medicine, Springfield, Illinois

DIMITRI J. ANASTAKIS, MD
Professor of Surgery, Chair, Division of Plastic and Reconstructive Surgery, University of Toronto, Toronto, Ontario, Canada

NINA BIEDERMANN, MD
ETHIANUM – Clinic for Plastic and Reconstructive Surgery, Aesthetic and Preventive Medicine at Heidelberg University Hospital, Heidelberg, Germany

CHANTAL BONNARD, MD
Service de Chirurgie Plastique et Reconstructive et Chirurgie de la main, Clinique de Longeraie, Université de Lausanne, Lausanne, Switzerland

KIRSTY U. BOYD, MD, FRCS(C)
Assistant Professor, Division of Plastic and Reconstructive Surgery, Department of Surgery, University of Ottawa, Ottawa, Ontario, Canada

REUBEN A. BUENO, MD
Associate Professor, Program Director, Division of Plastic Surgery, Institute for Plastic and Reconstructive Surgery, Southern Illinois University School of Medicine, Springfield, Illinois

JAMES CHANG, MD
Professor, Chief, Division of Plastic and Reconstructive Surgery, Department of Surgery, Stanford University Hospitals and Clinics, Palo Alto, California

KEVIN C. CHUNG, MD, MS
Professor of Surgery, Section of Plastic Surgery, Department of Surgery; Assistant Dean for Faculty Affairs, University of Michigan Medical School, Ann Arbor, Michigan

BRIAN M. DERBY, MD
Resident, Department of Plastic Surgery, Division of Plastic Surgery, Southern Illinois University School of Medicine, Springfield, Illinois

POUYA ENTEZAMI, BS
Research Assistant, Section of Plastic Surgery, Department of Surgery, The University of Michigan Health System, Ann Arbor, Michigan

JEFFREY B. FRIEDRICH, MD
Division of Plastic Surgery, Department of Orthopedics, University of Washington, Seattle, Washington

GÜNTER GERMANN, MD, PhD
Professor of Plastic Surgery, Chairman, ETHIANUM – Clinic for Plastic and Reconstructive Surgery, Aesthetic and Preventive Medicine at Heidelberg University Hospital, Heidelberg, Germany

WARREN C. HAMMERT, MD
Associate Professor of Orthopaedic Surgery
and Plastic Surgery, Department of
Orthopaedic Surgery, University of Rochester
Medical Center, Rochester, New York

THERESA HEGGE, MPH, MD
PGY IV Resident, Department of Plastic
Surgery, Division of Plastic Surgery, Southern
Illinois University School of Medicine,
Springfield, Illinois

MEGAN HENDERSON, MD
PGY IV Resident, Department of Plastic
Surgery, Division of Plastic Surgery, Southern
Illinois University School of Medicine,
Springfield, Illinois

JAMES P. HIGGINS, MD
The Curtis National Hand Center,
Baltimore, Maryland

MATTHEW L. IORIO, MD
The Curtis National Hand Center,
Baltimore, Maryland

NEIL F. JONES, MD
Professor and Chief of Hand Surgery, Division
of Plastic and Reconstructive Surgery,
Department of Orthopaedic Surgery, University
of California Irvine Medical Center, Orange,
California

DONALD H. LALONDE, MD, MSc, FRCSC
Professor of Surgery, Department of Plastic
Surgery, Dalhousie University, Saint John,
New Brunswick, Canada

**WEE-LEON LAM, MB ChB, MPhil,
FRCS (Plast)**
Microsurgical Fellow, Department of Plastic
and Reconstructive Surgery, Chang Gung
Memorial Hospital, Taoyuan, Taiwan

SCOTT L. LEVIN, MD, PhD
Chief of Orthopedics, Department of
Orthopedic Surgery, University of
Pennsylvania, Philadelphia, Pennsylvania

GUSTAVO R. MACHADO, MD
Hand Surgery Fellow, Department of
Orthopaedic Surgery, University of California
Irvine Medical Center, Orange, California

SUSAN E. MACKINNON, MD, FRCS(C)
Division of Plastic and Reconstructive Surgery,
Department of Surgery, School of Medicine,
Washington University, St Louis, Missouri

DEREK L. MASDEN, MD
The Curtis National Hand Center,
Baltimore, Maryland

**MICHAEL W. NEUMEISTER, MD,
FRCSC, FACS**
Professor and Division Chair, Department of
Plastic Surgery, Division of Plastic Surgery,
Southern Illinois University School of Medicine,
Springfield, Illinois

ANDRÉ S. NIMIGAN, MD, FRCS(C)
The Medical Centre, Peterborough, Ontario,
Canada

SHIMPEI ONO, MD, PhD
International Research Fellow, Section of
Plastic Surgery, Department of Surgery,
The University of Michigan Health System,
Ann Arbor, Michigan

WILLIAM C. PEDERSON, MD, FACS
The Hand Center of San Antonio and The
University of Texas Health Science Center,
San Antonio, Texas

ALEXANDER SEAL, MPhil, MD, FRCSC
Department of Orthopaedic Surgery, University
of Southern California, USC University
Hospital, LAC + USC Medical Center,
Los Angeles, California

MILAN STEVANOVIC, MD, PhD
Department of Orthopaedic Surgery, University
of Southern California, USC University
Hospital, LAC + USC Medical Center,
Los Angeles, California

NICHOLAS B. VEDDER, MD
Division of Plastic Surgery, Department of
Orthopedics, University of Washington,
Seattle, Washington

ANDREW J. WATT, MD
Division of Plastic and Reconstructive Surgery,
Department of Surgery, Stanford University
Hospitals and Clinics, Palo Alto, California

LAURENT WEHRLI, MD
Service de Chirurgie Plastique et
Reconstructive et Chirurgie de la main,
Clinique de Longeraie, Université de Lausanne,
Lausanne, Switzerland

FU-CHAN WEI, MD, FACS
Professor and Chancellor, Department of
Plastic and Reconstructive Surgery, Chang
Gung Memorial Hospital, College of Medicine,
Chang Gung University, Taoyuan, Taiwan

BRADON J. WILHELMI, MD, FACS
Leonard Weiner Endowed Professor and Chief
of Plastic Surgery, Residency Program Director,
Division of Plastic and Reconstructive Surgery,
Department of Surgery, University of Louisville
School of Medicine, Louisville, Kentucky

ELVIN G. ZOOK, MD
Professor Emeritus, Division of Plastic Surgery,
Department of Plastic Surgery, Southern
Illinois University School of Medicine,
Springfield, Illinois

Contents

Theresa Hegge and Michael W. Neumeister

The authors provide a review of treatment of the mutilated hand, discussing the effect of injury on soft tissue loss, intrinsic and extrinsic musculature, paravascular structures, tendons, and the bony skeleton. The authors review functional loss and restoration.

Wee-Leon Lam and Fu-Chan Wei

Microsurgical toe-to-hand transplantation remains a valuable reconstructive option for severe, mutilated hand injuries ever since its inception in the 1960s, allowing composite replacement of amputated digits through a single-stage procedure with minimal donor morbidity. Increased experience over the past 40 years has allowed establishment of certain principles that yield consistent results with optimal functional and esthetic outcomes. This article critically examines the latest innovations and refinements in the continual pursuit of excellence for microsurgical toe-to-hand transplantation.

Alexander Seal and Milan Stevanovic

Free functional muscle transfers are an excellent treatment option in patients when significant time has passed after a nerve injury. In addition, they are the treatment of choice for reconstruction of established Volkmann's ischemic contracture, muscle loss from trauma, or tumor resection, and in congenital muscle absence. In cases where there is both soft tissue and functional muscle loss, free functional muscle transfers can address these problems together. This article focuses on the key principles for functional reconstruction of the upper extremity with free functional muscle transfers.

Andrew J. Watt and James Chang

Proper hand function relies on a combination of strength and mobility. The intricate architecture that allows for hand mobility includes the articular surfaces of joints, periarticular ligamentous structures, tendon mechanisms, and the soft-tissue envelope. These structures are subject to injury and scarring. The net effect of a variety of etiologic factors is stiffness of the hand with diminution of hand function. This article reviews the biology of healing, pertinent anatomy of the hand, and operative and nonoperative treatment of the stiff hand.

Theresa Hegge, Megan Henderson, Ashley Amalfi, Reuben A. Bueno, and Michael W. Neumeister

This article discusses scar contracture of the hand. It contains a brief outline of the anatomy of the hand and upper extremities and the types of injuries involved. Hand reconstruction, including examination, nonoperative treatment, surgery, excision and skin grafting, flaps, postoperative management, and complications, are covered.

is an important part of caring for patients with hand fractures. The decision to intervene must be based on the likelihood of achieving the desired correction, and improving the function, of the hand. This article reviews principles of diagnosis and treatment of non-unions and malunions, including conditions affecting the thumb and pediatric patients.

anatomy, clinical challenges, and risk-benefit profiles of each option. The review is limited to salvage reconstructive procedures of the small joints of the hand.

Reconstruction of the Hand with Wide Awake Surgery   761

Donald H. Lalonde

Wide awake hand surgery means no sedation, no tourniquet, and no general anesthesia for hand surgery. The only medications given to the patient are lidocaine with epinephrine. Lidocaine is for anesthesia, and epinephrine provides hemostasis, which deletes the need for a tourniquet. The advantages are: (1) the ability of the comfortable unsedated tourniquet-free patient to perform active movement of the reconstructed structures during surgery so the surgeon can make alterations to the reconstruction before the skin is closed to improve the outcome of many surgeries; and (2) the deletion of all risks, costs, and inconveniences of sedation and general anesthesia.

Index   771

Erratum

In the July 2011 issue of *Clinics in Plastic Surgery,* the descriptive labels in Figure 22 in the article by Swift and Remington, BEAUTIPHICATION™: A GLOBAL APPROACH TO FACIAL BEAUTY, were incorrectly presented.

Figure 22 is reprinted here correctly: The Beauti"phi"ed Brow: Begins vertically in-line with the medial canthus (*a*); lies phi above the bony rim from the pupil; has a 10 to 20 degree climb from medial to lateral (*b*); is arched at a distance equal to the intercanthal distance (*x*) which is phi of the total eyebrow length [the point crossed by a line drawn from the alar base tangential to the lateral aspect of the pupil (*c*)]; has a lateral tip higher than the medial tip; is Phi of the medial canthus in length [delineated by a line drawn from the lateral alar base through the lateral canthus (*d*)]; and has tissue fullness over the lateral supraorbital rim.

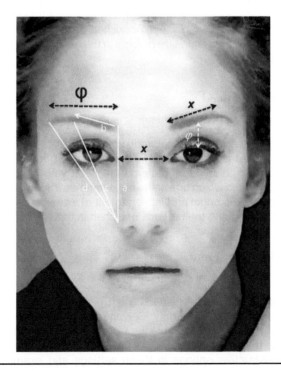

Clinics in Plastic Surgery

THE CLINICS ARE AVAILABLE ONLINE!

Access your subscription at:
www.theclinics.com

From Dysfunction to Function in Hand and Upper Limb Reconstruction

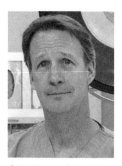

Michael W. Neumeister, MD, FRCSC
Guest Editor

Reconstruction of the upper extremity is designed primarily to restore function. The limb without function becomes a burden or liability to the patient. The challenges that surgeons face to restore that which was lost from injury, cancer resection, or disease are based on the principles of forefathers in hand surgery. Dysfunction may arise from soft tissue contractures, nerve or tendon loss or damage, amputations, ischemia, malunion or nonunion, stiffness, or pain. New innovation and improvements of established techniques are continuously updating the methods used for any given area of reconstruction.

As doctors, we are consummate learners and educators. This *Clinics in Plastic Surgery* title in Hand Reconstruction brings together world experts who have learned through research and clinical experience and who educate through sharing new information. Each expert focuses on a different aspect of functional reconstruction of the upper extremity. Many secondary procedures can be prevented or perhaps minimized if the initial treatment of the acute injuries follows sound principles. Residual loss of function is managed after the acute setting and usually after therapy has plateaued. This issue describes surgical procedures that provide reliable and consistent results. The collaborative efforts of the therapists and the surgeons are highlighted. My overall goal of this review in *Clinics in Plastic Surgery* was to illustrate the newest techniques and treatment algorithms for specific causes of upper limb dysfunction. All critical areas that can render the hand or upper extremity functionless are compiled in one focused publication and their treatment remedies are described in detail to offer a comprehensive understanding of the secondary procedures used today for reconstruction.

I would like to thank all of the esteemed contributors for their hard work, time, and gracious efforts in helping to make this review publication possible. Their pursuit of optimal function for their patients is reflected in the tremendous quality of their articles. A special thank you also goes out to Joanne Husovski and Elsevier for professional assistance and her positive attitude during the creation of this issue of *Clinics in Plastic Surgery*.

Michael W. Neumeister, MD, FRCSC
Department of Plastic Surgery
Division of Plastic Surgery
Southern Illinois University School of Medicine
747 North Rutledge, Third Floor
Springfield, IL 62702, USA

E-mail address:
mneumeister@siumed.edu

doi:10.1016/j.cps.2011.09.003
0094-1298/11/$ – see front matter

plasticsurgery.theclinics.com

Mutilated Hand Injuries

Theresa Hegge, MPH, MD,
Michael W. Neumeister, MD, FRCSC*

KEYWORDS

- Mutilated hand • Acute trauma • Crush injury
- Avulsion injury • Hand reconstruction • Hand function

Mutilated hand injuries are one of the most challenging reconstruction problems than can confront hand surgeons (**Fig. 1**).[1] Injuries occur by a variety of mechanisms, including crush, avulsion, friction, or sharp trauma. Because of the nature of the trauma and the intricate balance of hand structures, these injuries may result in devastating compromise of function of the entire extremity and impair the quality of daily living.[2] Mutilating injuries not only involve soft tissue loss but also damage the intrinsic and extrinsic musculature, paravascular structures, tendons, and the bony skeleton, requiring complex problem solving to restore function.

The American Medical Association has developed the guidelines for the evaluation of permanent impairment, which described the functional contribution of each digit to the hand, upper extremity, and the entire body. Loss of the thumb results in a 40% loss of function and 25% loss of total body function.[3] Although other digits are not rated as high, each one has its specific functional contribution. The radial digits are important for key and chuck pinch, whereas the ulnar digits are more important for grip strength and strong grasp. Compromise to any digit translates to a functional deficit with enormous implications for individuals who work with their hands.

The proper evaluation of outcomes includes not only the assessment of overall function but also the ability to perform the desired work and activities of daily living, pain, total range of motion, sensation, and grip strength.[2] These outcomes paired with patient and physician priorities direct the reconstructive efforts.[4]

INITIAL EVALUATION

Although the mangled extremity is often one of the most obvious of injuries, each patient should undergo an initial trauma evaluation to rule out more life-threatening injuries.[5] After stabilization and initial resuscitation, the physician can further address limb salvage and functional reconstruction. The functional restoration of the upper extremity relies on many factors. The patient's premorbid functional status, handedness, occupation, general medical status, and socioeconomic status are all important in treating the patient.[2] Comorbidation, such as diabetes and heart and pulmonary disease, can complicate acute medical and surgical care but can also be contributing factors to compliance with postoperative therapy.[6]

Functional Outcome

The functional outcome depends ultimately on various factors such as mechanism of injury, ischemia time, contamination, and tissue loss. The final outcome also depends on the ability of secondary procedures to reconstruct tissue, release contractures and adhesions, or restore nerve, muscle, or tendon responsibility.[7]

If tissue is amputated and replantation is contemplated, the ischemia time will be critical. An attempt should be made to instruct the field staff on proper care during transport of the

Department of Plastic Surgery, Division of Plastic Surgery, Southern Illinois University School of Medicine, 747 North Rutledge, Third Floor, Springfield, IL 62702, USA
* Corresponding author.
E-mail address: mneumeister@siumed.edu

Clin Plastic Surg 38 (2011) 543–550
doi:10.1016/j.cps.2011.08.004
0094-1298/11/$ – see front matter © 2011 Elsevier Inc. All rights reserved.

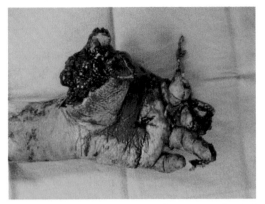

Fig. 1. Mutilating injuries can be extremely challenging due to the nature of the trauma. A surgical plan is formulated, pending requirements for reconstruction.

amputated part. Immediate cooling of any amputated parts should be achieved by wrapping the parts in moist saline gauze and placing them into a sealed bag on ice.[1] Those amputated parts that have less muscle can withstand greater ischemia times. The degradation products of muscle can be detrimental to life. These byproducts include high potassium and myoglobin levels that can disrupt cardiac and kidney function, respectively. There are no muscles within digits; therefore, ischemia is well tolerated in digits. The recommended ischemia times are 12 hours for warm and 24 hours for cold ischemic digits and 6 hours for warm and 12 hours cold ischemia for other more proximal replants that involve greater amounts of muscle.[8] Although longer times have resulted in success, such as 94 hours of cold ischemic digits,[9] 54 hours of cold ischemia in the hand,[10] and 42 hours of warm ischemia,[11] these prolonged ischemia times are not globally achievable or advisable.

SURGERY FOR THE MUTILATED HAND

The mainstay of the initial surgery should include irrigation, debridement, and treating the wound like a pseudotumor (**Fig. 2**).[1,5] The wound is thoroughly debrided of any devitalized tissue or contamination. The vascular status can be evaluated not only through color and skin turgor but also through direct bleeding of surrounding tissues. Reconstructive efforts can be delayed until a second- or third-look procedure is performed to make sure that contamination or infection is

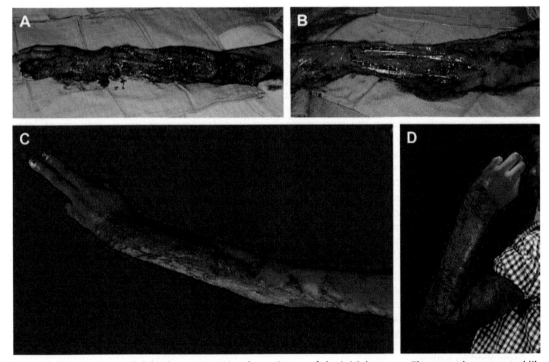

Fig. 2. (A–D) Irrigation and debridement remains the mainstay of the initial surgery. The wounds are treated like a pseudotumor, removing all devitalized tissue and contamination. Coverage can be delayed until the surgeon thinks the wound is stable with minimal risk of infection and viable tissue demarcation.

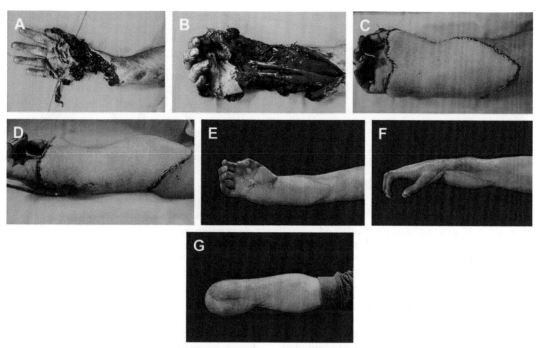

Fig. 3. (*A, B*) A 38-year-old man who sustained a severe near-amputation crush injury to his right hand. Segmental loss of tendons, nerves, and soft tissue were reconstructed using vein grafts for revascularization, tendon grafts, and nerve grafts. (*C, D*) A perforator anterolateral thigh free flap was used to cover the soft tissue defect. (*E, F*) Because of the severe crush injury mutilation to the hand, function was not restored. The hand was painful and motionless. (*G*) Patient opted for an amputation and prosthesis fitting instead of the useless dysfunctional hand.

minimized. Vascular compromise may require arterial repair or vein transplants to the initial surgery. Nerve repairs should also be performed with microsurgical assistance. Other aspects of microsurgical care can be delayed, including definitive coverage with free tissue transfer.[7]

Free Tissue Transfers

Free tissue transfers at the time of the initial surgery are rarely, if ever, indicated. The exceptions to that rule is the use of spare parts, in which amputated segments of the extremity can be used as a free tissue transfer to close exposed structures (**Fig. 3** A–C).[12] In this scenario, the amputated part was otherwise to be discarded, and, therefore, its potential as spare parts should be used. Replantation is another indication for emergent microsurgical techniques. In multiple digit replants, the current philosophy is to perform structure by structure as opposed to digit by digit.[13–15] This method seems to optimize operative time.

Reconstruction

The principles of reconstruction of the various tissues in the mutilated upper extremity should follow those principles identified for each indivial structure within the hand. That is, all the important principles of repair and reconstruction apply to individual tissues such as tendons, nerves, arteries, bone, and skin. Bony fixation proceeds soft tissue repair (**Fig. 4**). The optimum treatment of fractures is dictated somewhat by the pattern and location of the fracture.[2] However, surgeon preference and comfort level is probably the most important factor because each type of fixation affects its own inherent advantages and disadvantages (**Table 1**).[16] Tendon repair and/or reconstruction proceeds soft tissue coverage but need not be delayed for secondary surgery. Primary tendon transfers and repair affect early outcomes with fewer secondary procedures and foster return to function.

Devastating injury to multiple tissues usually portends a rather poor prognosis in terms of return to normal function (see **Fig. 3**).[2] Surgeons should adhere to the initial principles but fully understand and plan for secondary procedures that may be warranted. These secondary procedures may be required to release scar tissue, improve range of motion, provide soft tissue coverage, counteract

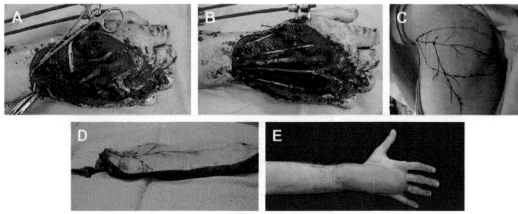

Fig. 4. (*A*) A 37-year-old man who sustained a significant devastating injury to the dorsal aspect of his hand. Multiple tendons were disrupted and segmental loss observed. (*B*) After debridement and irrigation, the tendons were repaired. The segmental loss is reconstructed immediately with extensor indices proprius and extensor digiti minimi tendons transfers. (*C*, *D*) A scapular flap was designed to offer a thin pliable skin for the dorsal aspect of the hand. (*E*) Final result with stable coverage.

contractures, restore sensation, and provide bony stabilization. The surgeon should start to formulate the definitive surgical architectural plan for subsequent reconstructions even at the initial surgery (**Figs. 5–7**).[7]

Although the initial management of the acute mutilating injuries should try to restore as much function as possible, if functioning muscle or nerve/tendon transfers are planned for future reconstruction, a fasciocutaneous flap for soft tissue coverage provides the most appropriate coverage. However, segmental bone loss and segmental loss of tendon, nerve, and soft tissue can be dealt with during the secondary reconstruction procedures to restore function if primary repair or reconstruction is not an option. A well-planned staged procedure is often better than trying to accomplish too much at the initial injury.

Table 1
Advantages and disadvantages of different types of bone fixation

Fixation	Advantages	Disadvantages
Kirschner wire & interosseous wire	Fast, easy, less foreign body load	Not a rigid fixation, requires prolonged immobilization to obtain bone healing, external Kirschner wire may serve as a portal to bacteria
Tendon band	Strong, fast	Restriction of motion, irritation from wire ends
Plates	Strong, able to contour to bone shape, can start range of motion early, stable, rigid fixation, permits primary healing	Periosteal stripping may devascularize bone fragments, larger foreign body load, restrictive in digits
Lag screws	Compressive and strong, allows early range of motion, permits stable rigid fixation and primary healing	Not all fractures amenable to screws, ie, transverse; requires greater technical expertise
External fixation	Stable fixation, bridges boney gaps, keeps digit out to length	Limits range of motion, bulky, pin tract infection

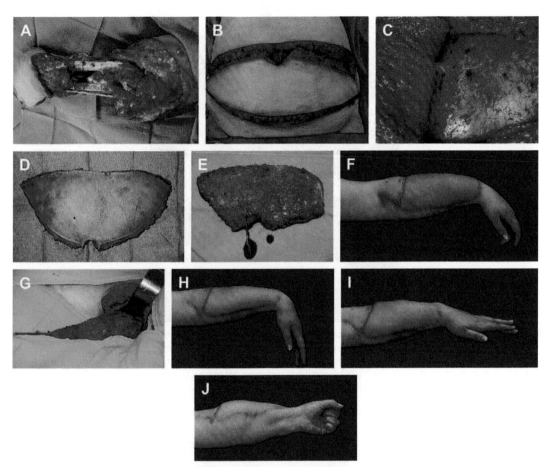

Fig. 5. (*A*) A 19-year-old women involved in a motor vehicle accident sustained a devastating injury in the left upper extremity. After debridement, irrigation, and osteosynthesis, the wound is ready for soft tissue closure. (*B–E*) Anticipating secondary procedures such as a functioning muscle transfer for the hand exterior muscles, a fasciocutaneous flap was designed. A deep inferior epigastric perforator flap was used because of the enormous amount of tissue that could be harvested with a minimal donor site. (*F*) After contouring of the flap, the patient lacked extension. (*G*) The flexor muscles had been injured at the original injury necessitating a functioning muscle gracilis flap to be used to restore extensor pollicis longus and extensor digiti communis function. The muscle was tunneled underneath the fasciocutaneous flap. (*H–J*) Contour was maintained and function restored in a staged reconstruction.

Fasciocutaneous Flaps

Coverage of defects in the upper extremity after mutilating injuries can be accomplished in many ways (**Figs. 8–10**).[17] Fasciocutaneous flaps, facial flaps, and muscle flaps are often used for definitive coverage (**Fig. 11**). It is often desirable to have fasciocutaneous flap for coverage if secondary reconstruction, such as tendon or ligament repair, is anticipated under the flap. Muscle flaps often become fibrotic, making secondary elevation somewhat difficult in prolonged procedures that require tendon, nerve, or ligament reconstruction. Fasciocutaneous flaps that are too bulky can be debulked easily at a third or fourth procedure.

POSTOPERATIVE CONCERNS

Complications and secondary procedures are common in mutilating hand injuries, but reconstruction is functionally more advantageous over upper extremity prosthesis. Complications include stiffness, contracture, cold intolerance, pain, scarring, loss of sensibility, and psychosocial implications. The process of reconstruction of mutilating injuries may take many years. This procedure requires significant patient compliance and surgical effort and represents one of the most challenging aspects of hand surgery. Innovation and perseverance have the potential to dramatically change the functional outcomes of patients with such injuries. The best practice of these

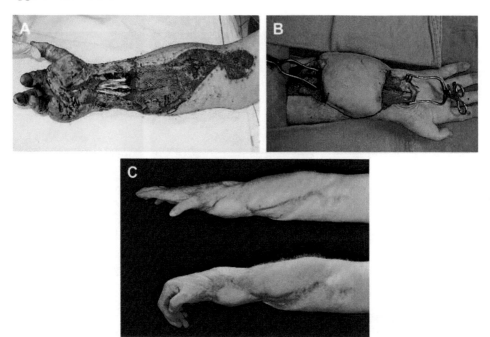

Fig. 6. (*A*) A 53-year-old electrical worker sustained an electrical burn. After stabilization of the patient's condition, exposed tendons and nerves were observed, as well as soft tissue defect circumferentially around the wrist. (*B*) An anterolateral thigh free flap was used to offer soft tissue coverage in anticipation of secondary procedures such as tendon grafts and nerve grafts. (*C*) Functional outcome after free tissue transfer for soft tissue coverage. Multiple secondary procedures, including tendon grafts, nerve grafts, capsulotomies, and tenolysis procedures, were done.

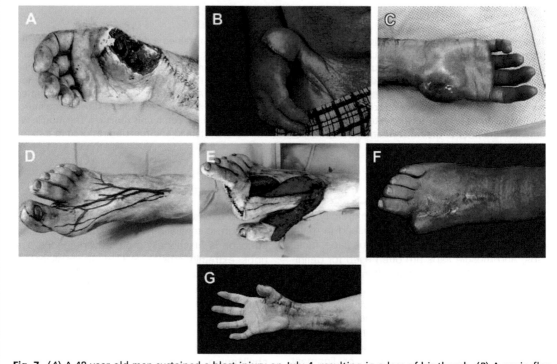

Fig. 7. (*A*) A 48-year-old man sustained a blast injury on July 4, resulting in a loss of his thumb. (*B*) A groin flap was used to provide stable coverage in anticipation of secondary procedures such as pollicization or toe-to-hand transfer. (*C*) The groin flap was divided and inset and allowed to mature. (*D, E*) A free toe-to-hand transfer was designed. (*F, G*) A functional result of a toe-to-hand transfer and the donor site.

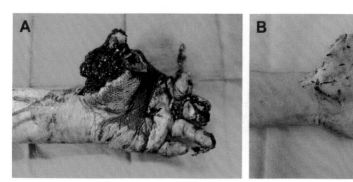

Fig. 8. (*A, B*) Coverage of defects in the upper extremity may be as simple as revision amputation and skin transplants.

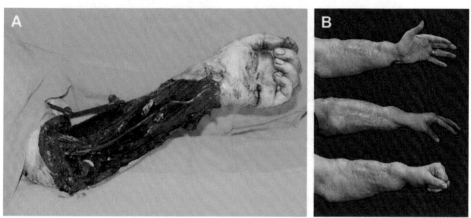

Fig. 9. (*A, B*) A 35-year-old woman with a devastating injury to the left upper extremity. Exposed vital structures necessitated flap closure. The size of the defect required a large amount of tissue. An anterolateral thigh free tissue transfer was used to provide appropriate coverage.

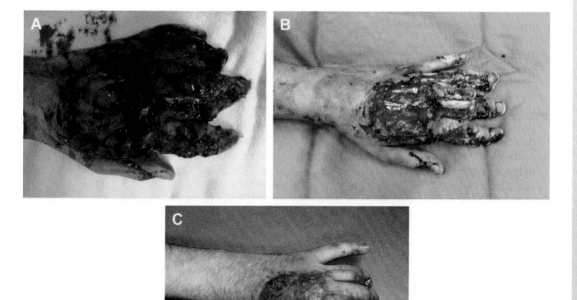

Fig. 10. (*A, B*) A 24-year-old girl with a mutilating injury to the dorsal aspect of the hand underwent debridement and irrigation. (*C*) Definitive coverage was obtained using a cellular dermal matrix skin substitute (Integra®).

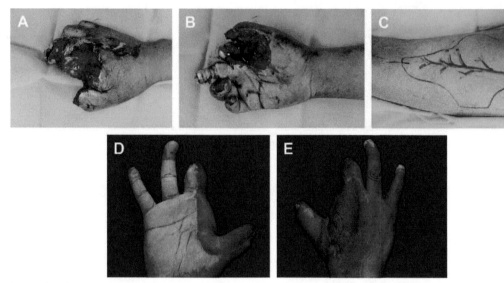

Fig. 11. (*A, B*) A 38-year-old man sustained a mutilating injury to his right hand involving amputation of his index finger and partial loss to the thumb and long finger. (*C*) An anterolateral thigh tissue transfer was designed on the left thigh. (*D, E*) The flap was thinned and contoured to the size of the defect. Further debulking procedures produced the final outcome.

mangled injuries should be elucidated and reconstructive efforts and outcomes improved.

REFERENCES

1. Neumeister MW, Brown RE. Mutilating hand injuries: principles and management. Hand Clin 2003;19(1):1–16.
2. Bueno RA, Neumeister MW. Outcomes after mutilating hand injuries: review of the literature and recommendations for assessment. Hand Clin 2003;19(1):193–204.
3. Rondinelli R, editor. Guides to the evaluation of permanent impairment, 19. 6th edition. Chicago: American Medical Association; 2007. p. 1–15, 2003.
4. Axelrod TS, Buchler U. Severe complex injuries to the upper extremity: revascularization and replantation. J Hand Surg 1991;164(4):574–84.
5. Vedder N, Hanel D. The mangled upper extremity. In: Green DP, Hotchkiss RN, Pederson WC, et al, editors. Green's operative hand surgery. Philadelphia: Elsevier; 2005. p. 1587–628.
6. Brown HC, Wiliams HB, Woodhouse FM. Principles of salvage in mutilating hand injuries. J Trauma 1968;8:318–21.
7. Russell RC, Bueno RA, Wu TT. Secondary procedures following mutilating hand injuries. Hand Clin 2003;19(1):149–64.
8. Wilhelmi B, Lee A, Pagensteert G, et al. Replantation in the mutilated hand. Hand Clin 2003;19:89–120.
9. Wei FC, Chen HC, Chuang CC. Three successful digital replantations in a patient after 84, 86, and 94 hours' cold ischemia time. Plast Reconstr Surg 1988;82(2):346–50.
10. VanderWilde RS, Wood MB, Zeng-gui S. Hand replantation after 54 hours of cold ischemia: a case report. J Hand Surg 1992;17(2):217–20.
11. Baek SM, Kim SS. Successful digital replantation after 42 hours of warm ischemia. J Reconstr Microsurg 1992;9:455.
12. Russell RC, Neumeister MW, Ostric SA, et al. Extremity reconstruction using nonreplantable tissue ("spare parts"). Clin Plast Surg 2007;34(2):211–22.
13. Medling BD, Bueno RA Jr, Russell RC, et al. Replantation outcomes. Clin Plast Surg 2007;34(2):177–85.
14. O'Brian BM. Replantation surgery. Clin Plast Surg 1974;1:405–26.
15. Graham B, Adkins P, Tsai TM, et al. Major replantation versus revision amputation and prosthetic fitting in the upper extremity: a later functional outcomes study. J Hand Surg 1998;123:783–91.
16. Freeland AE, Lineaweaver WC, Lindley SG. Fracture fixation in the mutilated hand. Hand Clin 2003;19(1):51–62.
17. Neumeister MW, Hegge T, Amalfi A, et al. The reconstruction of the mutilated hand. Semin Plast Surg 2010;24(1):77–102.

Toe-to-Hand Transplantation

Wee-Leon Lam, MB ChB, MPhil, FRCS (Plast)[a],
Fu-Chan Wei, MD[b],*

KEYWORDS

- Toe-to-hand transplantation • Metacarpal hand
- Thumb reconstruction

This article attempts to summarize some of these most recent innovations, many of which have been built on previous foundations that had remained surprisingly unchanged over the past four decades. Each section will generally describe what is accepted as current or established practice, examine what is new or controversial and finally offer concluding views on the subject. Ever since the first toe-to-hand procedure, as reported by Nicolandi with the use of a pedicled great toe,[1] the logic of using toes to replace digits was immediately appreciated but not widely practiced until the advent of microsurgery. The first successful microvascular toe-to-hand transplantations were carried out by Yang and Gu[2] and Cobbett[3] using the second toe and great toe, respectively, for thumb reconstruction. Since then, toe-to-hand transplantation has occupied a special role in the history of microsurgery, being among the first few free tissue transfers to be attempted in humans and also as a rich source of innovation and technical refinements for microsurgical procedures in general. The ever-growing wealth of literature bears testament to the increasing acceptance of toe-to-hand transplantation and also the ongoing innovations and refinements in the pursuit of excellence. This article attempts to summarize some of these most recent innovations, which are built on previously established foundations, many that remain surprisingly unchanged over the past 4 decades. Each section will generally describe what is accepted as current or established practice, examine what is currently new or controversial, and finally offer concluding views on the subjects.

INITIAL ASSESSMENT AND MANAGEMENT OF THE INJURED HAND
Established Practice

Following digital amputations, the replacement of "like-for-like" tissues that can potentially restore the exacting demands of different digits is achievable only by a successful replantation. In cases of nonreplantable or failed replantations, toe-to-hand transplantations remain the next-best option with a far superior result than the use of prosthesis or other nonmicrosurgical techniques.[4,5] Initial assessment of the injury may prompt a preemptive discussion with the patient regarding the possibility of toe-to-hand transplantations, especially if the success of replantation is in doubt, such as in cases of severely avulsed, crushed, or multiple amputations. Such a preemptive approach provides guidance for the initial management of the injured hand; the surgeon is reminded to maximally preserve all vital structures, such as neurovascular bundles, tendons, bones, joints, and soft tissues, which will greatly facilitate the subsequent toe-to-hand transplantation.[6,7] Any soft tissue defects can be temporarily covered using an interim groin flap with the following advantages:

1. It avoids the need for excessive shortening of vital structures by providing soft tissue protection.

The authors have nothing to disclose.
[a] Department of Plastic and Reconstructive Surgery, Chang Gung Memorial Hospital, Taoyuan, Taiwan
[b] Department of Plastic and Reconstructive Surgery, Chang Gung Memorial Hospital, College of Medicine, Chang Gung University, Taoyuan, Taiwan
* Corresponding author.
E-mail address: fcw2007@adm.cgmh.org.tw

Clin Plastic Surg 38 (2011) 551–559
doi:10.1016/j.cps.2011.07.001
0094-1298/11/$ – see front matter © 2011 Published by Elsevier Inc.

2. It avoids skin grafts in the hand.
3. It avoids the need to include a large amount of skin with toe harvest, thus facilitating primary closure in the donor site.
4. It avoids the need for local flaps in the hand, which may cause further scarring.
5. It provides redundant skin that can be used for web space reconstruction. ·

In the highly motivated and well-informed patient, primary toe-to-hand transplantation (before the wound is healed) can be reliably performed without an increased risk of complications or need for secondary revisions.[8]

Immediate, 1-Stage, and Total Reconstruction

Over the past 2 decades, increased experience in microsurgical toe-to-hand transplantation and free tissue transfers in general has led to a move toward immediate or primary, 1-stage, and total reconstruction. An increasing number of immediate toe-to-hand transplantations have recently been described for total thumb[9,10] or partial thumb defects,[11] reflecting perhaps an increasing comfort with the indications of toe-to-thumb transplantation and its growing establishment as the definitive choice of thumb reconstruction by patients and surgeons alike. Other than minimizing the number of operations, these immediate procedures shorten the rehabilitation period and provide great psychological benefits without compromising the functional or esthetic outcome. For similar reasons, 1-stage reconstructions offer the advantage of earlier return of function and avoid the need for multiple operations. Another recent area of development is the increasing reports for 1-stage reconstruction involving digit amputations with associated soft tissue defects. Although these soft tissue defects can be reliably covered with nonmicrosurgical loco-regional or pedicled flaps or with microsurgical workhorse flaps, the problem is multiplied when toe-to-hand transplantation is also required for replacing missing digits. The amount of soft tissue that can accompany the toe is limited, as is the number of recipient vessels in the hand for multiple microsurgical procedures. Various investigators have recently reported different approaches to tackle these limitations. Fan and colleagues,[12] for example, described the use of a second free flap in conjunction with the toe transplantation to re-create a contracted web space where the accompanying free flap was anastomosed to the donor vessels of the toe via a "chain-link" fashion to present a single unit of anastomosis in the recipient hand. Thomas and Tsai[13] described a case report where a combined second and third toe unit was anastomosed to a reversed radial forearm flap to resurface a dorsal-palmar hand defect with multiple finger

amputations. del Pinal and colleagues[14] described a dorsalis pedis fascio-subcutaneous toe free flap to reconstruct the missing digit, as well as overcome medium-size defects in the hand, with little donor morbidity. More recently, Zhang and colleagues[15] reported a series using a triple chimeric flap (including skin from the anterior tibial area, the dorsum of the foot, and a transplanted toe) based on the anterior tibial artery or resurfacing accompanying extensive defects in the hand. The donor defect subsequently required extensive skin grafting of the anterior tibial area and the dorsum of the foot.

A further area that has attracted interest is to achieve total reconstruction in one setting. Other than soft tissue defects, traumatic amputations of digits may be accompanied by component loss of bone, nerve, or tendon. As a logical choice, the foot represents a natural warehouse for replacing different missing components with "like-for-like" tissues. del Pinal and colleagues[16] described the use of neurocutaneous vascularized nerve grafts harvested from the tibial side of the second toe to reconstruct nerve defects of up to 4 cm for important finger contact surfaces (eg, ulnar side of thumb or radial side of index finger). Earlier, they also described the application of 1-stage vascularized toe bone blocks for complex intercalated bone defects in the fingers.[17] From our own institution, a new reconstructive strategy was designed using a combined harvest of the metatarsophalangeal joint and second toe extensor digitorum brevis muscle for simultaneous abductoplasty and joint reconstruction to restore opposition and thumb reconstruction in a single stage.[18]

These recent reports illustrate an increased move toward primary, 1-stage, and total reconstruction of the mutilated hand. Indeed, this reconstructive philosophy has been practiced and developed in our institution since the 1990s, where accumulated experience with adequate debridement followed by immediate or primary toe transplantation,[8] functional reconstruction, and continual refinements where different flaps are tailored for different defects have proven the safety and advantages of these approaches.[8,19,20] Some caution is warranted, however, when encountering the mutilated hand with extensive soft tissue defect. The upper extremity poses a reconstructive challenge for the surgeon because of the limitation of recipient vessels. In the traumatic situation, judicious use of available vessels becomes even more critical, as some of these vessels may be damaged. Sacrificing a set of potential recipient vessels for any reconstructive procedures other than toe transplantation should therefore be carefully considered. For similar reasons, sacrificing a major vessel, for example, by performing a reversed radial forearm flap to resurface hand defects in conjunction with a toe-to-hand transplantation should probably be contraindicated. Furthermore, any method to ensure survival of multiple free flaps (including the toe transplantation) on a single set of anastomosis should also be discouraged. In such a "flow-through" design with 2 microsurgical free tissue transfers including the toe transplantation, a single thrombotic event could potentially lead to the loss of both flaps with no chance to salvage either of the flaps.

In principle, whereas we advocate a single-stage reconstruction wherever possible in properly selected cases, a staged reconstruction may sometimes be the best choice to produce the best functional outcome. An example can be seen from our recent series of osteoplastic reconstructions for thumb defects.[21] Of 24 patients who received osteoplastic thumb reconstruction for amputations proximal to the metacarpophalangeal joint, 10 received subsequent toe transplantations as a secondary procedure with the primary osteoplastic reconstruction, avoiding the need for unnecessary toe transplantation in 14 patients who achieved good enough function without further reconstruction. This staged approach was also advantageous in augmenting the length of the remaining stump, thus limiting the length of toe that needed to be harvested and thus reducing donor morbidity. More importantly, it allowed a more strategic positioning of the subsequent transplanted toe by guiding the toe inset into a suitably abducted position as a result of the osteoplastic thumb reconstruction.

Considerations of Donor Site Morbidity

The key objective of any new method is, and always should be, to achieve optimum functional results. The pursuit of this objective should, however, be carefully balanced against the cost of donor site morbidity. Since its first description,[22] the combined dorsalis pedis flap in conjunction with toe transplantation has been a highly appraised option for resurfacing of associated soft tissue loss with digit amputation. The use of skin grafts to resurface the donor foot defect, however, is notorious in creating an unstable surface that is often painful and prone to wound break down. For this reason, primary closure of the donor site should always be achieved to prevent painful scars on the foot and also delays in ambulation. In our experience, the amount of skin to be harvested with the toe is always deliberately restricted. If additional skin is needed for resurfacing accompanying defects in the hand, it should be recruited from sources other than the foot. For this reason, and also for those mentioned previously, the pedicled groin flap is still our preferred option. It obviates the need for a second set of recipient vessels for micro-anastomosis and leaves an almost negligible donor scar. The amount of soft tissue that can be harvested is abundant to cover most defects and to recreate a new web space if necessary. The major drawback remains the inconvenience of a staged procedure and the need for hand attachment to the groin for a few weeks. However, those problems can be easily overcome with careful patient explanation and creative rehabilitation by the physiotherapists (**Fig. 1**).

DECISION MAKING FOR TOE-TO-HAND TRANSPLANTATIONS
Established Practice

The decision of whether to proceed with a toe-to-hand transplantation often needs to take into consideration factors "external" to the hand, such as the general condition of the patient, level of surgeon's microsurgical experience, and also the available resources. Once a decision has

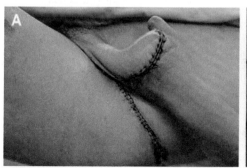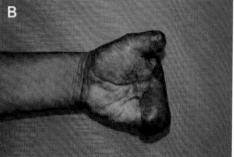

Fig. 1. The use of a pedicled groin flap to resurface accompanying coverage defect in a metacarpal hand obviates the need to use an extra pair of anastomoses with another free flap and also provides abundant tissues for web space creation. (*A*) Pedicled groin flap covering the hand defect. (*B*) Appearance of the injured hand after division of the pedicle and before toe transplantation reconstruction.

been made, the subsequent choice of toe or its variation depends on "internal" factors drawn from examination findings of the injured hand.

Thumb Amputations

The function of the thumb decreases by 50% once the amputation level is proximal to the proximal interphalangeal joint and approaches 100% once it crosses the metacarpophalangeal joint.[23] For this reason, the interphalangeal joint is usually considered the minimum functional length for adequate prehension. Patients who present with an amputation distal to the interphalangeal joint should be considered for toe-to-hand transplantations on a "case-by-case" basis, whereas it should always be offered for amputations proximal to this level. Other factors guiding the choice of toe flap include the functional and cosmetic requirements of the patient, the size of the contralateral normal uninjured thumb, and the condition of the thenar musculature or carpometacarpophalangeal joint. The various options for thumb reconstruction therefore include the total great toe, trimmed great toe, great-toe wrap-around flaps, and the second toe.[9,24]

Finger Amputations

Factors to consider in finger reconstruction include the level of amputation (proximal or distal) and the number of fingers involved (single or multiple). Perhaps more so than the thumb, finger reconstruction using toe transplantation is guided by the specific occupational or cosmetic needs of the patient. In general, toe transplantations for proximal amputations in a single finger are largely unacceptable because of the suboptimal functional and cosmetic outcomes. Distal finger reconstruction, however, seems to be enjoying increasing popularity with excellent outcomes reported (see later in this article). Multiple proximal finger amputations carry a morbidity approximating

that of thumb loss and should always be considered for reconstruction.

Metacarpal Hand

"Metacarpal hand" involves amputations of all fingers proximal to a functional level (middle of the proximal phalanx) with or without the involvement of the thumb. The significance of this injury lies in the loss of basic prehension abilities owing to missing opposable elements. At present, toe-to-hand transplantation represents the only option in these injuries capable of restoring any form of useful prehension. A classification system based on the level of finger amputations (type I) or thumb amputations (type II) has been widely used for the management of this condition (**Fig. 2**).[25–27] The different reconstructive options proposed in these 2 classifications offer clear management pathways that take into account not only the level of amputations, but also important factors like the status of the thenar musculature or carpometacarpophalangeal joint.

These established principles greatly facilitate decision making when considering the appropriateness of toe-to-hand transplantation and also the choice of toe flap for reconstruction. Whereas toe-to-hand transplantation was once confined mainly to the reconstruction of total thumb or multiple finger loss, there are now increasing numbers of reports using toe-to-hand transplantations for isolated distal partial thumb or finger defects. Woo and colleagues[11] reported a series of distal thumb reconstructions with different great toe flaps. Similar to our previous description of the great toe modified wrap-around flap,[28] recommendations were made to always include the distal phalanx when harvesting a partial or total great toe to prevent iatrogenic injury to the germinal matrix. For significant volar surfaces, toe pulp transplantations continue to be worthwhile options in providing a sensate, stable pulp

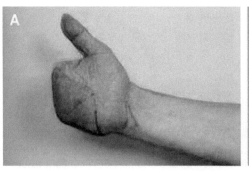
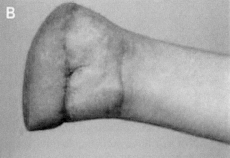

Fig. 2. Metacarpal Hand Classification Types I and II. (*A*) Type I: all 4 fingers amputated proximal to their functional levels. (*B*) Type II: all 4 fingers, as well as the thumb, amputated proximal to their functional levels.

surface, especially if the use of local flaps runs the risk of further restricting global hand function. Pulp flaps can be reliably harvested from the fibula side of the great toe, with primary closure of the donor site achievable if the width of the flap is less than 10 to 12 mm. Although the second toe has been proposed for the same purpose,[20] the limited width of flap available means that skin grafting is invariably necessary, which creates significant donor site problems. For dorsal thumb loss or combined dorsal-volar losses, the harvest of a bigger unit from the great toe, including the nail bed, as suggested by Woo and colleagues,[11] should be approached with caution because of the larger donor defects that have to be grafted or closed with cross-toe flaps.

Distal finger reconstruction has also gained popularity in recent years. Another report by Woo and colleagues[29] found great patient satisfaction when using toe transplantation for missing fingers at the distal interphalangeal joint level. This supports our previous concept[20,30] that toe-to-hand transplantation when performed purely for cosmetic or psychological reasons is justified in properly selected patients. Distal toe transplantation is not only able to replace the original length of the amputated digit, but also reproduce the cosmetic appeal of a nail. In our opinion, distal finger–toe transplantation should be considered

a good indication (**Fig. 3**). In contrast, proximal finger–toe transplantation (proximal to the proximal interphalangeal joint) for isolated finger amputation continues to be an area of difficult decision making, as it is nearly always impossible for the transplanted toe to match the length of the original digit and to resume the same finger cascade. We recommend that proximal finger–toe transplantation for single finger amputation be offered only to patients who are very clear about their goals and who are willing to accept the limitations of a shorter reconstructed finger. Furthermore, it should be offered only for radial digit (index or middle finger) amputations because of the possible functional gain of pulp-to-pulp pinch from these fingers.

Recent work has also been reported for multiple finger amputations. del Pinal[31] proposed the concept of the "balanced" or "acceptable" hand as a guide to decision making for achieving the final aim of a harmonious digital arcade. Strong recommendations are made for reconstruction of central finger losses (the unbalanced hand) or to reconstruct at least 1 of 2 distal finger losses,[31] reinforcing the importance of the tripod pinch, which has previously been reported from our series of multiple finger amputations.[32] Although the number of true metacarpal hand injuries has decreased in number owing to improved

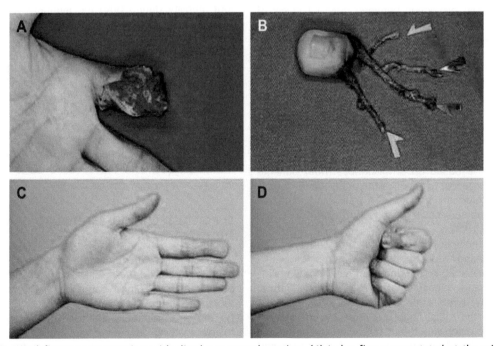

Fig. 3. Distal finger reconstruction with distal toe transplantation. (*A*) Index finger amputated at the middle phalanx. (*B*) Harvested distal second toe; note skeletonized neurovascular structures. (*C, D*) Postoperative appearance.

standards in industrial safety, interesting points are still being raised in recent reports[33,34] with regard to classification and management of such injuries. Fan and colleagues[34] attempted to confine the donor defect of a metacarpal hand (type IIA) reconstruction to one foot by harvesting a great toe wrap-around flap and combined second and third toe based on a single arterial pedicle. Kotkansalo and colleagues[33] used different configurations of toe transplantations for metacarpal hand defects with an alternative classification: level A refers to amputations with resultant intact finger metacarpophalangeal joints and thumb amputation distal to the metacarpophalangeal joint; level B refers to amputations proximal to the finger metacarpophalangeal joints and thumb amputations with resultant thenar or carpometacarpophalangeal joint disruption (analogous to Wei's classification of IIC and IID); level C refers to a transcarpal amputation; and level D refers to a more proximal wrist level or distal antebrachial amputation. This classification is useful in providing information for more proximal or antebrachial amputations where the usefulness of toe-to-hand procedures has been previously demonstrated.[35] However, with experience drawn from a relatively small number of patients, many of their philosophies contrasted sharply with ours for reconstruction of the metacarpal hand. The major differences between this classification[33] and that described by Wei and colleagues[27] is the absence of a clear distinction between different levels of finger amputations (Wei's type I) and also a separate classification for metacarpal hand defects focusing on thumb reconstruction (Wei's type II). The reasons for the contrasts are observable from differences in emphasis for thumb and finger reconstruction. For thumb reconstruction, the second toe was preferred in most of this study[33] instead of the great toe. In addition, single-digit pulp-to-pulp pinch was always preferred to the reconstruction of a tripod pinch. These strategies could be based on unwillingness (both patients and surgeons) to sacrifice the great toe for thumb reconstruction and also a reluctance to use a combined second and third toe for finger reconstruction.

For multiple finger amputations, we have been advocating reconstruction of a tripod pinch, wherever possible, for the dominant hand or the unilateral hand injury to achieve increased lateral stability, pinch strength, and width span,[27,36,37] where the radial finger provides the main pulp-to-pulp pinch with the thumb, while the additional finger plays the important role of a buttress and stabilizer (**Fig. 4**). Despite concerns over donor morbidity following combined second and third

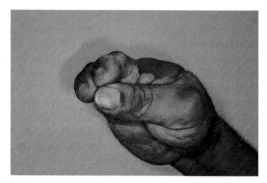

Fig. 4. Tripod pinch achieved with combined second and third toe transplantations in a type I metacarpal hand.

toe harvest, our experience with more than 200 cases has proved the safety and efficacy of this reconstructive option with an acceptable donor foot morbidity. Our experience with a large volume of thumb reconstruction has also convinced us that the great toe (total or trimmed) is the ideal and superior choice over the second toe. Despite concerns from Kotkansalo and colleagues[33] and others regarding the donor morbidity of losing the great toe, the donor morbidity is generally acceptable if at least 1 cm of the proximal phalanx of the great toe is preserved to protect the integrity of the foot and the windlass mechanism (tightening of the plantar fascia) to enable better push-off and foot stability during both the stance and swing phases of walking. For defects involving the first thumb metacarpal where a longer length of bone is needed, we prefer to use a bone block or a staged reconstruction with an initial osteoplastic ray reconstruction, as described previously.[21] In addition, the left foot is always chosen because of its less dominant role in walking, running, or sport activities. By carefully choosing the donor toes and observing certain surgical principles (see the following section), foot function is well maintained even after the harvest of up to 5 toes, as is necessary for bilateral injuries.[26]

SURGICAL TECHNIQUES IN TOE-TO-HAND TRANSPLANTATIONS

Our experience with more than 1800 cases over 30 years has allowed the distillation of certain reproducible principles and concepts in the surgical technique of toe-to-hand transplantation that can be applied to most types of toe flap. These serve to alleviate anxiety over anatomic variations, lessen donor site morbidity, improve functional and esthetic outcomes, and allow quick mastery over the entire range of flaps available. The reader is referred to other sources for an elaboration of these principles, as outlined in **Table 1**. Consistent and predictable results can be achieved by the application of these principles. Surprisingly little has been mentioned in the recent literature regarding the actual techniques of toe harvest and inset since the 1990s. However, continuous practice of these applications, as listed in **Table 1**, has resulted in further evolution of more recent concepts in our department as presented in the following sections.

Managing the Extensor Lag

Extensor lag following toe-to-hand transplantations continue to be challenging owing to the natural clawing of toes. Previous methods to improve extension of fingers have included K-wire splinting, tight extensor repair, and long-term night splinting.[28] A few studies have highlighted several extrinsic and intrinsic differences between the toe joint and finger joint,[38] although detailed

comparative anatomic studies for the benefit of improving outcomes for toe-to-hand transplantations are lacking. Future efforts may be directed to reinforcing the central slip of the proximal interphalangeal toe joint and also reconstructing the intrinsic muscles of the hand.

Refinements in the Great Toe Wrap-Around Flap

The original description of the wrap-around flap, as described by Morrison and colleagues,[39] involves removing a subtotal circumferential toe flap and "wrapping" it around an iliac bone graft to simulate a toe. We have recently modified our technique to include the dorsal half of the distal phalanx together with the entire nail width to preserve the paronychium (lateral nail folds), as we have found that routine trimming of the nail leads to a loss of nail fold definition and increased incidence of nail deformities. Concerns about the wider nail diameter are often unfounded; the

---

Table 1
Different emphases of surgical techniques and the importance of their contribution to the overall outcome of toe-to-hand transplantation

Principles or Concepts	Main Aims and Objectives	Specific Key or Technical Points
Two-team approach	• Reducing operative time • Reducing surgeon fatigue	• Constant communication between recipient and harvest team with regard to length of pedicle, tendon, and nerve
Retrograde dissection of arterial pedicle	• Alleviating anxiety and confusion over anatomic variation • Facilitating easier and quicker dissection • Avoiding the need for angiogram	• Identification of the dominant arterial pedicle in the first web space • Early division of the nondominant pedicle allows easier harvest
Correct placement of incisions	• Creation of adequate web spaces in the hand • Avoiding tension in closure • Avoiding skin grafts	• Incision on the inside of web space midpoints for combined second- and-third toe harvest • Incisions on the outside of midpoints for isolated lesser toe harvest • "V"-shaped incision situated proximal 1 cm to osteotomy site
Recipient site incision	• Avoiding a bulbous appearance at toe-thumb or toe-finger junction	• Cruciate incision with creation of 4, equal triangular flaps
Inset and osteosynthesis	• Achieving a stable, yet "flexible," fixation that allows early manipulation of malunion or malrotation	• Bony fixation using parallel intraosseous wires
Tendon repair	• Reducing the extensor lag and natural tendency of toes to claw	• Extensor tendon repair first with finger in full extension • Flexor tendon repair against extensor tension to restore digital arcade

overall size of the thumb is usually more noticeable than the actual nail width.

Refinements with the Use of the Combined Second-and-Third Toe Flap

The use of combined second-and-third toe flap is a useful reconstructive option for multiple finger amputations proximal to the web spaces. With regard to the donor foot, we have previously made recommendations to reconstruct radial amputations using combined toe units from the contralateral foot, whereas ipsilateral combined units are used for ulnar amputations.[40] This appears to be a logical choice, as the natural toe arrangements mimic the corresponding lengths of the missing fingers, with the second toe always placed in the most central position. We now prefer to harvest toes from the left foot regardless of which hand is injured if they are the only toes to be used for reconstruction, because of its lesser functional demand. The right foot is selected only when the left foot is unsuitable, eg, when the left great toe has already been removed for thumb reconstruction. With regard to positioning of the toes, we have also previously recommended replacing the radial digits (index and middle) for patients with occupations that require fine manipulation and replacing the ulnar digits (ring and middle) for patients with more manual work who require a powerful grasp.[40] We have recently shifted our preference to reconstructing the central digits (middle and ring fingers) rather than the ulnar digits (ring and little fingers), as we have found that even the most perfect ulnar construct may not re-create the necessary power grasp owing to the limited range of motion of the transplanted toes.

Another modification pertains to the actual inset. During osteosynthesis, we prefer to orient each toe individually and rotate it radially toward the thumb rather than simply letting it point downward, as this seemed to produce a better tripod pinch, especially if the circumduction of the opposable thumb is compromised. Contrary to popular descriptions, we have also found osteotomizing the metatarsal heads at an angle (in transmetatarsal toe harvest) to be unnecessary; the angular osteotomy may confer a theoretical correction of the extensor lag but this is not actually transferable to actual improvements in functional outcome. Finally, we have also changed our original idea of using bone blocks to fill the dead space in the donor foot following transmetatarsal combined second-and-third toe harvests, as we have found no increased problems with gait or foot stability even without these additional procedures.

SUMMARY

Toe-to-hand transplantations are reliable and worthwhile operations that restore useful prehension that are lost through hand injuries. Their development has led to wider clinical applications, better functional outcome, and also improved esthetic results. There is also an increasing move in the timing of toe transplantations from secondary to immediate reconstruction while the wound is still open to achieve a total, 1-stage reconstruction. In addition, more reports are emerging of distal reconstructions, reflecting increased patient demands and surgeons' mastery of the techniques. In the exciting pursuit of innovations, it is important to ensure that solid principles that have already been built are not abandoned, and certain boundaries are not crossed, especially in areas of more "secondary" considerations, such as donor site morbidity. Future areas of development are likely to focus on reducing these donor morbidities and also on improving outcomes, such as sensory recovery through cross-specialty nerve research. Until the problem of immunosuppression is solved to usher in routine, safe composite tissue allotransplantation, toe-to-hand transplantation continues to remain the best option next to a successful replantation.

REFERENCES

1. Nicolandi C. Daumenplastik. Wien Klin Wochenschr 1897;10:663.
2. Yang DY, Gu YD. The report of free second toe transfer for thumb reconstruction in 4 cases. Chinese Journal of Surgery 1977;15:1–3.
3. Cobbett JR. Free digital transfer. Report of a case of transfer of a great toe to replace an amputated thumb. J Bone Joint Surg Br 1969;51:677–9.
4. Michon J, Merle M, Bouchon Y, et al. Functional comparison between pollicization and toe-to-hand transfer for thumb reconstruction. J Reconstr Microsurg 1984;1:103–12.
5. Morrison WA, O'Brien BM, MacLeod AM. Experience with thumb reconstruction. J Hand Surg Br 1984;9:223–33.
6. Wallace CG, Wei FC. Posttraumatic finger reconstruction with microsurgical transplantation of toes. Hand Clin 2007;23:117–28.
7. Cheng MH, Wei FC, Santamaria E, et al. Single versus double arterial anastomoses in combined second- and third-toe transplantation. Plast Reconstr Surg 1998;102:2408–12 [discussion: 2413].
8. Yim KK, Wei FC, Lin CH. A comparison between primary and secondary toe-to-hand transplantation. Plast Reconstr Surg 2004;114:107–12.

9. Ray EC, Sherman R, Stevanovic M. Immediate reconstruction of a nonreplantable thumb amputation by great toe transfer. Plast Reconstr Surg 2009;123:259–67.

10. Huang D, Wang HG, Wu WZ, et al. Functional and aesthetic results of immediate reconstruction of traumatic thumb defects by toe-to-thumb transplantation. Int Orthop 2011;35(4):543–7.

11. Woo SH, Lee GJ, Kim KC, et al. Immediate partial great toe transfer for the reconstruction of composite defects of the distal thumb. Plast Reconstr Surg 2006;117:1906–15.

12. Fan CY, Jiang J, Zeng BF, et al. Reconstruction of thumb loss complicated by skin defects in the thumb-index web space by combined transplantation of free tissues. J Hand Surg Am 2006;31:236–41.

13. Thomas BP, Tsai TM. Primary reconstruction of a degloved hand using multiple toe transfers on a single pedicle and a reversed radial artery flap. J Reconstr Microsurg 2004;20:3–6.

14. del Pinal F, Garcia-Bernal FJ, Delgado J, et al. Overcoming soft-tissue deficiency in toe-to-hand transfer using a dorsalis pedis fasciosubcutaneous toe free flap: surgical technique. J Hand Surg Am 2005;30: 111–9.

15. Zhang YX, Wang D, Zhang Y, et al. Triple chimeric flap based on anterior tibial vessels for reconstruction of severe traumatic injuries of the hand with thumb loss. Plast Reconstr Surg 2009;123:268–75.

16. del Pinal F, Garcia-Bernal FJ, Regalado J, et al. The tibial second toe vascularized neurocutaneous free flap for major digital nerve defects. J Hand Surg Am 2007;32:209–17.

17. del Pinal F, Garcia-Bernal FJ, Delgado J, et al. Vascularized bone blocks from the toe phalanx to solve complex intercalated defects in the fingers. J Hand Surg Am 2006;31:1075–82.

18. Lin CH, Tang PL, Lin CH. Second toe extensor digitorum brevis provides a simultaneous abductorplasty to free vascularized metatarsophalangeal joint transfer for posttraumatic thumb composite metacarpophalangeal joint defect. J Trauma 2009;66:1374–8.

19. Wei FC. Tissue preservation in hand injury: the first step to toe-to-hand transplantation. Plast Reconstr Surg 1998;102:2497–501.

20. Wei FC, Epstein MD, Chen HC, et al. Microsurgical reconstruction of distal digits following mutilating hand injuries: results in 121 patients. Br J Plast Surg 1993;46:181–6.

21. Lin CH, Mardini S, Lin YT, et al. Osteoplastic thumb ray restoration with or without secondary toe transfer for reconstruction of opposable basic hand function. Plast Reconstr Surg 2008;121:1288–97.

22. Chang T, Wang W, Wu J. Free transfer of the second toe combined with dorsalis pedis flaps using microvascular technique for reconstruction of the thumbs and other fingers. Ann Acad Med Singapore 1979;8:404–12.

23. American Medical Association. Guides to the evaluation of permanent impairment. Chicago: American Medical Association; 1990. p. 14–55.

24. Wei FC, Chen HC, Chuang CC, et al. Microsurgical thumb reconstruction with toe transfer: selection of various techniques. Plast Reconstr Surg 1994;93: 345–51 [discussion: 52–7].

25. Buck-Gramcko D, editor. The metacarpal hand. London: Martin Dunitz; 1997.

26. Mardini S, Wei FC. Unilateral and bilateral metacarpal hand injuries: classification and treatment guidelines. Plast Reconstr Surg 2004;113:1756–9.

27. Wei FC, el-Gammal TA, Lin CH, et al. Metacarpal hand: classification and guidelines for microsurgical reconstruction with toe transfers. Plast Reconstr Surg 1997;99:122–8.

28. Wei FC. Toe to hand transplantations. In: Green D, Hotchkiss R, Pederson WC, et al, editors. Green's operative hand surgery. Philadelphia: Churchill Livingstone; 2005. p. 1835–63.

29. Woo SH, Lee GJ, Kim KC, et al. Cosmetic reconstruction of distal finger absence with partial second toe transfer. J Plast Reconstr Aesthet Surg 2006;59:317–24.

30. Wei FC, Colony LH. Microsurgical restoration of distal digital function. Clin Plast Surg 1989;16:443–55.

31. del Pinal F. The indications for toe transfer after "minor" finger injuries. J Hand Surg Br 2004;29:120–9.

32. Wei FC, Chen HC, Chuang CC, et al. Simultaneous multiple toe transfers in hand reconstruction. Plast Reconstr Surg 1988;81:366–77.

33. Kotkansalo T, Vilkki SK, Elo P. The functional results of post-traumatic metacarpal reconstructions with microvascular toe transfers. J Hand Surg Eur Vol 2009;34:730–42.

34. Fan CY, Liu XD, Cai PH, et al. Modification of hand reconstruction with unilateral foot donation. Chin Med J (Engl) 2007;120:1206–8.

35. Vilkki SK, Kotkansalo T. Present technique and long-term results of toe-to-antebrachial stump transplantation. J Plast Reconstr Aesthet Surg 2007;60:835–48.

36. Wei FC, Coessens B, Ganos D. Multiple microsurgical toe-to-hand transfer in the reconstruction of the severely mutilated hand. A series of fifty-nine cases. Ann Chir Main Memb Super 1992;11:177–87.

37. Wei FC, Colony LH. Microsurgical reconstruction of opposable digits in mutilating hand injuries. Clin Plast Surg 1989;16:491–504.

38. Sarrafian SK, Topouzian LK. Anatomy and physiology of the extensor apparatus of the toes. J Bone Joint Surg Am 1969;51:669–79.

39. Morrison WA, O'Brien BM, MacLeod AM. Thumb reconstruction with a free neurovascular wrap-around flap from the big toe. J Hand Surg Am 1980;5:575–83.

40. Wei FC, Colony LH, Chen HC, et al. Combined second and third toe transfer. Plast Reconstr Surg 1989;84:651–61.

Free Functional Muscle Transfer for the Upper Extremity

Alexander Seal, MPhil, MD, FRCSC,
Milan Stevanovic, MD, PhD*

KEYWORDS

- Free functional muscle transfer • Upper extremity
- Nerve injury • Volkmann's ischemic contracture

Injuries to the brachial plexus, or those to the upper extremity resulting in Volkmann's ischemic contracture, can cause devastating functional loss. Nerve transfers for brachial plexus and peripheral nerve injuries have become the cutting-edge reconstructive options for loss of distal function in the upper extremity.[1–7] Nerve transfers, direct nerve repair, or nerve grafting should be used in acute cases of plexus and/or peripheral nerve loss during the first 6 to 9 months following injury; this can allow adequate time to reinnervate distal motor targets. It is known that by 18 to 24 months, irreversible changes in muscle cells occur and limit the chance of motor recovery.[8–10] Free functional muscle transfers are an excellent treatment option in patients when significant time has passed after a nerve injury. In addition, they are the treatment of choice for reconstruction of established Volkmann's contracture, muscle loss from trauma or tumor resection, and in congenital muscle absence. These procedures are indicated only if functional deficits cannot be restored by local muscle rotation or tendon transfers. In cases where there is both a soft tissue and functional muscle loss, free functional muscle transfers can address these problems together. The focus of this article is to highlight the key principles for functional reconstruction of the upper extremity with free functional muscle transfer.

HISTORY

In 1970, Tamai and colleagues,[11] using a canine model, were able to successfully transfer a rectus femoris muscle to the forelimb. Free functional muscle transfer (FFMT) was first done clinically by Harii and colleagues[12] for facial reanimation using the gracilis muscle. At the same time, surgeons at Six People's Hospital in Shanghai transferred a portion of the pectoralis major muscle to the forearm to restore finger flexion in a patient with Volkmann's Ischemic Contracture.[13] In Japan, Ikuta and colleagues,[14] used free functional gracilis muscle transfers for the same functional reconstruction. In North America, credit should be given to Manktelow and Zucker for pioneering FFMTs.[15,16] Since the reports in the 1970s, the literature has increased with an expanded application of FFMT demonstrating improvement in function of the upper extremity.[9,17–22] In recent publications, larger case series have been reported that include functional outcomes.[10,23–26]

PATIENT SELECTION

Reconstructive surgeons involved in the care of patients who may benefit from FFMT should first consider less complicated options for reconstruction. These procedures would commonly include local muscle and/or tendon transfers. In severe cases of Volkmann's ischemic contracture, often the flexor and extensor compartments are damaged to a varying degree, limiting the local reconstructive options.[27] In these situations a FFMT is the best option. Other patients who would potentially benefit from FFMT include, those with muscle loss from direct trauma, electrical injuries, long-standing neurologic injury, congenital

Department of Orthopaedic Surgery, University of Southern California, USC University Hospital, LAC + USC Medical Center, 2025 Zonal Avenue, GNH 3900, Los Angeles, CA 90089-9312, USA
* Corresponding author.
E-mail address: stevanov@usc.edu

Clin Plastic Surg 38 (2011) 561–575
doi:10.1016/j.cps.2011.09.001

absence and, now with the increase in limb salvage surgery, those with functional deficits after tumor excision (**Box 1**).[25,28]

For all of these indications, a compliant and motivated patient is perhaps the most important component to successful functional transfers, as the rehabilitation programs can be complex and time consuming. Patients and families must have detailed explanations of the commitment, as well as, realistic expectations for outcomes. Patients should be encouraged to meet with other patients that have had the same procedure and have successfully completed rehabilitation. It is equally important to ensure the patient does not have any other underlying medical conditions that would compromise the functional transfer or put the patient at risk by performing these procedures. In the authors' experience, the most successful outcomes with FFMT have been when the patients are younger than 45 years of age.

PRINCIPLES

The common problem for patients who require FFMT is loss of function of one muscle, or a group of muscles. The most important reconstructed function in the upper extremity is elbow flexion. In addition, FFMTs are also used for deltoid reconstruction, elbow extension, and wrist and finger flexion and extension. With functional loss in the forearm, it is important to evaluate both the flexor and extensor muscles to determine whether an antagonistic force exists to the proposed transferred muscle.[29] If there is no opposing muscle function, the patient may require a double transfer, or other procedures, such as wrist arthrodesis or tenodesis, to obtain this balance. The authors agree that finger extension should be reconstructed prior to finger flexion to allow for a more rapid return of function and faster rehabilitation.[30] A prerequisite for a successful FFMT is a healthy recipient bed to allow tendon gliding. If this does not exist, the patient may require a staged procedure to prepare the arm for an FFMT, such

as, local tissue rearrangement, tissue expansion, or free tissue transfer.

Success also depends on the patients having mobile joints and gliding tendons. If this mobility does not exist, the patient requires contracture release, tenolysis, and/or capsulotomies. It is essential to combine these initial procedures with aggressive physiotherapy, to achieve full passive range of motion before the planned FFMT (**Box 2**).

Viability of the transferred muscle is achieved using meticulous microsurgical technique. Successful FFMT requires a pure motor nerve to power the transfer with an appropriate size match to the donor nerve. The nerve coaptation should be as close as possible to the transferred muscle to minimize the reinnervation distance. Good sensation of the hand is important for optimal functional results, and this often may require sensory nerve reconstruction at the same time as, or before, the motor reconstruction.[6] To ensure successful FFMT, the resting length of the muscle must be correctly restored. These key principles are summarized in **Box 3**.

FFMT requires a great deal of preoperative planning; however, the care of these patients requires a multidisciplinary team with the ability to support the intensive and long postoperative rehabilitation.

MUSCLE SELECTION

There have been many muscles studied for their suitability to be used as FFMT (**Box 4**). Desirable characteristics include a reliable neurovascular pedicle, as well as, having minimal or no donor site deficit. The muscle should have adequate strength and have a range of excursion that will meet the needs of the site to which it is being transferred (**Box 5**). A good example meeting these criteria is the gracilis muscle, which is the

---

Box 1
Indications for FFMT

Volkmann's ischemic contracture

Direct traumatic loss of muscle

Electrical injury involving the upper extremity

Long-standing neurologic injury

Upper extremity tumor excision

Congenital muscle absence

Box 2
Key principles for FFMT

Good soft-tissue coverage for the reconstruction site

Full passive range of motion of the joints the transfer will act across

Pure, undamaged donor motor nerve at the site of transfer

Reliable recipient vessels

Adequate tendon glide

Antagonistic muscle function

Motivated, compliant patient

Adequate physical therapy

Box 3
Key points for functional transfer

Plan incisions for exposure and tendon coverage

Prepare tendon for muscle insertion with normal cascade

Select healthy vessels close to the muscle pedicle

Select healthy motor nerve

Perform a nerve repair as close to muscle as possible to minimize time of denervation

Secure fixation at origin and insertion to minimize stretching

Ensure correct resting length of the muscle

Box 5
Guidelines for muscle selection

Desirable neurovascular anatomy

Adequate strength

Suitable range of excursion

Suitable gross anatomy to fit defect

Adequate fascia or tendon to allow secure attachment

Minimal donor deficit and limited cosmetic donor defect

---

most commonly transferred muscle to the upper extremity because of its functional and anatomic fit. The muscle can be used for deltoid reconstruction, elbow flexion, as well as finger flexion and extension. A review of 71 free gracilis functional transfers, supports the consensus that this muscle is useful for reconstruction of both finger flexion and extension.[26] This muscle is also commonly used for reconstruction of elbow flexion. Kay and colleagues[10] reviewed 33 patients that underwent free functional gracilis transfers for elbow flexion over a 14-year period.[10] In their series, 70% of the patients obtained a successful result with elbow flexion M3 or greater. Using intercostal nerves as donor nerves in their series appeared to have better outcomes than using other nerves, such as ulnar fascicles or the spinal accessory nerve.

There have been many techniques described for reconstruction of elbow flexion. When no local option, such as latissimus dorsi and pectoralis major pedicled transfers are available, or the use of a proximal advancement of the flexor-pronator

origin (Steindler procedure),[33] FFMT remains the only choice. Options for restoring elbow flexion with FFMT include gracilis, latissimus dorsi, or rectus femoris muscles. In the authors' practice the gracilis muscle is most commonly used, followed by the latissimus dorsi. In 2010, Muramatsu and colleagues[25] published their case series, which included 7 patients requiring reconstruction after oncologic sarcoma resection in the upper extremity using free latissimus dorsi, with good results. Kay and colleagues[10] highlight the importance of a learning curve for FFMT.

Muscle Physiology

An understanding of the length-tension curves for muscle contraction is required when planning functional muscle transfers. The contraction of a muscle is a dynamic process involving coordinated contraction of thousands of muscle fibers consisting of overlapping actin and myosin filaments.[34] The force of contraction generated by a muscle is directly proportional to the amount of overlap of these thick and thin fibers, in a calcium-dependent process known as the sliding filament mechanism of contracture.[34] This process is influenced by the length the muscle is stretched before it contracts. With the muscle stretched beyond its normal limits, there is the least amount of overlap between the actin and myosin fibers, and therefore the muscle contraction is weak. As the muscle shortens and the amount of overlap is increased between the fibers, the strength of muscle contraction increases to a maximum point found at the resting length in its most elongated position.[34] This point is the peak of the length-tension curve for the muscle after which, if the muscle continues to shorten, there is less optimization of the overlap of myosin fibers relative to actin, resulting in less force of muscle contraction.[34] The goal of tensioning a functional muscle transfer is to allow the muscle

---

Box 4
Common FFMTs

Gracilis

Latissimus dorsi

Rectus femoris

Tensor fascia lata

Gastrocnemius

Serratus anterior

Gracilis with adductor longus[31,32]

to act at its peak length-tension point for contraction at its resting length.

It must be noted that the connective tissue framework surrounding the muscle fibers contributes to the contraction force. The connective tissue provides a recoil tension when the muscle is in full extension, adding to the contractile force, and limiting the maximal extension of the muscle. Muscle contraction relates to the number of muscle fibers that are activated by a neural stimulus, and contraction strength is increased as more fibers are recruited to contract.[34] Maximal innervation of the muscle is therefore important for functional transfers to ensure that the maximum strength is obtained from the muscle.

VASCULAR CONSIDERATIONS

It is of paramount importance to use meticulous technique for the vascular anastomoses for FFMT, and the reconstructive surgeon must carefully plan the location of these to ensure there is no tension on the pedicle with muscle excursion. Standard options for vascular anastomosis include end-to-end suturing to existing, healthy named vessels. If there is a large mismatch between the donor and recipient vessels, end-to-side anastomosis should be performed.

For successful FFMT, the recipient vessels ideally should be of equivalent caliber to the donor vessels. In addition, the anastomosis should be in healthy tissue away from the site of injury. The vena comitantes in the upper extremity, especially in cases of previous trauma and ischemic injuries, can often be damaged. Venous outflow problems are more common than arterial inflow problems for complications with FFMT; therefore, the vena comitantes should always be flushed with heparinized saline to ensure they are draining well. If there is any resistance in these veins, other deep veins or superficial veins should be used. It is important to look for and protect superficial arm veins during the initial incisions and flap elevation in the upper arm and forearm for this reason. When using superficial veins there is often a mismatch in size between the donor and recipient vein, making them more difficult to use.

The most common vascular pedicle used at the shoulder for deltoid reconstruction, or elbow flexion, is the thoracoacromial artery, with either the associated vena comitantes or a branch of the cephalic vein. This is due to the excellent size match between the donor and recipient vessels and its anatomic location. Alternatively, the thoracodorsal artery and vena comitantes can be used.

For finger flexion and extension reconstruction, if the ulnar artery is present the authors' preference is to use the radial artery and vena comitantes. If it is not present, the anterior interosseous artery is a viable option, or an end-to-side anastomosis to the radial artery can also be performed.

NERVE CONSIDERATIONS

A preoperative physical examination should always be performed to identify which nerves are functioning in the upper extremity. For successful FFMT, the donor nerve must be a pure motor nerve, with no surrounding scar tissue, and ideally with a synergistic function to the muscle the transfer is replacing. If there is any question on the viability of the donor nerve, an intraoperative biopsy should be performed to confirm its health.[35] This action is undertaken before the functional muscle is harvested.

For deltoid or elbow flexion reconstruction, preference is to use either the musculocutaneous or axillary nerves if they are present. Alternatively, the spinal accessory nerve or 3 intercostal motor nerves can be used, usually the third, fourth, and fifth branches. Chuang and colleagues[23] found that if the original musculocutaneous nerve is present, the results are better than intercostal reinnervation. It is important to perform direct repair without intervening nerve grafts to maximize the functional outcome. For triceps reconstruction and elbow extension, a branch of the radial nerve to the long head of the triceps is preferred. If this is not present, motor fascicles from either the median or ulnar nerve can be used.

The anterior interosseous nerve is the best choice for reconstruction of finger flexion. If this is not a viable option, fascicles of the median nerve to the flexor digitorum superficialis (FDS), or a fascicle of the ulnar nerve to the flexor carpi ulnaris muscle, can be used if available. For finger extension reconstruction, the posterior interosseous nerve is ideal. If this is not possible, again, branches of the median nerve to the FDS can be used.

In patients with complete brachial plexus palsy, the only motor nerve options for reconstruction on the side of injury are the spinal accessory nerve, intercostal nerves, and phrenic nerve. In the authors practice, only the spinal accessory and intercostal nerves are used. The authors agree with other investigators that it is important to keep in mind that when there is preceding chest trauma, these nerves should be used with caution.[10,23,35] In a case series of elbow reconstruction presented by Kay and colleagues,[10] a better motor outcome was achieved when the intercostal nerves were used as donor nerves as opposed to ulnar fascicles.

Other investigators have reported successfully using the contralateral C7 and the contralateral medial pectoral nerve with nerve grafting for reconstruction.[10,23,24,26,29,36] In a modest series of a dozen cases using these two procedures, the authors were unable to obtain useful functional outcomes, and because of this, in their practice, these procedures are no longer used. This result is supported by Terzis and Kostopoulos,[26] who in their recent review of 74 functional muscle transfers found that for finger flexion, intercostals, upper ipsilateral plexus, and distal accessory gave better results than the contralateral C7.

PREOPERATIVE PLANNING

The preoperative planning for these patients starts with a detailed history outlining the mechanism of injury, previous investigations, interventions, and the remaining functional impairment of the patient. A detailed physical examination should include the vascular system, as well as, evaluation of the nerves, muscles, joints, and soft tissues of the upper extremity.

Formal nerve conduction studies are often not indicated or helpful. Electromyography (EMG) can be useful to assess muscle function. In the distal forearm EMG evaluation of the pronator quadratus can give information about the status of the anterior interosseous nerve function.[29]

Magnetic resonance imaging (MRI) is required to assess viability of the affected muscles in the upper extremity. With the newer higher-powered MRI studies (3 Tesla and above), information can be obtained about the conditions of the nerves, and this can help for preoperative planning and decisions on the need for nerve grafting to restore sensation.

Angiography is recommended to provide valuable information about the arterial inflow for the extremity, especially after significant traumatic injuries.[29] It is useful to assess interosseous vessels in these studies, as these can serve as key recipient vessels for functional transfers.[29] Often an intact anterior interosseous artery will correlate with an uninjured anterior interosseous nerve.[29]

Muscle selection is based on the functional requirements at the recipient site; these include the muscle length and expected excursion. Ideally the transferred muscle will span from a selected origin to insertion, optimizing its resting length. The muscle should also have adequate fascia and tendon to facilitate a secure attachment to the origin and insertion. The vascular and nerve anatomy should be considered to ensure the orientation to the recipient vessels and nerve is optimized. Finally, the functional and cosmetic deficit of the donor site should be minimized.

Adequate soft-tissue coverage is essential for a successful transfer, and may require staging the reconstruction with a first-stage local, regional, or free tissue transfer. It is always preferable to use a myocutaneous flap for the functional transfer. The benefit of this is it provides a reliable skin paddle to monitor the muscle postoperatively, and, in addition, provides a healthy gliding surface and coverage over the muscle. Myocutaneous flaps can, however, be bulky, and result in a less desirable cosmetic result. Skin grafts over the muscle belly proximal to the musculocutaneous junction can be used initially and heal well cosmetically; however, the authors recommend these to be replaced secondarily and covered with a skin flap to improve gliding. Incisions should always be planned for access and exposure of the donor vessels and nerves to facilitate the microsurgery, as well as, to ensure adequate coverage for the musculotendinous junctions.

SPECIFIC MUSCLE DISSECTION
Gracilis Elevation

The gracilis muscle is anatomically located in the medial thigh, posterior to adductor longus, superficial to adductor magnus, and with sartorius laterally and semimembranosus and semitendinosus posterior. The muscle originates from the pubic tubercle, and inserts on the medial side of the tibial tubercle. The gracilis is a Type II muscle with the dominant vascular supply being the ascending branch of the medial circumflex femoral artery, originating from the profundus femoral artery.[37] The dominant pedicle enters the superior one-third of the muscle, approximately 8 to 12 cm inferior to the origin of the muscle at the pubic tubercle.[37] There are usually at least 1 or 2 perforators entering the distal half of the muscle. The motor innervation to the muscle is from the anterior division of the obturator nerve, which enters the muscle just proximal to the main pedicle. There are usually 2 to 3 fascicles, which with intraoperative stimulation can be used to identify different motor territories.[29,38]

The patient is placed supine on the operative table, in a frog-leg position. It is important to keep in mind that the gracilis muscle is located more posteriorly in the thigh than often is the initial impression. It is the authors' preference to use a contralateral gracilis muscle for elbow flexion and finger extension, and an ipsilateral muscle for finger flexion reconstruction. This decision is made based on the position of the recipient vessels.

The axis of the myocutaneous flap is designed 2 to 3 cm posterior to a line drawn between the pubic tubercle and medial femoral condyle. The adductor longus in the upper medial thigh can also be palpated as a landmark, and a longitudinal incision can be made inferior to this. Until recently, the authors were only able to harvest a skin paddle that successfully covered the proximal half of the gracilis muscle. With better understanding now of the blood supply to the skin through the superficial fascia, it has been possible to harvest a skin paddle that covers the entire muscle by taking all of the superficial fascia with the gracilis muscle from the medial thigh (**Fig. 1**).[39] This factor is very important in cases of finger flexion and extension reconstruction because of a lack of skin coverage in the forearm. In addition, a branch of the superficial saphenous vein that drains the skin paddle is dissected and included with the flap to allow augmentation of venous outflow once the muscle is transferred (see **Fig. 1C**). This

is done to help prevent venous congestion of the large volume of tissue transferred.

On skin incision, if the saphenous vein is encountered it can be used as a landmark to suggest the incision is too anterior and dissection should proceed more posterior and inferior. The subcutaneous tissue should be beveled away from the muscle to prevent shearing injury of the perforating branches from the fascia to the skin. If one intends to take a large skin paddle that covers the entire muscle, all of the superficial fascia of the muscles of the medial thigh should be harvested, keeping the gracilis muscle within the fascia (see **Fig. 1C**). To better define the location of the gracilis muscle, a distal incision can first be made at the medial side of the thigh, close to the knee, to identify the gracilis tendon. A Penrose drain can be wrapped around the tendon, and traction is used to make locating the muscle proximally easier.

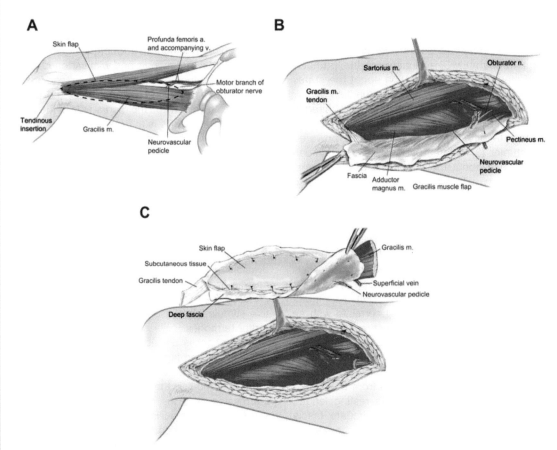

Fig. 1. Harvest of a free functional gracilis with skin paddle and extended superficial fascia. (*A*) Outline of skin paddle over the gracilis muscle. (*B*) Dissection of skin paddle and gracilis muscle with extended superficial fascia. (*C*) Free functional gracilis harvested with extended fascia and superficial vein included for venous outflow augmentation. a, artery; m, muscle; n, nerve; v, vein.

Once the pedicle is identified, it can be dissected back to branches going upward into the adductor longus. These branches are divided, and further length on the pedicle can be obtained by tracing it deeper to its origin from the profunda femora artery.[40] Usually at this level, the two vena comitantes will have come together into one originating from the profunda femoral vein. A vascular pedicle length of 4 of 6 cm can be easily obtained.[41]

Before the origin and insertion of the muscle are divided and the pedicle is ligated, the resting length of the muscle should be marked; this is done with the hip maximally abducted and the knee extended. Markings are placed at 5-cm intervals with a silk suture for easy recreation of the resting length once the muscle is transferred (**Fig. 2**). The microscope should be brought to the recipient site after the origin and insertion for the muscle have been prepared, and the neurovascular pedicle should be divided only when the recipient site is completely ready to receive the muscle.

The insertion of the gracilis is divided first, identifying the tendinous insertion at the medial tibial tubercle. Following this, the origin is divided, and then the vascular pedicle. The length of the obturator nerve is maintained long enough so that no nerve grafts are needed for coaptation in the upper extremity.

Gracilis Revascularization

The gracilis is brought to the recipient site, and the vascular pedicle is prepared under the microscope. It is important to test the freedom of the pedicle in relation to the intended site of anastomosis by placing the muscle under full stretch, restoring muscle resting length. This action is taken to ensure the anastomosis will not be stretched or kinked with motion. It is also important to thoughtfully place the muscle at the recipient site to allow coaptation of the nerve as close to the muscle as possible to reduce the time to reinnervation.[29] Minimal suturing

with the augmentation of fibrin glue is the authors' preference for the coaptation. Meticulous microvascular anastomosis is performed before the neurorrhaphy.

Before the muscle is secured proximally and distally, and after the anastomosis is completed, the muscle is allowed 5 minutes to revascularize. After this time, the comitant vein should not appear engorged or have a dark color to it. One of the best indicators for good flap perfusion is the size and color of the draining vein. In addition, the muscle should become pink with bright bleeding from its cut edges. The muscle should be revascularized within 30 minutes to maximize functional outcome. In the authors' experience, if there are difficulties with muscle perfusion and establishing good flow takes longer than 2 hours, the functional outcomes are poor.

The superficial vein from the skin paddle is anastomosed at the recipient site to a superficial vein after the origin and insertion of the muscle is completed.

Latissimus Dorsi Elevation

The latissimus dorsi muscle is a large type V triangular muscle covering the posterior-inferior trunk. The muscle originates from the T6 through T12 vertebrae, the posterior iliac crest, the lower 4 ribs, and some minor attachments to the scapula.[42] There is a strong tendinous confluence that inserts into the medial border of the intertubercular groove of the humerus. The superior fibers of the muscle are deep to the trapezius muscle, and the remaining muscle is superior to the muscles of the posterior trunk, including erector spinae, serratus posterior inferior, and serratus anterior.[42] It is important to note that the deep surface of the lateral border of the muscle merges with the serratus anterior and must be carefully elevated to isolate the latissimus muscle. As a type V muscle, inferiorly, there are posterior lumbar perforators medially, and posterior intercostal perforators laterally. The dominant blood supply is through the thoracodorsal artery, which enters the muscle approximately 10 to 15 cm inferior to its insertion, and originates from the subscapular artery.[42] The motor innervation of the muscle is from the thoracodorsal nerve, which travels with the vascular pedicle. The average size of the muscle can be up to 25 × 30 cm.[42]

To harvest the muscle, the patient is placed in the lateral decubitus position and draped in the standard fashion. A longitudinal incision is designed parallel to the lateral border of the latissimus dorsi, extending from the posterior axillary line to the posterior inferior iliac crest. A skin

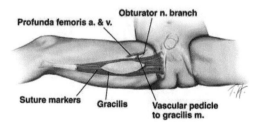

Fig. 2. Resting length of the gracilis muscle with the leg positioned in maximal abduction with knee extension. Sutures are placed at 5-cm intervals from the origin to the musculotendinous junction.

paddle is designed, centered on the middle of the muscle, starting 6 to 8 cm inferior to the axilla and extending distally as far as necessary to completely cover the transferred muscle. The width of the skin paddle should be 8 to 10 cm or less to allow primary closure of the donor site. This width is adequate to cover the muscle, as during the insetting of the FFMT the latissimus dorsi muscle is rolled on itself to maximize its strength.

The subcutaneous dissection should be beveled away from the incision and the fascia should be preserved over the muscle to facilitate muscle contracture and minimize scarring. To mark the resting tension of the muscle, the arm is positioned in 180° of abduction and forward flexions. In this position, the muscle is marked with sutures at 5-cm intervals starting from the musculotendinous junction.

The muscle is elevated from origin to insertion, and from the lateral to medial border. Special care should be taken to ligate the large posterior lumbar and intercostal perforators. As elevation continues superiorly, the branch to the serratus anterior muscle is visualized, and alerts the surgeon that the common thoracodorsal pedicle is near. This branch is ligated close to the bifurcation to the thoracodorsal artery and venae comitantes. Special care should be taken to avoid injury to the long thoracic nerve, which runs close to this pedicle. The elevation is performed more proximally, and several more perforating branches from the thoracodorsal artery should be ligated. Stretching or injury to the neurovascular pedicle should be avoided.

The dissection of the tendinous portion of the latissimus muscle is continued to its insertion on the humerus, where it will be divided. As already described for the gracilis muscle transfer, the neurovascular pedicle should be divided only when the recipient site is completely ready to receive the muscle.

Latissimus Dorsi Revascularization

The same principles for revascularization and insetting already described for the gracilis muscle apply to the latissimus dorsi muscle functional transfer. It is important to highlight that the latissimus dorsi muscle does not have a tendinous origin, and coaptation of the tendons to the muscle is much more challenging. The authors' preference for reconstruction of elbow flexion is to wrap the muscle around the biceps tendon if it is present; otherwise suture anchors are used to secure the muscle to the radial tuberosity. For finger flexion and extension, the muscle is wrapped around all

of the distal tendons, and secured with mattress suturing using a nonabsorbable suture.

Deltoid Reconstruction

For deltoid reconstruction the origin of the muscle should be from the distal half of the clavicle to the acromion. The insertion of the muscle should be at the anatomic site where the deltoid inserts on the humerus. To tension the muscle correctly, the arm is placed in hyperextension to recreate the resting length. In this position, the length of the muscle is identified; however, the repair of the transfer at the insertion is completed with the arm in forward flexion and abduction to relieve tension on the repair site. The arm should be immobilized in the same position for 8 weeks postoperatively.

Elbow Flexion

With elbow flexion reconstruction, the origin of the FFMT is from the distal third of clavicle to the acromion (**Fig. 3**). Chuang and colleagues[23] reported in their series that the proximal attachment of the muscle appears to relate to the patient's functional outcome. When the corocoid was used, all of the patients had equal or greater strength than when the FFMT was attached to the second rib.[23]

Tensioning is performed with the elbow in full extension. The distal tendon repair is ideally sutured to the biceps tendon, and the position for this is marked with the arm in full extension; however, the repair is performed with elbow flexion to ensure there is no tension on the repair site (see **Fig. 3**). Another option is to fixate the muscle distally using suture anchors in the radial tuberosity or a drill hole at the same level in the

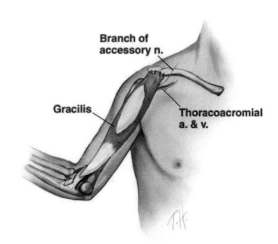

Fig. 3. Insetting of free functional gracilis muscle for elbow flexion reconstruction.

ulna. Following completion of the procedure, the arm is maintained at 90° of elbow flexion for 7 to 8 weeks. If intercostal nerves are used for the FFMT, the arm should be maintained in adduction.[10]

Chuang and colleagues[23] describe using the intercostal nerves to power functional muscle transfers, and their preference is for two nerves coapted to the muscle motor nerve, with one nerve embedded into the muscle for direct necrotization. In addition, the brachioradialis is used as a proximally based muscle flap to create a pulley for the muscle.[23]

Gousheh and Arasteh[24] describe using the contralateral medial pectoral nerve as a staged procedure with a sural nerve graft, rather than other donor options, and report good results in 17 of 19 patients. These investigators describe a staged reconstruction, where in the first stage sural nerve grafts are attached to the contralateral medial pectoral nerve and tunnelled across the chest. Approximately 1 year later, a free functional gracilis is transferred for elbow flexion.[24] The timing for the second stage is planned based on following an advancing Tinel sign across the chest. The authors of this chapter have used this technique 4 times with less successful results. Gousheh and Arasteh[24] also describe a third stage for these patients, which consisted of transferring the biceps tendon to the finger flexors using a tensor fascia lata spanning graft. In doing so, the fingers are tensioned so that elbow extension provides finger flexion.

In 1993, Doi and colleagues[19] also described their successful reconstructive approach with FFMT to restore more than one function in patients with brachial plexus palsy. Their original technique focused on simultaneous finger and elbow flexion reconstruction; however, they expanded this to include shoulder abduction and elbow flexion, and elbow flexion and wrist extension.[19]

Muscle Transfers for Triceps

The gracilis muscle can be used for elbow extension reconstruction using the same principles described for elbow flexion, except that the resting length of the muscle should be restored when the elbow is in full flexion. Vascular anastomosis options include the profunda brachii artery with venae comitantes, or the thoracodorsal pedicle. Innervation is ideally through branches from the radial nerve. If these are not available, intercostal nerves can be used, or the spinal accessory nerve with a sural nerve graft if needed. The new origin for the muscle is the lateral aspect of the scapula, with the muscle inserted into remnants of triceps tendon distally or into the olecranon directly. After the resting length has been restored in the position of full elbow flexion, the elbow can be brought to approximately 20° of flexion to allow for fixation of the muscle distally.

Finger Flexion

The origin for the FFMT for finger flexion is the medial epicondyle (**Fig. 4**). The tendon insertion should be performed without tension. To achieve this the elbow, wrist, and fingers are first placed into full extension, and the location of the tendon repair is marked. This action is performed with the muscle lying at its resting length as marked by the sutures. The wrist and fingers are then

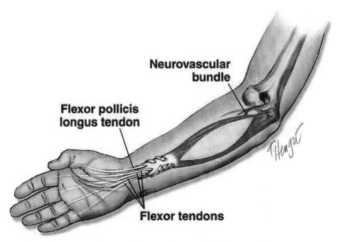

Neurovascular bundle

Flexor pollicis longus tendon

Flexor tendons

Fig. 4. Insetting of a free functional gracilis muscle transfer to the forearm for restoration of finger flexion with proper resting length.

brought into flexion, allowing the repair to be performed without tension. The authors' preference is to do this as a Pulvertaft weave to the flexor digitorum profundus (FDP) tendons (see **Fig. 4**). The FDP tendons are initially prepared as a single unit with side-to-side suturing. In doing so, there should be a slight progressive flexion of digits from radial to ulnar. It should be noted that the FDS tendons should be excised at the level of the wrist to limit adhesions.

If no tendon transfers are available to restore thumb flexion, it is possible for the gracilis to power both the thumb and finger flexors. If this is done as single unit, the flexor pollicis longus tendon must not be as tight as the finger flexors, so that the fingers will flex before the thumb moves. This allows the thumb to pinch against the radial side of the index finger for key pinch. The gracilis can also be divided for independent finger and thumb movement. To achieve this, the muscle must be split into two separate neuromuscular territories and innervated with two donor nerve branches with separate function.[36]

Postoperatively, the hand should be splinted with the wrist flex 20° to 30°, the fingers with the metacarpophalangeal (MCP) joints flexed at 70° to 90°, and full extension of the proximal interphalangeal (PIP) and distal interphalangeal (DIP) joints. The thumb should be splinted in full abduction with some interphalangeal joint flexion. This position is maintained for 4 weeks, during which time the elbow should also be maintained in up to 90° of flexion. During this period passive range of motion (ROM) flexor tendon protocols should be used.

Finger Extension

The origin of the muscle is sutured to the lateral epicondyle and common extensor fascia. Following this, the muscle is pulled distally until the resting length is achieved. Proper tensioning of the muscle requires the wrist and fingers to be placed in maximum flexion. To facilitate coordinated finger extension, the extensor digitorum communis (EDC) tendons should be woven together. The extensor pollicis longus (EPL) tendon can be rerouted along the radial side of the first metacarpal to provide extension and abduction. The position of tendon overlap is noted. Tension is then removed by placing the wrist in extension, and the tendon-to-tendon repairs are performed between the EDC and gracilis with a Pulvertaft weave. If there are no appropriate tendon transfers for thumb extension reconstruction, the EPL should be woven into the radial side of the gracilis tendon. Postoperatively, the elbow is immobilized at 90° flexion for 4 weeks.

The wrist is extended 30° to 45°, with the MCP joints flexed to 70° and full extension of the PIP and DIP joints for 6 weeks.

POSTOPERATIVE MANAGEMENT

Patients should have close monitoring for free tissue transfer 3 to 5 days postoperatively. The first 8 hours postoperatively are the most critical, when the highest incidence of vascular complications occurs. In the authors' practice, monitoring is performed every 30 minutes during the first 8 hours, followed by hourly checks for the next 16 hours. Paramount to the success of these procedures is a dedicated patient and therapist team for the often demanding and labor-intensive rehabilitation protocols. In the early period, the goal is to prevent contractures and to improve and maintain tendon gliding. For deltoid reconstruction, the arm is maintained in its splinted position; however, the therapist works on elbow, wrist, and finger ROM. For elbow flexion reconstruction, the elbow is maintained at 90°, as already described, for 6 to 8 weeks. During this time shoulder, wrist, and finger motion is preserved with ROM exercises. For finger flexion and extension reconstruction, passive stretching of the wrist and fingers is initiated 1 week after surgery, and is performed for 4 to 6 weeks postoperatively.

Once spontaneous contraction is observed, the patient is encouraged to actively contract the muscle frequently throughout the day. When intercostal nerves are used as the donor nerve, initially the transfer will be activated when the patient takes a deep breath.[23,34] Specific therapy for intercostal transfers involves exercises incorporating breathlessness, and then breathing retraining should be done.[31]

No resistance exercises are allowed for at least 3 to 4 months to prevent easy rupture of the muscle fibers. Following this, a graduated strength program for resisted exercise is initiated, and the patient should follow this for at least 2 years. In the authors' experience, swimming programs are an excellent way to optimize outcomes.

Electrical stimulation is used by some centers throughout the rehabilitation process[23]; however, its contribution to the success of the transfer is controversial. A 24-hour continuous passive motion machine incorporated into a custom splint postoperatively to limit adhesions has also been described,[26] however, the authors do not use this in their practice. Regardless of the use of these modalities, it is believed by many groups that it is important to incorporate activities of daily living into the rehabilitation training. In addition, patience awaiting the final outcome is important,

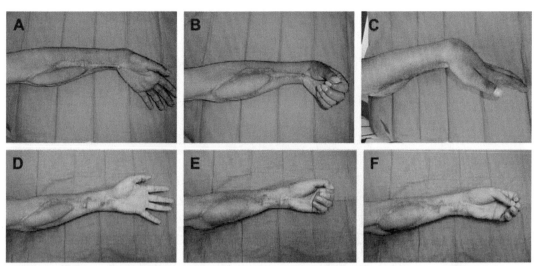

Fig. 5. A 4-year-old boy with severe Volkmann's contracture post supracondylar fracture. The patient had a free functional muscle transfer (FFMT) using a gracilis muscle at age 6 years. At 1.5 years post transfer, the patient demonstrated excellent flexion of his fingers. (*A–C*) Six years following the transfer development of severe flexion contracture of the wrist was treated with wrist fusion. (*D–F*) Functional outcome 1 year following wrist fusion as shown.

as the authors agree with other investigators that the rehabilitation program may not plateau for as long as 2 years following surgery.[29]

COMPLICATIONS

Complications with these complex procedures can occur, and these can be divided into acute surgical complications and more subacute or long-term complications. The acute complications include bleeding from the scarred tissue planes, infection, and wound breakdown with delayed healing. The most serious complication is problems with venous outflow and arterial inflow. Even if this is identified early and the muscle vascularity can be restored by returning to the

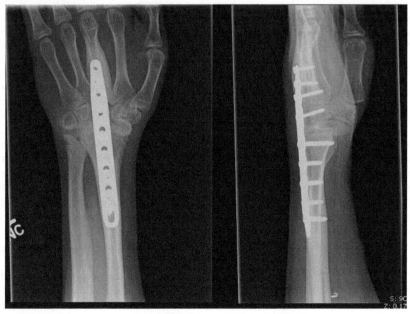

Fig. 6. Radiograph of the patient presented in **Fig. 5**, demonstrating successful correction of wrist flexion deformity with wrist fusion.

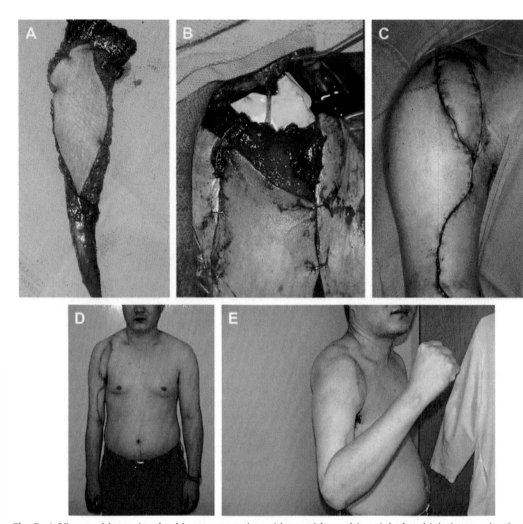

Fig. 7. A 27-year-old man involved in a motorcycle accident, with resulting right brachial plexus palsy. Supraclavicular exploration and intercostal nerve transfer were performed in another country. The patient was seen in the authors' clinic at age 30, with good hand function but no elbow flexion. Reconstruction was done with gracilis FFMT, using the spinal accessory nerve as a donor nerve with direct coaptation. (*A*) Free functional gracilis muscle harvest. (*B*) Direct nerve repair of obturator nerve to spinal accessory nerve. (*C*) Final insetting of musculocutaneous gracilis flap. (*D, E*) Follow-up at 2 years with excellent functional results showing greater than 140° elbow flexion.

operating room, the functional outcome will be poor if the ischemic period is longer than 1 hour. It would be more beneficial to remove the transferred muscle and perform a second FFMT.

More delayed complications include tendon adhesions and wrist flexion deformities.[26] In patients reconstructed for Volkmann's contracture, the two main reasons for wrist flexion deformities are weak extensor muscles and, in the pediatric patient population, ongoing growth of the extremity. In these cases, the bone grows at a faster rate than the muscles and soft tissues, creating a deforming force on the wrist, and because of this the authors recommend the patients are maintained with diligent splinting of the wrist in slight extension until bony maturity.[29] For correction of a permanent wrist flexion deformity, wrist fusion with partial proximal row carpectomy is the treatment of choice (**Figs. 5** and **6**). In cases of tendon adhesions, tenolysis is necessary to improve ROM.

RESULTS OF FREE FUNCTIONAL TRANSFERS

These procedures are very rewarding for both the patient and the multidisciplinary team involved in their care. The outcomes generally measured for FFMT are tip-to-palm distance, grip strength, and pinch strength. Because the group of patients

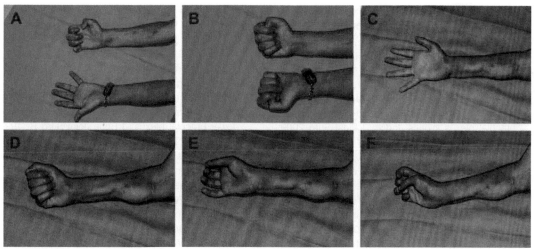

Fig. 8. (*A, B*) A 3-year-old boy with previous supracondylar fracture and development of Volkmann's ischemic contracture showing extension and flexion. The patient was referred for reconstruction at age 5. Functional gracilis was performed for finger flexion. The extensor carpi radialis longus was used at the same time as a tendon transfer for flexor pollicis longus reconstruction. (*C–F*) One-year follow-up with excellent finger extension, flexion, and thumb opposition.

requiring these procedures is so heterogeneous in their presentation and existing function, comparison of outcomes is variable. Predictors of good functional outcomes include the presence of intrinsic function in the hand, as well as, good pronation and supination.

Excellent results would include, for deltoid reconstruction, the ability to abduct the shoulder 80° or more. One of the main improvements with deltoid reconstruction is help with chronic subluxation and decreased shoulder pain.[29]

A patient with excellent results for elbow flexion reconstruction should be able to flex at least 120°. Other investigators have described a reasonable goal to achieve Medical Research Council (MRC) 4/5 strength, with full flexion and the ability to lift a 5-lb (2.27-kg) weight.[29] The authors have found that some patients with excellent results have been able to demonstrate greater than 140° of elbow flexion, though they have had difficulty lifting more than 3 lb (1.36 kg) of weight (**Fig. 7**). In a review, Kay and colleagues[10] found 70% of their patients to have a successful result, defined by a gain of greater than 1 MRC grade to 3 or greater.

Chuang and colleagues,[23] reported their 6-year experience with 38 FFMTs for elbow flexion. The majority of cases used the intercostal nerves as donor nerve (32 cases), versus only 4 cases using the spinal accessory and 3 cases using the musculocutaneous nerve. Success was graded as MRC strength of 4 or greater, and this was seen in 100% of the musculocutaneous nerve donor cases, 78% (18/23) of the intercostal nerve donor cases, and none of the spinal accessory cases (who only achieve MRC 2+).[23]

With finger flexion reconstruction, an excellent result is obtained when the fingers can touch the proximal palmar crease and have balanced flexion and extension with functional pinch (**Fig. 8**).

Muscle contraction can be present usually 2 months after surgery[29]; however, in the authors' experience, in the majority of patients this occurs at between 3 and 6 months. It is again important to highlight that the functional outcome can continue to improve up to 2 years postoperatively. Grip strength compared with the contralateral side has been shown to be 38% in adults and 25% in children.[29] These investigators believe the functional difference between these two groups may reflect testing techniques and difficulties in children, and the authors of this chapter have found similar outcomes.

SUMMARY

Brachial plexus injuries, and other conditions resulting in devastating loss of function in the upper extremity, have several well-described reconstructive options. These procedures include direct nerve repair, nerve transfer, tendon transfer, and/or local muscle transfer. In cases where these options are not suitable, FFMT is the treatment of choice. FFMTs require a great deal of preoperative planning and are technically demanding procedures; however, with the appropriate multidisciplinary support and the correct patient indications, they can provide excellent functional reconstruction in the upper extremity.

REFERENCES

1. Bhandari PS, Sadhotra LP, Bhargava P, et al. Surgical outcomes following nerve transfers in upper brachial plexus injuries. Indian J Plast Surg 2009; 42(2):150–60.

2. Brown JM, Yee A, Mackinnon SE. Distal median to ulnar nerve transfers to restore ulnar motor and sensory function within the hand: technical nuances. Neurosurgery 2009;65(5):966–77 [discussion: 977–8].

3. Chuang DC. Nerve transfers in adult brachial plexus injuries: my methods. Hand Clin 2005;21(1):71–82.

4. Gutowski KA, Orenstein HH. Restoration of elbow flexion after brachial plexus injury: the role of nerve and muscle transfers. Plast Reconstr Surg 2000; 106(6):1348–57 [quiz: 1358; discussion: 1359].

5. Mackinnon SE, Colbert SH. Nerve transfers in the hand and upper extremity surgery. Tech Hand Up Extrem Surg 2008;12(1):20–33.

6. Teboul F, Kakkar R, Ameur N, et al. Transfer of fascicles from the ulnar nerve to the nerve to the biceps in the treatment of upper brachial plexus palsy. J Bone Joint Surg Am 2004;86(7):1485–90.

7. Tung TH, Mackinnon SE. Nerve transfers: indications, techniques, and outcomes. J Hand Surg Am 2010;35(2):332–41.

8. Bishop AT. Functioning free-muscle transfer for brachial plexus injury. Hand Clin 2005;21(1):91–102.

9. Doi K, Muramatsu K, Hattori Y, et al. Restoration of prehension with the double free muscle technique following complete avulsion of the brachial plexus. indications and long-term results. J Bone Joint Surg Am 2000;82(5):652–66.

10. Kay S, Pinder R, Wiper J, et al. Microvascular free functioning gracilis transfer with nerve transfer to establish elbow flexion. J Plast Reconstr Aesthet Surg 2010;63(7):1142–9.

11. Tamai S, Komatsu S, Sakamoto H, et al. Free muscle transplants in dogs, with microsurgical neurovascular anastomoses. Plast Reconstr Surg 1970;46(3):219–25.

12. Harii K, Ohmori K, Torii S. Free gracilis muscle transplantation, with microneurovascular anastomoses for the treatment of facial paralysis. A preliminary report. Plast Reconstr Surg 1976;57(2):133–43.

13. Free muscle transplantation by microsurgical neurovascular anastomoses. report of a case. Chin Med J (Engl) 1976;2(1):47–50.

14. Ikuta Y, Kubo T, Tsuge K. Free muscle transplantation by microsurgical technique to treat severe Volkmann's contracture. Plast Reconstr Surg 1976;58(4):407–11.

15. Manktelow RT, McKee NH. Free muscle transplantation to provide active finger flexion. J Hand Surg Am 1978;3(5):416–26.

16. Manktelow RT, Zuker RM, McKee NH. Functioning free muscle transplantation. J Hand Surg Am 1984; 9(1):32–9.

17. Chuang DC, Carver N, Wei FC. Results of functioning free muscle transplantation for elbow flexion. J Hand Surg Am 1996;21(6):1071–7.

18. Doi K, Hattori Y, Kuwata N, et al. Free muscle transfer can restore hand function after injuries of the lower brachial plexus. J Bone Joint Surg Br 1998; 80(1):117–20.

19. Doi K, Sakai K, Ihara K, et al. Reinnervated free muscle transplantation for extremity reconstruction. Plast Reconstr Surg 1993;91(5):872–83.

20. Ercetin O, Akinci M. Free muscle transfer in Volkmann's ischaemic contracture. Ann Chir Main Memb Super 1994;13(1):5–12.

21. Favero KJ, Wood MB, Meland NB. Transfer of innervated latissimus dorsi free musculocutaneous flap for the restoration of finger flexion. J Hand Surg Am 1993;18(3):535–40.

22. Liu XY, Ge BF, Win YM, et al. Free medial gastrocnemius myocutaneous flap transfer with neurovascular anastomosis to treat Volkmann's contracture of the forearm. Br J Plast Surg 1992;45(1):6–8.

23. Chuang DC, Yeh MC, Wei FC. Intercostal nerve transfer of the musculocutaneous nerve in avulsed brachial plexus injuries: evaluation of 66 patients. J Hand Surg Am 1992;17(5):822–8.

24. Gousheh J, Arasteh E. Upper limb functional restoration in old and complete brachial plexus paralysis. J Hand Surg Eur Vol 2010;35(1):16–22.

25. Muramatsu K, Ihara K, Taguchi T. Selection of myocutaneous flaps for reconstruction following oncologic resection of sarcoma. Ann Plast Surg 2010; 64(3):307–10.

26. Terzis JK, Kostopoulos VK. Free muscle transfer in posttraumatic plexopathies: part III. The hand. Plast Reconstr Surg 2009;124(4):1225–36.

27. Stevanovic M, Sharpe F. Management of established Volkmann's contracture of the forearm in children. Hand Clin 2006;22(1):99–111.

28. Doi K, Kuwata N, Kawakami F, et al. Limb-sparing surgery with reinnervated free-muscle transfer following radical excision of soft-tissue sarcoma in the extremity. Plast Reconstr Surg 1999;104(6): 1679–87.

29. Zuker RM, Manktelow RT. Functioning free muscle transfers. Hand Clin 2007;23(1):57–72.

30. Chuang DC, Epstein MD, Yeh MC, et al. Functional restoration of elbow flexion in brachial plexus injuries: results in 167 patients (excluding obstetric brachial plexus injury). J Hand Surg Am 1993;18(2):285–91.

31. Chuang DC, Strauch RJ, Wei FC. Technical considerations in two-stage functioning free muscle transplantation reconstruction of both flexor and extensor functions of the forearm. Microsurgery 1994;15(5): 338–43.

32. Sananpanich K, Tu YK, Pookhang S, et al. Anatomic variance in common vascular pedicle of the gracilis and adductor longus muscles: Feasibility of double functioning free muscle transplantation with single pedicle anastomosis. J Reconstr Microsurg 2008; 24(4):231–8.

33. Mayer L, Green W. Experiences with the Steindler flexorplasty at the elbow. J Bone Joint Surg Am 1954;36(4):775–89, passim.

34. Functional anatomy and contraction of muscle. In: Guyton AC, editor. Anatomy and physiology. Philadelphia: Saunders College Publishing; 1985. p. 199–217.

35. Hattori Y, Doi K, Ohi R, et al. Clinical application of intraoperative measurement of choline acetyltransferase activity during functioning free muscle transfer. J Hand Surg Am 2001;26(4):645–8.

36. Chen L, Gu YD, Hu SN, et al. Contralateral C7 transfer for the treatment of brachial plexus root avulsions in children—a report of 12 cases. J Hand Surg Am 2007;32(1):96–103.

37. Mathes SJ, Nahai F. Gracilis flap. In: Reconstructive surgery: principles, anatomy and technique. New York: Churchill Livingstone; 1997. p. 1173–91.

38. Manktelow RT, Zuker RM. Muscle transplantation by fascicular territory. Plast Reconstr Surg 1984;73(5): 751–7.

39. Chuang DC. World Congress of Microsurgery Meeting. Okinawa, Japan, June 24–27, 2009.

40. Addosooki AI, Doi K, Hattori Y. Technique of harvesting the gracilis for free functioning muscle transplantation. Tech Hand Up Extrem Surg 2006; 10(4):245–51.

41. Barrie KA, Steinmann SP, Shin AY, et al. Gracilis free muscle transfer for restoration of function after complete brachial plexus avulsion. Neurosurg Focus 2004;16(5):E8.

42. Mathes SJ, Nahai F. Latissimus dorsi flap. In: Reconstructive surgery: principles, anatomy and technique. New York: Churchill Livingstone; 1997. p. 565–615.

Functional Reconstruction of the Hand: The Stiff Joint

Andrew J. Watt, MD*, James Chang, MD

KEYWORDS

- Stiff finger • Hand trauma • Flexor • Extensor
- Tenolysis • Capsulotomy

Proper hand function relies on a unique combination of strength, stability, discriminate sensation, and mobility. Disruption of this delicate balance results in diminution of hand function and loss of the ability to perform not only fine tasks but also basic activities of daily living. Joint contracture and stiffness of the hand are the net effect of several underlying etiologic factors including congenital abnormalities, neurologic disease, traumatic injury, prolonged immobilization, arthritis, and regional pain syndromes. These etiologic elements are often interrelated and multifactorial. Stiffness of the hand represents a challenging problem for surgeons and therapists, and remains the key impediment to achieving desired surgical outcomes in joint and soft-tissue reconstruction of the hand including tendon repair, replantation, and joint arthroplasty.

Evaluation and treatment of the stiff hand requires application of a systematic approach that integrates an understanding of the mechanism of injury, anatomic structures involved, and the modalities and proper timing of treatment available. Successful management relies on a cooperative effort, integrating the expertise of hand surgeons and therapists with patient education and diligence. This article provides an overview of the etiology, evaluation, and treatment of the stiff joint.

ETIOLOGY OF JOINT STIFFNESS
Wound Healing and Scar Formation

Joint motion is reliant on a balance between the rigid bony and ligamentous structures and the supple gliding of the joint surface, tendons, and the overlying soft tissues. Following a traumatic injury, infection, or surgical procedure, a predictable cascade of events is set in motion that seeks to restore tissue integrity. Although intricate, this wound-healing cascade cannot perfectly replicate or replace the damaged structures of the hand; rather, bone, tendon, synovium, and skin are replaced with callous and scar. An understanding of this wound-healing progression provides a framework for the application a variety of treatment modalities including splinting, mobilization, and operative intervention.

Wound healing comprises 3 overlapping phases: inflammatory, proliferative, and remodeling or maturation. The inflammatory phase begins with vascular disruption and the exposure of subintimal collagen. This insult leads to the activation of both the clotting and complement cascades.[1] Cytokines and chemokines released from platelets and neutrophils trigger vascular dilation, increased vascular permeability, and cell migration to the region of injury. Increased capillary permeability allows for protein-rich exudate to accumulate within the interstitial space. Coupled with decreased

Funding: No external funding was utilized in the preparation of this article.
Disclosure: The authors have no financial interests or conflicts to disclose.
Division of Plastic & Reconstructive Surgery, Department of Surgery, Stanford University Hospitals & Clinics, 770 Welch Road, Suite 400, Palo Alto, CA 94304, USA
* Corresponding author.
E-mail address: awatt@stanford.edu

Clin Plastic Surg 38 (2011) 577–589
doi:10.1016/j.cps.2011.07.006

lymphatic outflow, this increased permeability results in localized edema and is itself a primary contributor to stiffness. Edema results in direct, hydrostatic joint capsular distension and resistance to the normal gliding movements of the joints and tendons throughout the hand. If chronic, interstitial edema may become fibrotic as the fibrinogen-rich exudate is converted into interstitial scar, resulting in direct adhesion between normally mobile tissues.[2,3]

Inflammatory leukocytes (neutrophils and macrophages) are recruited to the site of injury. These cells produce matrix metalloproteinase enzymes that act to degrade extracellular matrix components, clearing necrotic debris and laying the foundation for fibroblast-dependent collagen synthesis and subsequent scar formation.[4] This second, proliferative phase is marked by the synthesis of disorganized type III collagen, and angiogenesis. Collagen is deposited along the joint capsule and collateral ligaments as well as along the flexor and extensor tendons. Wound healing progresses from the proliferative phase to the third phase of wound maturation and remodeling. Scar maturation is characterized by breakdown of the disorganized type III collagen and replacement with highly organized, cross-linked type I collagen. This scar is indiscriminate, providing necessary strength while obliterating the normal anatomic architecture and distinct tissue planes that facilitate joint motion.[5] Scar maturation is also characterized by scar contracture or tightening as a direct result of myofibroblast activity. The net effect is one of distorted anatomic structures, destruction of normal anatomic planes, and the direct connection of typically mobile structures to fixed ones.

Articular, Periarticular, and Tendon Anatomy

Alterations in the articular surface, periarticular ligamentous structures, and the flexor and extensor tendon mechanisms act alone or in concert to contribute to joint stiffness. Joint surfaces within the hand are analogous to larger articular surfaces found throughout the body. These surfaces are characterized by smooth yet durable articular cartilage with an intervening synovial space. Loss of this architecture through mechanical degradation in the form of osteoarthritis or secondary to traumatic events including intra-articular fractures can lead to deterioration in joint mobility. Intra-articular anatomy is closely aligned with periarticular structures that provide stability about the joint. These periarticular structures are highly specialized in the hand, and deserve particular attention when considering the etiology of joint stiffness.

The metacarpophalangeal (MCP) joint is a multi-axial condyloid joint. Motion about this joint includes flexion, extension, abduction, adduction, and a limited degree of circumduction.[6] The joint is stabilized by a taut volar plate that serves to prevent hyperextension, and a redundant dorsal capsule that allows for full flexion. Collateral and accessory collateral ligaments are present on the radial and ulnar sides of the joint coursing from metacarpal head to the base of the proximal phalanx in a dorsal to volar direction. These ligaments stabilize the joint against radially and ulnarly directed forces (**Fig. 1**). The consequence of this tangential orientation is that the collateral ligaments and capsule are taut with the MCP joint in flexion. This position also minimizes the intra-articular volume. Edema in the setting of inflammation about the MCP joint has a tendency to force the joint into extension, maximizing intra-articular volume and placing the collateral ligaments in a position of laxity. If this position persists throughout the phases of wound healing, the MCP joint will become stiff in this position of extension, with shortened collateral and accessory collateral ligaments.

In comparison with the MCP joint, the proximal interphalangeal (PIP) joint is significantly more restricted. The PIP joint is a hinge or ginglymus joint allowing for a wide arc of flexion, with motion restricted to the coronal plane. The configuration of the joint surface and the periarticular ligamentous structures is highly stable. Analogous to the MCP joint, the volar plate of the PIP joint is taut in extension and prevents hyperextension while allowing full flexion. The volar plate of the PIP joint, however, differs from that of the MCP joint, in that it is thin or membranous proximally. The proximal portion of the PIP joint volar plate also gives rise to two distinct structures that course proximally, crossing the transverse digital artery just proximal to the PIP joint, anchoring the volar plate to the proximal phalanx. These structures have been variously referred to as check ligaments or checkreins, and can be a significant source of joint stiffness if shortened or fibrosed.[7,8] Two soft-tissue layers define the radial and ulnar aspects of the PIP joint. The superficial layer consists of a thin complement of transverse and oblique fibers known as the retinacular ligament of Landsmeer. This structure contributes very little to the stability of the joint; however, scarring and fibrosis of this ligament can restrict joint motion substantially. Deep to Landsmeer's ligament are the proper and accessory collateral ligaments. These substantive structures course from the proximal phalangeal head to the middle phalangeal base in a dorsal to volar direction, inserting on the lateral

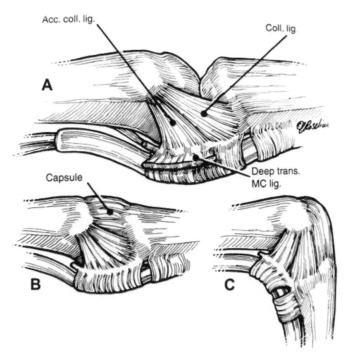

Fig. 1. Anatomy of the metacarpophalangeal (MCP) joint. (*A*) The accessory and proper collateral ligament provide resistance to radial and ulnar deviation. (*B*) MCP joint in extension; the dorsal capsule and proper collateral ligament are lax. (*C*) MCP joint in flexion; the dorsal capsule and proper collateral ligament are taut. (*From* Shin AY, Amadio PC. Stiff finger joints. In: Green DP, Hotchkiss RN, Pederson WC, et al, editors. Green's operative hand surgery. 5th edition. Philadelphia: Elsevier Churchill Livingstone; 2005. p. 418; with permission.)

aspects of the volar plate (**Fig. 2**). Although the course is similar to that taken by the MCP collateral ligaments, the proximal phalangeal head has no volar flare and the PIP collateral ligaments are taut throughout the full arc of PIP motion. Direct injury to or immobilization of these structures in a position of laxity can result in significant stiffness and consequent functional impairment.

Finger stiffness can arise not only from the articular and periarticular structures but also from the mobile components or tendons acting across these joints. The musculotendinous units of the

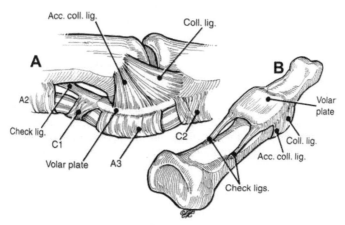

Fig. 2. Anatomy of the proximal interphalangeal (PIP) joint. (*A*) The accessory and proper collateral ligament provide resistance to radial and ulnar deviation. (*B*) PIP joint in extension; the volar plate and proper collateral ligament are taut. (*From* Shin AY, Amadio PC. Stiff finger joints. In: Green DP, Hotchkiss RN, Pederson WC, et al, editors. Green's operative hand surgery. 5th edition. Philadelphia: Elsevier Churchill Livingstone; 2005. p. 419; with permission.)

hand may be subdivided into intrinsic and extrinsic groups. The intrinsic system is powered by muscles taking their origin within the hand itself, and includes the palmar and dorsal interossei, the lumbricals, and the thenar and hypothenar units. The extrinsic system, by contrast, is powered by muscles taking their origin within the forearm.

The extrinsic extensor system comprises extra-synovial tendons, and includes extensors of the thumb (extensor pollicis longus [EPL], extensor pollicis brevis [EPB]) and fingers (extensor digitorum communis [EDC], extensor indicis proprius [EIP], and extensor digiti minimi [EDM]). The EDC components to the index through small fingers share a common muscle of origin, and are often linked by tendinous juncturae. These shared structures tend to propagate restricted motion to adjacent tendons; consequently, if the EDC to the long finger is restricted, motion of the EDC to the ring finger may be restricted as well. The extensor tendons glide over the periosteum of the metacarpals and phalanges, and lack an associated fibro-osseous sheath. At the level of the MCP joint, the extrinsic extensor tendons are centralized by the sagittal bands. Over the PIP joint the extensor tendons are joined by the dorsal and volar interossei and the lumbricals. This interconnection serves as a biomechanical link between the intrinsic and extrinsic musculotendinous systems. Insertion of the extensor tendon into the middle phalanx occurs via a central slip, just distal to the PIP joint, and into the distal phalanx via two lateral slips that join to insert at the base of the distal phalanx.

The extrinsic flexor system comprises synovial tendons and includes the thumb flexor (flexor pollicis longus [FPL]) and finger flexors (flexor digitorum superficialis [FDS], flexor digitorum profundus [FDP]). These tendons course through a synovial lined fibro-osseous canal consisting of a series of annular and cruciate pulleys. These pulleys provide a biomechanical advantage, allowing the flexor tendons to exert their distal effects without the need for excessive excursion or bowstringing.

The intrinsic system of the hand serves to fine-tune motor movements and modulate the activity of the less precise extrinsic tendons, and affords a greater degree of dexterity by facilitating composite motions. This intrinsic system consists of the thenar and hypothenar musculature as well as the interossei and lumbrical muscles. The interossei muscles are divided into volar and dorsal groups. The 3 volar interossei are responsible for digital adduction across the MCP joint. The 4 dorsal interossei are responsible for digital abduction. Damage to these muscles with subsequent

scarring, tethering of the flexor or extensor mechanisms, and shortening of the interosseous or lumbrical tendons all contribute to stiffness of the hand and present with characteristic functional deficits that must be recognized to ensure proper correction.

EVALUATION OF THE STIFF HAND

Evaluation and treatment of the stiff hand requires application of an organized approach. The surgeon's primary objective is to properly identify the factors contributing to joint stiffness, and to specifically and systematically target these factors with the treatment plan. Consideration is given as to whether the stiffness is manifest as primarily an inability to flex, an inability to extend, or both. This knowledge is coupled with a comparison of active and passive motion and tests of both intrinsic and extrinsic tightness.

The factors contributing to joint stiffness may be organized in a superficial to deep manner. This method provides a framework for evaluation and corresponds with a logical sequence of surgical interventions. Examination begins with inspection and palpation of the skin. Scar and scar contracture are often a significant source of limited mobility. Dorsal scars tend to restrict flexion, whereas volar scars result in flexion contractures and restrict extension. The next level of analysis involves distinguishing the degree to which stiffness is related to musculotendinous pathology. A direct comparison of active and passive motion across a joint is performed. If passive motion exceeds active motion the etiology is, at least in part, musculotendinous. In other words, if the joint across which the tendons are acting is supple (passive motion) but the tendons across that joint do not affect the same degree of joint motion (active motion), the musculotendinous unit is either incompetent or adherent. If active and passive motion are equal, the tendons acting across a joint are able to affect maximal movement allowed by that joint. In this case, articular and periarticular origins are most likely responsible for the limited motion. In this case, radiographic imaging including plain radiography and computed tomography are helpful in evaluating articular congruence and in identifying bony impediments to movement. The presence of a joint that exhibits no motion, either active or passive, is particularly problematic with regard to diagnosis. This type of finger represents a key principle: the etiology of restricted motion is often multifactorial, and certain elements contributing to contracture may become apparent only after other contributing factors are addressed.

In addition to careful examination of both active and passive joint motion, the effect of joint position on motion should be carefully noted. Evaluation of joint motion with the hand and wrist in a variety of positions can add valuable information regarding intrinsic and extrinsic tightness. Sterling Bunnell described the physical examination findings associated with intrinsic tightness. Knowing the intrinsic muscles cross both the MCP and PIP joints acting as flexors of at the level of the MCP joint and extensors at the level of the PIP joint, Bunnell described the effect of MCP joint position on PIP joint motion. The Bunnell intrinsic tightness test consists of placing the MCP joints in flexion, thereby shortening the intrinsic musculature, and comparing PIP joint motion obtained with the MCP joints in flexion and extension. If PIP flexion is greater with the MCP joints flexed (positive intrinsic test), then there is some element of intrinsic tightness contributing to finger stiffness.[9,10] Similar tests of extension and flexion with the wrist in neutral, flexed, and extended positions provide information as to extrinsic sufficiency and possible extrinsic tightness.

TREATMENT

Treatment of the stiff hand is guided by a thorough knowledge of normal anatomy coupled with an appreciation for the mechanism of injury, and an understanding of the pathologic anatomy following injury (**Table 1**). Three basic principles guide treatment of the stiff hand. First, no operative intervention should be undertaken until maximal gains have been achieved via nonoperative modalities. Second, the patient must have an understanding of their critical role both in preparation for and rehabilitation from surgical intervention. Third, operative treatment must be well planned, focused, and logical.

Nonoperative Treatment

Nonoperative treatment of the stiff finger is of paramount importance in maximizing recovery from the initial injury, preparing the patient for surgical intervention, and in rehabilitation following any surgical intervention. Basic interventions include strict elevation above the level of the heart to minimize interstitial edema and proper splinting at the time of the initial injury. The vast majority of hand injuries may be splinted in the position of safety with the wrist in 30° of extension, the MCP joints flexed at 90°, and the PIP joints in full extension. This position places the MCP and PIP collateral ligaments at their maximum stretch, straightens the volar plate of the PIP joint, and minimizes the intra-articular space of the MCP joint. These effects are all beneficial in minimizing

Table 1
Anatomy and treatment of the stiff hand

	Anatomic Components	Treatment

First web space adduction contracture	Skin
	First dorsal interosseous
	
	Adductor pollicis
		Skin only:
		    4-Flap Z-plasty
		    "Jumping man" Z-plasty
		Skin and musculature:
		    Reverse radial forearm flap
		    Lateral arm flap
		    ALT fascial flap

Flexion contracture	Volar skin
	Palmar/digital fascia
	Flexor tendon sheath
	Flexor tendon
	Collateral ligaments
	
	Transverse retinacular ligaments (PIP joint only)
	Checkrein ligaments (PIP joint only)
	Volar plate
		Z-Plasty, skin graft, cross-finger flap
		Excision of fascia
		Release of tendon sheath
		Flexor tenolysis
		Collateral ligament division
		    Accessory collateral
		    Proper collateral
		Division of transverse retinacular ligament
		
		Checkrein release
		Volar plate release

Extension contracture	Dorsal scar Extensor tendon Dorsal joint capsule Collateral ligaments	Z-Plasty, skin graft, reverse cross-finger flap Extensor tenolysis Dorsal capsular release Collateral ligament division

Abbreviations: ALT, anterolateral thigh; PIP, proximal interphalangeal.

postimmobilization stiffness. Immobilization should be performed only as long as is necessary to allow for adequate healing. Early, protected motion is always favorable if the injury pattern or fixation will allow. Care should also be taken to avoid unnecessarily immobilizing joints or digits that are uninvolved in the injury.

Beyond preventive measures, hand surgeons and therapists have a host of modalities, exercises, and splinting methods at their disposal to address the stiff finger. Modality therapy including ultrasound, heat, and cold all strive to reduce inflammation and edema. Once the hand has become stiff, active and passive range of motion exercises and a multiple splinting techniques are used to maximize function. These techniques rely on the principle that living tissue will reorganize and differentiate in response to mechanical stress.[11] These tissues can be induced to reorganize in a favorable anatomic configuration, conducive to increased motion. Refinements in these techniques have demonstrated that low-load, prolonged stress is more effective than high-load, brief stretch in inducing tissue remodeling, and that increase in the passive range of motion of a joint is directly proportional to the duration at which the joint is held at the end of its range.[12,13] In summary, motion therapy is maximized with long duration, low-load stress adequate to position the shortened tissue at or near the end of its currently available length.[14] This principle provides the basic foundation of range of motion therapy and splinting.

Splinting plays a central role in acute injury management as well as in preoperative and postoperative therapy. Splints may be static, serial static, static progressive, or dynamic. Each splint type has a specific function and is correlated with the phase of wound healing. Static splints are a mainstay in acute management, immobilizing injured structures, providing rest and pain relief, and maintaining tissue length to prevent joint stiffness and contractures. Serial static splints are molded to achieve a specific position, and adjusted to provide gentle prolonged stretch. These splints are useful in correcting existing contractures and improving passive joint range of motion. Dynamic splints apply a passive force across a joint in one direction while permitting active motion in the opposite direction. These splints work by employing energy-storing materials (rubber bands, springs) to counteract tissue resistance while still allowing active motion. Dynamic splints are particularly useful in allowing for early protected tendon range of motion after injury or repair, supplanting absent or existing motor functions and providing gentle, persistent stretch across contracted joints. In contrast to dynamic splints, static progressive splints are composed of inelastic components that position a joint close to the end range of motion, and are adjusted as passive range of motion gains are achieved.[3]

Nonoperative treatment modalities are often successful in improving joint range of motion and alleviating stiffness. It has been estimated that 87% of MCP and PIP joint contractures, arising from a variety of underlying etiologic factors, can be fully managed nonoperatively.[15] Nonoperative treatment should continue as long as there are continued positive gains. Surgical intervention is indicated if a plateau is reached and the net motion and hand function are still unacceptable.

Operative Treatment

Operative treatment of the stiff finger affords the surgeon the opportunity to restore function to the debilitated hand; however, this opportunity is tempered by the fact that any operation initiates an inflammatory cascade that may exacerbate existing stiffness. This risk is minimized via meticulous surgical technique, proper patient education, and aggressive postoperative hand therapy. To avoid repeated trauma, surgical intervention should be focused, avoid excessive dissection, and be properly sequenced. Staged procedures should be separated by 3 to 4 months to allow the tissues to reach equilibrium before proceeding with the subsequent stage. The extensor elements contributing to stiffness should be addressed first. Extensor mobility can be effectively maintained with passive motion regimens. The flexor elements contributing to stiffness should be addressed after the extensor elements are freed, as unrestricted active motion will be necessary to maximize results following flexor tenolysis. Attention should be paid to ensuring that the overlying soft-tissue envelope is sufficient and supple. Provision for adequate soft-tissue reconstruction should precede any attempt to restore finger motion.

Surgical treatment may be performed under local, regional, or general anesthesia. Local, infiltrative anesthesia with distal peripheral nerve blocks is preferred, as the awake patient can participate by providing active motion following the sequential release of structures. A tourniquet is useful in allowing for adequate visualization; however, longer tourniquet times result in temporary paralysis of the arm, and an upper arm tourniquet is often poorly tolerated by the awake patient. These effects can be minimized with the use of a forearm tourniquet. Infiltrative anesthesia with epinephrine may also be used to minimize bleeding, and has been demonstrated to be safe and effective in the finger.[16,17] Regional and general anesthesia are reserved for patients undergoing extensive tenolysis, typically on multiple fingers, and in those patients who may require forearm dissection.

Soft-tissue reconstruction

The skin of the hand is highly specialized. The dorsum of the hand is covered by thin, pliable, nonglabrous skin while the palm is covered by durable yet pliable glabrous skin. The skin alone may act as a significant source of limited mobility if extensively scarred (**Fig. 3**). Provision for soft-tissue reconstruction should precede or be combined with the first surgical stage of reconstruction. Soft-tissue reconstruction ranges in complexity from scar release or lengthening via Z-plasty, to skin grafting, local and regional flaps, and free tissue transfer. The majority of skin contractures can be addressed with scar excision and skin grafting. Indications for higher-level reconstruction include exposure of neurovascular structures, tendon, bone, or prosthetic hardware.

Contracture of the first web space deserves particular attention. First web space contractures are common, particularly following hand burns and trauma. In most cases a 4-flap Z-plasty or "jumping man" Z-plasty is sufficient to widen the web space (**Fig. 4**). In cases where there has been a significant crush component to the injury, the musculature of the first web space is often quite scarred, restricting motion. In these cases soft-tissue provision with a reverse radial forearm flap or a free tissue transfer (lateral arm flap, anterolateral thigh fascia flap) is necessary to restore adequate adduction (**Fig. 5**).

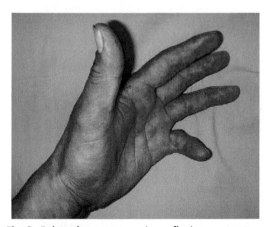

Fig. 3. Palmar burn scar causing a flexion contracture of the metacarpophalangeal joint.

Extensor tenolysis

Extensor contractures can result from dorsal scar, dorsal capsular fibrosis, contracted or adherent intrinsic muscles, articular deformity, and extensor tendon adhesion. Extensor tendon adhesions are the most common cause of extensor contracture. The extensor mechanism is most easily approached via a longitudinal incision placed directly over the site of suspected adherence. The incision should extend into uninjured anatomic regions both proximally and distally to allow for accurate identification of normal tissue planes.

The proper plane of dissection preserves the paratenon, and raises a composite skin and subcutaneous tissue skin flap. Residual adhesions between the skin and tendon should be released sharply. Once the tendon mechanism has been cleared along its dorsal surface, the volar surface is then approached. The sagittal bands are preserved as best as possible. If access to the joint requires release of a sagittal band, the ulnar sagittal band is released to prevent ulnar subluxation of the extensor tendon. Dissection is then performed distally along the undersurface of the lateral bands. The transverse retinacular ligament is divided by placing a Freer elevator between the ligament and the underlying collateral ligaments. A combination of dissection with a #15 blade and a Freer elevator is used to disrupt any adhesions between the extensor mechanism and the underlying bone. Dissection is facilitated by working alternately on the radial and ulnar aspects in regions where exposure is facile, then connecting these regions of dissection. On the dorsal aspect of the finger, dissection should be done distally to the base of the middle phalanx, taking care to avoid disruption of the central slip insertion. Laterally, the dissection may be performed to the level of the distal interphalangeal joint (DIP), if necessary, to restore motion.

Dorsal capsular release

If full passive flexion is not restored following extensor tenolysis, dorsal involvement of the periarticular soft tissues must be addressed. At the level of the MCP joint, the periarticular structures are concealed beneath the sagittal bands. These bands should be preserved to prevent extensor tendon subluxation; however, the ulnar sagittal band may be partially divided in the direction of their fibers without disrupting continuity. A #15-blade, passed under the sagittal band, can be used to sharply divide the dorsal capsule of the MCP joint (**Fig. 6**). Division of the collateral ligaments at this level is rarely necessary, and if performed, preservation of the proper collateral ligament is prudent. At the level of the PIP joint,

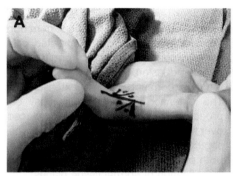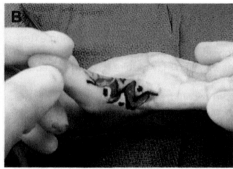

Fig. 4. Four-flap Z-plasty. (*A*) First web space adduction contracture. Note the design of a 4-flap Z-plasty. The long arm of the Z-plasty is placed within the plane of restriction. Equivalent-length dorsal and volar limbs are drawn at 90° angles to this axis. The resultant angle is then bisected to create 4 opposing flaps each with an angle of 45°. (*B*) Release of first web space adduction contracture with 4-flap Z-plasty. Note the interdigitation of the skin flaps.

the periarticular structures may be exposed by retracting the lateral bands. Division of the dorsal joint capsule is performed under direct vision. Intra-articular adhesions may be gently disrupted with a Freer elevator placed within the joint space; however, care should be taken to avoid damaging the delicate articular cartilage. PIP collateral ligament shortening is a cause of residual contracture, and may be performed under direct vision. Division of the collateral ligaments should be performed sparingly. The accessory ligaments should be divided bilaterally, before any division of the proper collateral ligaments. If division of the accessory collateral ligaments remains insufficient, the proper collaterals may be partially divided to facilitate motion. Every effort should be made to preserve at least a portion of the radial and ulnar proper collateral ligaments to prevent lateral instability of the joint.

Flexor tenolysis

Flexion contractures can result from palmar scarring, contracture of the superficial palmar or digital

fascia, shortening of the fibro-osseous flexor sheath, adhesions of the flexor tendon and associated musculature, adherence of the transverse retinacular ligaments to the collateral ligaments, contracture of the volar plate, or shortening of the accessory and proper collateral ligaments. Patients with restricted extension or with passive flexion in excess of active flexion who have plateaued as regards functional gains may benefit from flexor tenolysis and volar capsulotomy. The flexor mechanism may be approached through either a volar Bruner incision or a midlateral incision. A Bruner approach allows for greater exposure and facilitates proximal and distal dissection when necessary. This incision places a painful incision in the palm, which may restrict postoperative therapy. In addition, should wound complications arise, the underlying flexor mechanism may become directly exposed. The midlateral approach prevents these palmar complications; however, exposure is limited and extending the dissection proximal to the proximal phalanx becomes difficult. A midlateral approach is preferred in the

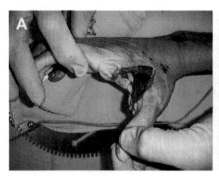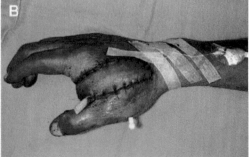

Fig. 5. First web space reconstruction. (*A*) First web space soft-tissue deficit following release of adduction contracture. (*B*) Reconstruction of the first web space with a free lateral arm fasciocutaneous flap.

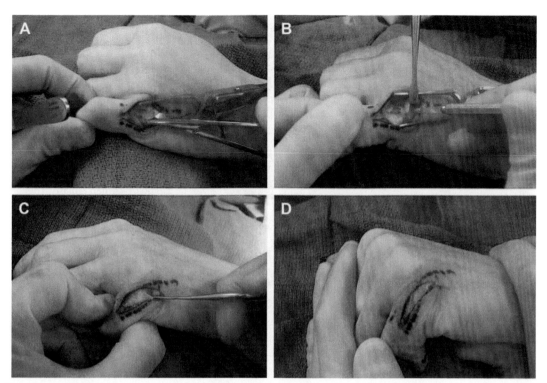

Fig. 6. Dorsal MCP capsulotomy. (*A*) Extensor mechanism overlying the MCP joint is exposed; a portion of the ulnar sagittal band is released to gain access to the joint. (*B*) The dorsal capsule is exposed. (*C*) A Freer elevator is used to ensure that all extensor adhesions have been taken down. (*D*) Full passive flexion is obtained following dorsal capsulotomy.

treatment of isolated PIP contractures, as functional outcomes have been proved to be superior.[18]

Analogous to extensor tenolysis, composite cutaneous flaps are elevated. The flexor tendon sheath is cleared of overlying adipose tissue and scar, preserving the fibro-osseous network of annular and cruciate pulleys. The A-2 and A-4 pulleys are preserved to prevent bowstringing of the flexor mechanism. Dissection proceeds in a proximal to distal fashion. A window in the flexor tendon sheath is made proximal to the A-1 pulley, and the FDS and FDP tendons are clearly identified. Once free at this level, a second window is made between the distal border of the A-2 pulley and the proximal border of the A-4 pulley. The superficialis and profundus tendons are freed from the overlying pulleys and underlying bone. The FDS and FDP are then separated from one another (**Fig. 7**). Differential traction on each tendon in the proximal palm aids in separation of these two tendons. This dissection is facilitated by the use of a Freer elevator and atraumatic "twirling" of the tendon using an Allis clamp. Suture-passing techniques are also helpful in connecting the inconspicuous regions of adhesion with easily exposed regions. A 2-0 silk suture can

be passed around the flexor tendons proximal to the A-1 pulley. The ends of the suture are then passed along the radial and ulnar aspects of the tendon and brought out through the distal sheath window. These ends are then pulled alternately, and disrupt weak adhesions while delivering strong adhesions distally so that they may be divided under direct vision. The FDS should be adequately freed at its decussation and traced dorsally toward its insertion. Intertendinous dissection is facilitated by applying differential traction on the FDS and FDP tendons. First the FDS is pulled distally while the FDP is pulled proximally, then this differential pull is reversed to expose occult adhesions. An additional sheath window may need to be created distal to the A-4 pulley if the FDP remains tethered at the level of the DIP joint.

It is often useful to supplement direct tenolysis with traction of the tendons from a proximal vantage point. In patients with extensive adhesions, a counter incision in the distal forearm allows for identification of the appropriate flexor tendons and the application of gently, longitudinally directed traction to supplement direct dissection within the palm and fingers.

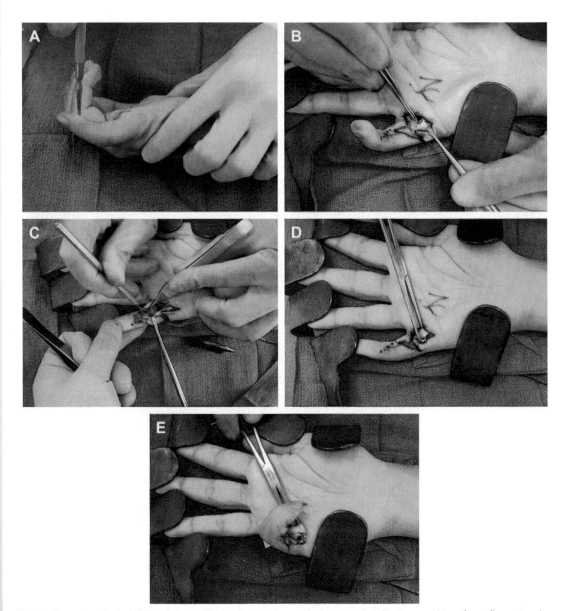

Fig. 7. Flexor tenolysis. (*A*) Small-finger limited extension and absent active flexion resulting from flexor tendon scarring. (*B*) Scarred flexor tendons distal to the A-1 pulley. (*C*) Checkrein release to achieve full PIP joint extension. (*D*) Allis clamp used to atraumatically "twirl" the flexor tendons. (*E*) Full flexion is obtained following tenolysis.

Volar capsular release

If adequate extension is not achieved with flexor tenolysis, attention is turned to the volar plate complex. The volar complex of the PIP joint is unique, and is often the final common restrictive element preventing full extension. Following even minor trauma and immobilization, the volar plate and associated checkrein ligaments are prone to thickening, tethering the volar plate to the proximal phalanx. The volar plate complex is exposed by retracting the flexor tendon mechanism at the level of the PIP joint. The checkrein ligaments are identified coursing from the volar plate to the proximal phalanx. The transverse digital artery courses deep to the checkrein ligaments 2 mm proximal to the PIP joint. This artery should be preserved as the checkrein ligament is sharply divided (**Fig. 8**). If restricted extension persists, formal capsular release is indicated. The volar plate is sharply divided at its distal insertion onto the middle phalanx. Extension is once again assessed. The accessory collateral ligament is

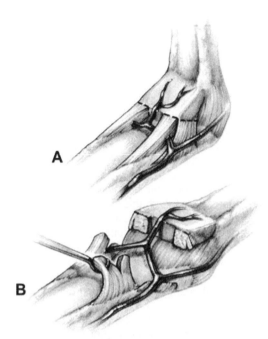

Fig. 8. Pathologic checkrein bands and checkrein release. (*A*) The checkrein ligaments anchor the volar plate to the proximal phalanx. The transverse communicating vessel traverses the checkrein ligaments 2 mm proximal to the volar plate. (*B*) Complete release of the checkrein ligaments with preservation of the transverse communicating vessel. (*From* Shin AY, Amadio PC. Stiff finger joints. In: Green DP, Hotchkiss RN, Pederson WC, et al, editors. Green's operative hand surgery. 5th edition. Philadelphia: Elsevier Churchill Livingstone; 2005. p. 431; with permission.)

identified and divided, preserving the proper collateral ligament. Every effort should be made to preserve the proper collateral ligament. It is prudent to accept up to 20° of residual contracture if necessary to preserve the proper collateral ligament. If extension remains markedly restricted, partial or complete release of the proper collateral ligament may be performed.

Articular replacement
Patients with articular injuries and those with long-standing contracture may have underlying articular incongruence or bony exostoses that restrict joint motion. Soft-tissue reconstruction may also convert a relatively painless stiff joint into a painful mobile joint. In these patients with an adequate soft-tissue envelope, surface replacement arthroplasty with a pyrolytic pyrocarbon prosthesis or silicone joint replacement arthroplasty may be indicated.

Wound closure and postoperative care
Skin closure following extensor tenolysis is performed with 4-0 nylon mattress sutures. These sutures must withstand early motion and are dressed daily with Xeroform gauze. Skin closure following flexor tenolysis and volar capsular release is analogously performed with 4-0 nylon sutures in the finger and 3-0 nylon sutures in the palm. These sutures remain in place 10 to 14 days depending on wound healing. A splint is placed for brief postoperative immobilization, and serves primarily to facilitate comfort. Patients then begin a supervised active and passive range of motion protocol on postoperative day 1. At this visit, the operative splint is removed and a removable splint is fashioned to allow the patient to perform hourly range of motion exercises. Strict elevation and edema control are reinforced. Patients who are able to adhere to this strict regimen typically maintain much of the intraoperative gains in mobility.

OUTCOMES ANALYSIS

Operative and nonoperative outcomes in the treatment of the stiff finger have been well studied. The nonoperative management of MCP flexion contractures has been documented by Weeks and colleagues,[15] who examined 336 MCP joint contractures in 212 patients treated with a combination of passive range of motion exercise and dynamic splinting. Average gains in range of motion were 35°, 40°, 11°, and 42° in the index, long, ring, and small finger, respectively. Four hundred and fifty-three PIP joint flexion contractures were studied within this population of 212 patients treated with a combination of active and passive range of motion exercises in addition to static and dynamic splinting. Average gains in range of motion were 34°, 35°, and 32° in the long, ring, and small finger, respectively. Overall, 173 (87%) patients responded favorably within 2 weeks of therapy, obviating the need for further intervention.

Prosser examined the effect of dynamic splinting for PIP joint contractures, comparing a Capener splint and a low-profile outrigger splint in 20 patients with PIP flexion contractures. No statistical difference was found between splint types; however, there was a significant relationship between longer splinting times and improved final range of motion.[19]

Operative outcomes of MCP and PIP contracture release have been well documented in the literature. Gould and Nicholson[20] examined the outcomes of 105 MCP joint capsulotomies performed in 37 patients through a dorsal approach, noting an improvement in average active flexion of 21°. Although this gain was modest and only a fraction of the motion gained intraoperatively, the investigators concluded that this gain was worthwhile and resulted in improvement in hand function.

Curtis[21] reported initial results in the operative treatment of 25 patients with PIP flexion contractures. These patients underwent surgical capsulotomy, collateral ligament excision, and volar plate elevation, followed by placement of a transarticular Kirschner wire for 1 week. Curtis' general conclusions remain valid. He noted that poorer results corresponded directly with an increasing number of structures involved in the contracture.[21] The explanation for this conclusion is twofold, with these patients having more severe contractures prior to surgical release, and with increased inflammation and scarring arising from more extensive surgical intervention. Curtis also noted that approximately 50% of the intraoperative gain in passive motion translates into retained active motion.

Bruser and colleagues[18] compared 45 PIP contracture releases performed either via a midaxial or volar approach. The midaxial group retained and average gain of motion of 50° at 1.5-year follow-up compared with an average gain of motion of 30° in the volar group. This difference was statistically significant.

Ghidella and colleagues[22] retrospectively reviewed 68 PIP contracture releases in an effort to determine predictive demographic, preoperative, and operative factors influencing functional outcomes. These investigators found an average of 7.5° of improvement in total arc of PIP motion at 2-year follow-up. It was concluded that the best candidates for surgical release of PIP contractures are younger than 28 years with an uncomplicated or isolated contracture, with maximal preoperative flexion of less than 43°.

For patients with articular disease, silicone implant arthroplasty provides reliable pain relief; however, joint range of motion is limited, varying between 27° and 60° in most outcomes analyses.[23–29] Patients often note significant instability against radial and ulnarly directed forces, which limits its application in the index finger, and the durability of silicone arthroplasty is poor. Surface replacement arthroplasty theoretically offers greater durability and stability, acting as a true joint rather than a flexible spacer. Outcomes analyses thus far have generally shown preservation of preoperative range of motion from 47° to 58°[30–32]; however, one-third of patients require revisional surgery including tenolysis, contracture releases, and revision arthroplasty.[30] These results underscore the fact that although encouraging, surface replacement arthroplasty of the small joints of the hand remains a challenge.

SUMMARY

Stiffness of the hand results from disruption of the delicate balance between the static and mobile components of the hand. Disruption of this balance primarily results from traumatic causes; however, neurologic injury, Dupuytren disease, infection, and prolonged immobilization may also contribute to decreased hand mobility. Stiffness and loss of motion remain the primary impediment to achieving functional outcomes in nearly every aspect of hand surgery and yet clinicians' ability to treat this stiffness remains limited. Sterling Bunnell adeptly identified this challenge: "An ever present menace in hand surgery is the decided tendency for the hand to stiffen and to stiffen in the position of nonfunction."[33] An understanding of the pathologic etiology and anatomic elements involved in the development of hand stiffness is critical for all practitioners who treat patients with hand injuries.

Hand stiffness remains the net effect of inflammation, immobilization, and scarring between normally mobile and nonmobile structures. Edema reduction, proper splinting, and early range of motion therapy coupled with appropriate use of progressive splinting remain the initial, and undoubtedly the most critical step in the management of the stiff hand. These measures not only help to prevent stiffness, but remain the most reliable means toward improving function in the already stiff hand. Surgical treatment is reserved for those patients who have plateaued with nonoperative therapy and have residual restricted hand function. Surgical treatment is guided by an accurate identification of the anatomic articular, periarticular, tendinous, and soft-tissue structures responsible for limiting motion. Surgical intervention is performed to precisely address only those components contributing to contracture while preserving the uninvolved structures. Meticulous surgical technique is critical in avoiding damage to uninvolved structures and minimizing postoperative inflammation.

A cooperative effort between the patient, hand therapist, and surgeon maximizes the potential outcomes. The results of surgical intervention for the stiff finger are modest and, at times, unpredictable. In general, motion gained intraoperatively is preserved only by the most motivated patients who undergo strict, goal-directed postoperative therapy following surgical intervention. The majority of patients can expect some improvement significant enough to restore acceptable function; however, normal motion is not a reasonable expectation. Incremental gains have been made in the treatment of the stiff finger with refined surgical technique and the evolution of a variety of splinting and distraction devices. Substantial gains will likely result from advances in our understanding of inflammation, and scar formation and remodeling. The ability to directly modulate these processes and to alter the biomechanical properties of scar likely hold the key to future advances in the treatment of the stiff finger.

REFERENCES

1. Singer AJ, Clark RA. Cutaneous wound healing. N Engl J Med 1999;341(10):738–46.
2. Brand PW, Hollister A. Clinical mechanics of the hand. 3rd edition. St Louis (MO): Mosby Year Book; 1999.
3. Wong JM. Management of stiff hand: an occupational therapy perspective. Hand Surg 2002;7(2): 261–9.
4. Reisch RG, Eriksson E. Scars: a review of emerging and currently available therapies. Plast Reconstr Surg 2008;122(4):1068–78.
5. Meals RA. Posttraumatic limb swelling and joint stiffness are not causally related experimental observations in rabbits. Clin Orthop Relat Res 1993;287: 292–303.
6. Kaplan EB. Functional and surgical anatomy of the hand. Philadelphia: Lippincott; 1965.
7. Eaton RG, Littler JW. Joint injuries and their sequelae. Clin Plast Surg 1976;3(1):85–98.
8. Watson HK, Light TR, Johnson TR. Checkrein resection for flexion contracture of the middle joint. J Hand Surg Am 1979;4(1):67–71.
9. Bunnell S, Doherty DW, Curtin RM. Ischemic contracture, local, in the hand. Plast Reconstr Surg 1948;3:424–33.
10. Bunnell S. Ischaemic contracture, local, in the hand. J Bone Joint Surg Am 1953;35(1):88–101.
11. Arem A, Madden J. Effects of stress on healing wounds: intermittent noncyclic tension. J Surg Res 1976;20:93–102.
12. Light K, Nuzik S, Personius W. Low-load prolonged stretch vs. high-load brief stretch in treating knee contractures. Phys Ther 1984;64:330–3.
13. Flowers KR, LaStayo P. Effects of total end-range time on improving passive range of motion. J Hand Ther 1994;7(3):150–7.
14. Schultz-Johnson K. Static progressive splinting. J Hand Ther 2002;15(2):163–78.
15. Weeks PM, Wray RC Jr, Kuxhaus M. The results of non-operative management of stiff joints in the hand. Plast Reconstr Surg 1978;61(1):58–63.
16. Lalonde D, Bell M, Benoit P, et al. A multicenter prospective study of 3,110 consecutive cases of elective epinephrine use in the fingers and hand: the Dalhousie Project clinical phase. J Hand Surg Am 2005;30(5):1061–7.
17. Fitzcharles-Bowe C, Denkler K, Lalonde D. Finger injection with high-dose (1:1,000) epinephrine: does it cause finger necrosis & should it be treated? Hand (N Y) 2007;2(1):5–11.
18. Bruser P, Poss T, Larkin G. Results of proximal interphalangeal joint release for flexion contractures: midlateral versus palmar incision. J Hand Surg 1999;24(2):288–94.
19. Prosser R. Splinting in the management of proximal interphalangeal joint flexion contracture. J Hand Ther 1996;9(4):378–86.
20. Gould JS, Nicholson BG. Capsulectomy of the metacarpophalangeal and proximal interphalangeal joints. J Hand Surg Am 1979;4(5):482–6.
21. Curtis RM. Capsulectomy of the interphalangeal joints of the fingers. J Bone Joint Surg Am 1954; 36(1):1219–32.
22. Ghidella SD, Segalman KA, Murphey MS. Long-term results of surgical management of proximal interphalangeal joint contracture. J Hand Surg Am 2002;27(5):799–805.
23. Swanson AB, Maupin BK, Gajjar NV, et al. Flexible implant arthroplasty in the proximal interphalangeal joint of the hand. J Hand Surg Am 1985;10(6): 796–805.
24. Herren DB, Simmen BR. Palmar approach in flexible implant arthroplasty of the proximal interphalangeal joint. Clin Orthop Relat Res 2000;371:131–5.
25. Conolly WB, Rath S. Silastic implant arthroplasty for post-traumatic stiffness of the finger joints. J Hand Surg Br 1991;16(3):286–92.
26. Dryer RF, Blair WF, Shurr DG, et al. Proximal interphalangeal joint arthroplasty. Clin Orthop Relat Res 1984;185:187–94.
27. Iselin F, Conti E. Long-term results of proximal interphalangeal joint resection arthroplasties with a silicone implant. J Hand Surg Am 1995;20(3):S95–7.
28. Pellegrini VD Jr, Burton RI. Osteoarthritis of the proximal interphalangeal joint of the hand: arthroplasty or fusion? J Hand Surg Am 1990;15(2):194–209.
29. Swanson AB, Bayne LG, Cracchiolo A, et al. Symposium: the use of silicone implants in orthopaedic surgery. Contemp Orthop 1994;29(5):363–75.
30. Bravo CJ, Rizzo M, Hormel KB, et al. Pyrolytic carbon proximal interphalangeal joint arthroplasty: results with minimum two-year follow-up evaluation. J Hand Surg Am 2007;32(1):1–11.
31. Jennings CD, Livingstone DP. Surface replacement arthroplasty of the proximal interphalangeal joint using the PIP-SRA implant: results, complications, and revisions. J Hand Surg Am 2008;33(9): e1–11.
32. Tuttle HG, Stern PJ. Pyrolytic carbon proximal interphalangeal joint resurfacing arthroplasty. J Hand Surg Am 2006;31(6):930–9.
33. Bunnell S. Surgery of the hand. 3rd edition. Philadelphia: JB Lippincott; 1956.

Scar Contractures of the Hand

Theresa Hegge, MPH, MD[a], Megan Henderson, MD[a],
Ashley Amalfi, MD[a], Reuben A. Bueno, MD[b],
Michael W. Neumeister, MD, FRCSC[a],*

KEYWORDS

- Scar contracture • Hand injury • Hand anatomy
- Hand reconstruction

The hand represents one of the most powerful sensory and functional organs of the body and separates us from other vertebrate animals through our ability to perform complex tasks. It represents a key component of almost all interactions with our environment, and serves an important role in social functioning, self-expression, productivity, and aesthetics. The hand is highly susceptible to injury. A variety of injuries may lead to contracture of the digits, wrist, and elbow. The contracture may result from simple lacerations that cross the flexion crease or web space, a postoperative infection, full-thickness skin loss, composite tissue injury, burns, crush injuries, avulsions, or amputations. Contractures across joints limit the ability to perform many of the tasks of daily living, including grasping, gripping, pinching, opening doors, getting dressed, or obtaining gainful employment.

Even small or partial functional deficits may compromise the function of the entire extremity and the quality of daily living. Scar management and revision represents a common challenge for reconstructive surgeons in the restoration of form and function.

ANATOMY OF THE HAND AND UPPER EXTREMITIES

The many specialized structures of the hand and upper extremity work in intimate synchrony to provide a harmonious interplay of precision motor biomechanics with fine tactile senses. Owing to the intricate nature these structures, there are often several components to hand stiffness and scar contracture. To appropriately treat any hand injury, one must understand each component's involvement.

The skin of the hand is a complex organ that not only covers the underlying structures but also has specialized functional and sensory components.[1] The glabrous palm skin can withstand shear forces and provides fine tactile sensation,[2] whereas the dorsal skin remains mobile and permits a wide range of motion in the wrist and digits. The periarticular stabilizing structures are essential to normal joint function. These ligamentous structures, however, are prone to contracture with even limited periods of immobilization. The volar plate, collateral ligaments, tendon sheaths, and intrinsic muscles all contribute to this process.[3] In addition, any decrease in excursion of gliding or mobile tissues, such as tendons, can result in significant compromise.[4] Splinting, edema control, and early motion guided by hand therapy are the key to the prevention and treatment of contractures of the hand and upper extremity.

At the core of hand function is the bony support and articular surfaces. Any fractures or articular injury can lead to tendon imbalance, alteration of joint biomechanics, and mechanical obstruction.[2,5] Proper treatment and healing is necessary to allow early range of motion and hand therapy. Both are keys in preventing and treating soft tissue contraction and subsequent contracture.

Joints are the areas of greatest motion in the hand. The metacarpal phalangeal (MCP) joint is

[a] Department of Plastic Surgery, Division of Plastic Surgery, Southern Illinois University School of Medicine, 747 North Rutledge, Third Floor, Springfield, IL 62702, USA
[b] Division of Plastic Surgery, Institute For Plastic and Reconstructive Surgery, Southern Illinois University School of Medicine, PO Box 19653, Springfield, IL 62794-9653, USA
* Corresponding author.
E-mail address: mneumeister@siumed.edu

Clin Plastic Surg 38 (2011) 591–606
doi:10.1016/j.cps.2011.08.005
0094-1298/11/$ – see front matter © 2011 Elsevier Inc. All rights reserved.

a condyloid joint with three planes of motion, including flexion or extension, adduction or abduction, and rotation. The collateral ligaments arise dorsal to the axis of rotation, and with the volar flare of the metacarpal head, provide a cam effect.[3] Thus, there is the least amount of joint space and the most stretch on the collateral ligaments during flexion and the greatest amount in extension. Swelling increases the volume of fluid within the joint and forces the MCP joint into extension in which the collateral ligaments contract to their shorter position and make flexion difficult. Following acute trauma, therefore, the MCP joint should be splinted in flexion to prevent collateral ligament contracture.

The proximal interphalangeal (PIP) joint is a hinge joint with 0° to 100° of flexion.[2] Here, the collateral ligament originates at the center of rotation, so there is no Cam effect and tension is equal throughout the arc of motion (**Fig. 1**). The accessory collateral ligament inserts onto the volar plate, so there is the least amount of joint space and the most stretch on the ligaments during extension. The volar plate is also at greatest stretch during extension of the PIP joint.[6] The PIP joint should be splinted in extension following acute trauma or in conditions of acute or chronic swelling.

INITIAL EXAMINATION FOR HAND AND UPPER EXTREMITY INJURY

The history and cause of the injury are important in assessing the potential structural involvement and previous interventions. This will provide the framework in which to begin treatment. Also important is the patient's medical and social history, which may reveal potential factors contributing to wound healing problems and increased scar propensity **Box 1**.

The physical examination of the scarred hand and upper extremity involves a systematic evaluation.

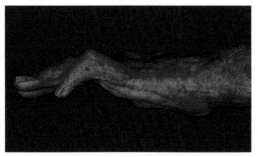

Fig. 1. A contracture of the proximal interphalangeal joint that involves soft tissue, but may also involve volar plate and collateral ligament contracture.

Box 1
An extended scheme of treatment of stiffness proposed by Kaplan

Factors and Conditions in Wound Healing and Scar Formation

Wound

    Contamination

    Infection

    Delayed closure

    Wound tension

    Wound location (trunk, chest)

    Sun exposure and UV damage

    Immobilization

    Swelling

Host

    Skin type

    Keloid history

    Radiation history

    Malnutrition

    Vascular disease

    Smoking

    Diabetes

    Connective tissue disorders (Dupuytren disease)

    Arthritis

    Autoimmune disorders

    Patient compliance/therapy

The neurovascular status should be examined throughout the able range of motion. Structural integrity is also assessed, first clinically by deformity, palpation, tenderness, and then radiographically though radiograph, CT scanning, and angiography, as necessary. Most important in the secondary scar release is a functional assessment, including a detailed motor and sensory examination.[7] First, passive and active ranges of motion are evaluated. A greater composite range of motion is required on the ulnar aspect of the hand for power grip, while less can be tolerated in the thumb and index and long fingers where key pinch is required.[3] Initially, an assessment of the skin should be performed and any areas of tightness or limited mobility documented. Next, testing of intrinsic tightness with the Bunnell-Francescetti intrinsic tightness test[8] will elucidate the cause of any additional limitations in range of motion, such as intrinsic or extrinsic musculotendinous tightness. This test assesses the

MCP motion's effect on PIP motion. If PIP motion is improved with MCP flexion, the test is positive for intrinsic tightness. If PIP motion is improved with extension, the limitation can be attributed to the extrinsic extensors.

TREATMENT OF SCAR CONTRACTURE

The initial treatment of any soft tissue scar contracture is optimization through nonoperative management and aggressive physical therapy. The nonoperative interventions include scar massage, compression therapy, silicon sheeting, static or progressive casting, steroid injection, assisted range of motion, and a variety of orthosis techniques, such as serial casting.[9] Surgical intervention is discussed when no additional improvement is expected with the conservative methods. Typically soft tissue equilibrium has been achieved for at least 6 months.[4]

SURGICAL INTERVENTION

The goal of procedures designed to release contractures of soft tissue are to improve the motion, sensibility, durability and overall function of the hand. The contracture release procedures should be timed appropriately with consideration given to other potential interventions that may require splinting or immobilization that may interfere with the release. Attempting to address too much in one stage carries a significantly higher risk of postoperative pain, edema, and poor outcomes.[10] The most common releases permit extension of the digits, wrist, elbow, or axilla, widening of the first web space, resurfacing of unstable scars, or restoring a sensate pad to finger tips.

EXCISION AND SKIN GRAFTING

Scar incision or excision may result in a significant soft tissue defect that extends beyond the capacity of local flaps. Skin grafts are often used to cover the wound bed following scar excision. Full-thickness grafts are usually used on the volar aspect of the hand to limit the recurrence of contractures.[11]

TRANSPOSITION FLAPS

Many minor or moderate contractures can be corrected with local skin flaps, avoiding the need for skin grafts or more extensive procedures. Transposition flaps are commonly used to correct these contractures. Z-plasties are normally oriented at 60° for each limb, which provides a 75% increase in length of the central limb; however, many angle modifications exist (**Fig. 2**). The larger the angle at

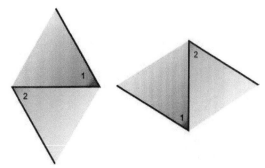

Fig. 2. Z-plasty is one of the standard transposition flaps used to lengthen and breakup scar tissue allowing release of contractures. The classic Z-plasty is 60°, lengthening the area of contracture by approximately 75%.

the apex of the Z-plasty, the more gain in length is achieved in the contracture release. The increase in this angle, however, puts greater the tension on closure and greater is laxity needed in the perpendicular plane.[12] It is often better to use multiple Z-plasties in sequence (**Figs. 3–5**). When the two limbs are unequal or nonparallel, it is more properly called a transposition flap.

Square, double, 4-flap, 5-flap, 6-flap (**Fig. 6**), and jumping man (**Fig. 7**) Z-plasties are all modifications of this procedure and are demonstrated below with additional information on length gain **Table 1**.

ADVANCEMENT FLAPS

V-Y advancement flaps have been used in several types of soft tissue deficiencies of the hand and upper extremity.[13–15] Minimal length gains can be achieved with a V-Y flap of a linear scar. These are often used when transposition flaps are not appropriate because of local scar or inadequate tissue availability. The V-Y flaps rely on laxity that exists at the proximal or distal end on the V (**Fig. 8**).

Just like Z-plasties, V-Y advancements can be used in sequence. Multiple V-Y flaps in succession resemble the result of a 5-flap Z-plasty (**Fig. 9**).

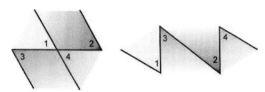

Fig. 3. Multiple Z-plasties can be arranged in a row of even greater length.

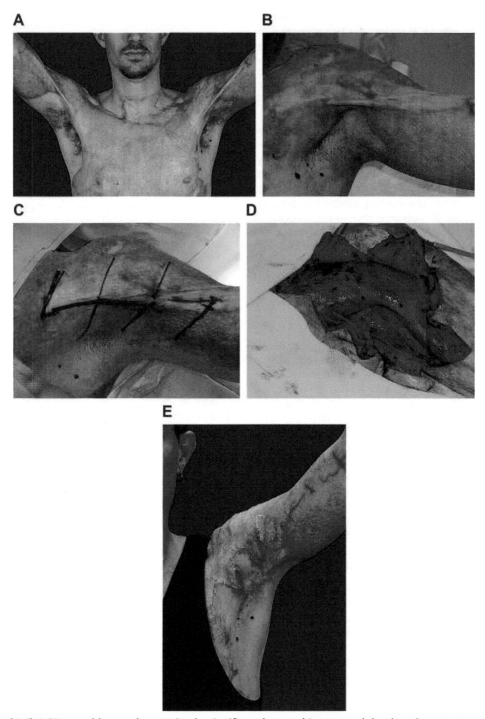

Fig. 4. (*A–E*) A 27-year-old man who sustained a significant burn to his torso and developed contractures in the anterior axillary line. Multiple Z-plasties were planned, transposed, and imbedded unimpaired to improve range of motion.

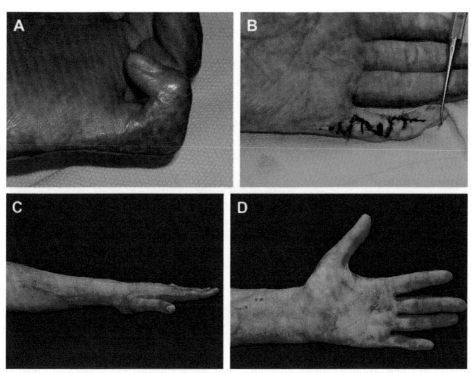

Fig. 5. A flexion contracture in a 19 year old male as are result of a previous burn to his hands. (*A*) Following multiple z-plasty (*B*) the digit was able to be actively extended and flexed in normal range (*C, D*).

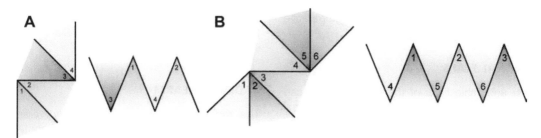

Fig. 6. (*A, B*) Multiple Z-plasties can be arranged to provide greater length or take advantage of laxity of soft tissue in the area. Areas of contour similar to a saddle, such as the first web space and axilla, are particularly amendable to these types of flaps.

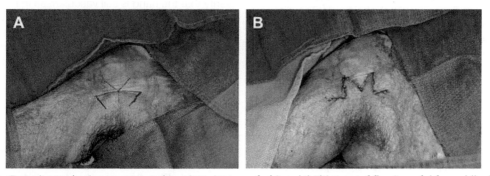

Fig. 7. Opposing z-plasties are arranged in a jumping man fashion. (*A*) This type of flap is useful for saddle shape areas such as the first web space or axilla (*B*).

Table 1
Z-plasty types and theoretical gains in length

	Theoretical Increase in Central Limb for Various Z-Plasties	
Type of Z-Plasty	Percentage Increase in Central Limb (%)	New Length of Central Limb[a] (cm)
Simple Z-plasty with 45°	50	1.5
Simple Z-plasty with 60°	75	1.75
Simple Z-plasty with 75°	100	2
4-flap Z-plasty with 45°	100	2
4-flap Z-plasty with 60°	150	2.5
6-flap Z-plasty with 45°	150	2.5
Double-opposing Z-plasty	75	1.75
2 Z-plasties in series	75	1.75
5-flap Z-plasty	125	2.25

[a] Gain in length is for a central limb originally 1 cm long.

Other modifications, such as V-M advancement flaps, provide additional options for closure (**Fig. 10**), but significantly increase the number of incisions and potential areas of future scarring. The increase in complexity of the flap inherently limits its size and, thus, use on the hand. Many soft tissue contractures of the fingers can be treated with Z-plasties. Aggressive physical therapy is initiated within 1 week postoperative to maintain extension.

REGIONAL FLAPS

Other adaptable flaps of the hand can be used for reconstruction of contractures. The first dorsal metacarpal artery flap is a very versatile flap used mostly for distal thumb reconstruction (**Fig. 11**). The reverse dorsal metacarpal artery flap is an island flap based on connections between the dorsal metacarpal artery and palmar arterial system.[16] The skin paddle for the first dorsal metacarpal artery flap is elevated over the dorsum of the index finger proximal phalanx.[17] The dissection incorporates the first dorsal metacarpal artery and superficial veins. The artery lies below the fascia of the first dorsal interosseous muscle.

The fascia should be elevated with the pedicle to protect it during the dissection. The skin paddle is sensate and innervated by the terminal branch of the superficial radial nerve.[18] Once elevated, the flap is transferred to the first web space or to volar contractures of the thumb either through a tunnel or open incision.[17] The donor site is skin grafted. Similar flaps are described over the second and third metacarpal arteries, but the fourth and fifth have a more unreliable blood supply.[16]

RADIAL FOREARM

The radial forearm flap is extremely versatile readily available flap that provides coverage to the first web space and digits as well as the dorsal hand (**Fig. 12**). The flap is based on retrograde flow of the radial artery.[11,19,20] It is a distally based flap and the surgeon must take the opportunity to perform an appropriate Allen test to verify that the hand is still vascularized in the ulnar artery. The radial artery is situated between the flexor carpi radialis and the brachial radialis muscle bellies. These two muscles are retracted to identify the pedicle and the perforators to the overlying skin in the proximal forearm are preserved. The flap can be elevated in superficial fashion to the level of the perforators from the radial artery and the superficial veins are harvested with the flap. The proximal radial artery and its venae comitantes are ligated and the flap is elevated in a retrograde fashion toward the hand. The flap can be tunneled or inset though an open incision. The other side is usually

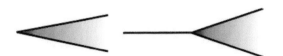

Fig. 8. V-Y flaps or advancement flaps that can be closed primarily at one end of the flap and allow tissue advancement in the area end.

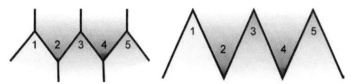

Fig. 9. Multiple V-Y flaps can be used in a similar fashion that multiple Z-plasties provide added length.

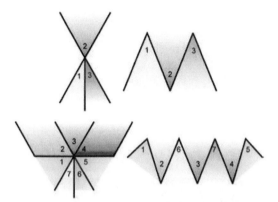

Fig. 10. V-M flaps are another variant of multiple V-Y flaps and incorporate the same principles as multiple Z-plasties.

closed with a split-thickness skin graft. The radial forearm flap can be harvested as a fasciocutaneous, a facial, or an osteocutaneous flap.[15,19] The pivot point of pedicle is usually at a level just proximal to the wrist before the bifurcation of the radial artery into a more superficial branch in the branch that travels through the anatomic snuff box.

ULNAR ARTERY FLAP

Similar to the radial forearm flap, the ulnar artery island flap provides thin and pliable skin for coverage of hand defects. The artery is relatively superficial in the distal arm and is bordered on the ulnar side by the flexor carpi ulnaris (FCU) and radially by the flexor digitorum superficialis of the ring and small fingers. The skin paddle is marked with the FCU in the longitudinal axis of the flap. The pedicle is dissected at the wrist and separated from the ulnar nerve and the ulnar side is dissected first. After location and visualization of the pedicle, the radial and deep surfaces are

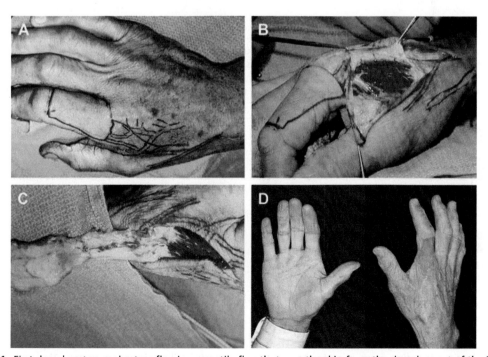

Fig. 11. First dorsal metacarpal artery flap is a versatile flap that uses the skin from the dorsal aspect of the index finger (A). This can be transposed down to the volar aspects of the thumb and also into the first web space if needed (B). There is a sensate flap if the superficial branches of the radial nerve are preserved (C). Postoperative result (D).

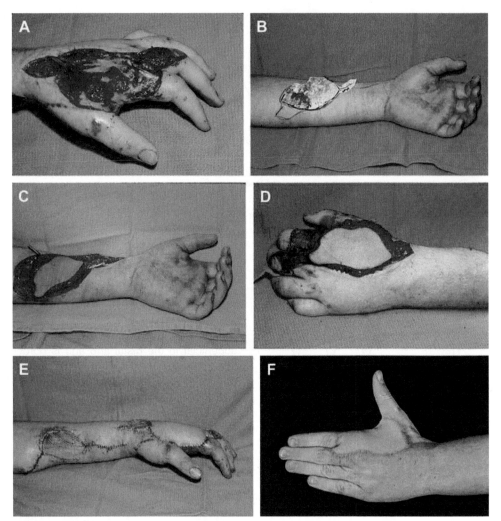

Fig. 12. The reverse radial forearm flap is a very versatile flap that can be utilized for coverage of areas of the dorsum of the hand, volar aspect of the hand, as well as the first web space for contractures. (*A*) The flap is based distally and the other side is usually skin grafted. (*B, C, D, E*) Appropriate flow through the ulnar artery must be assessed prior to ligating the proximal radial artery to prevent ischemia to the hand. Postoperative results (*F*).

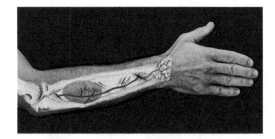

Fig. 13. The posterior interosseous artery flap is a distally based pedicle based on the communications with the anterior osseous artery at the wrist level. The interosseous artery courses from the volar to the dorsal aspect to a water shed area with the posterior interosseous artery. The interosseous artery travels between the extensor digiti minimi and the extensor carpi ulnaris originating from a perforator at the distal end of the supinator. This perforator can be identified at the proximal one-third, distal two-thirds of the extensor forearm. The flap is useful for coverage of defects for the dorsum of the hand and first web space, as well as volar areas of the hand.

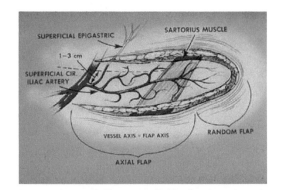

Fig. 14. The groin flap is a reliable flap based on the superficial iliac circumflex vessels. The groin flap is used in a staged procedure keeping the pedicle still attached to the groin while the skin paddle is inset onto the hand after contracture release. Three weeks later the pedicle is divided and the rest of the flap is inset to the hand.

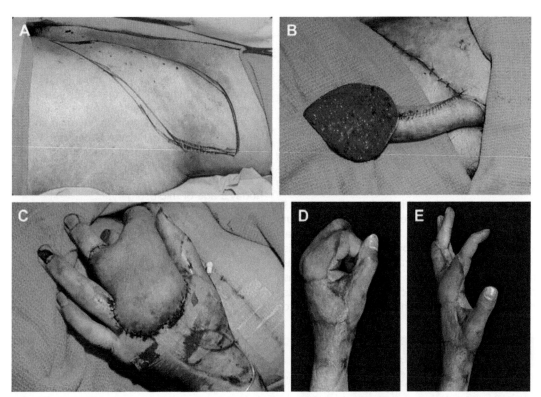

Fig. 15. The groin flap can be used as a pedicle flap or a free tissue transfer (*A, B*). The patients hand must be kept in the groin area while the skin paddle matures on the hand itself (*C*). In three weeks time the flap can be divided and inset (*D, E*).

also freed. Once elevated, the proximal portion of the pedicle is ligated and the flap is rotated into the defect. The flap can be innervated by a branch of the medial antebrachial cutaneous nerve and the defect is often closed primarily.[19] Because the ulnar artery is the dominant supply to the hand in most individuals, preoperative Allen testing is mandated. Close proximity of the ulnar nerve also make the dissection more tedious. The ulnar flap has less hair, a greater arc of rotation than the radial pedicle, and better donor cosmesis; therefore, it represents another option for coverage of hand defects, especially in radially dominant individuals.

POSTERIOR INTEROSSEOUS ARTERY FLAP

The posterior interosseous artery flap is a pedicled fasciocutaneous flap from the dorsal forearm that is supplied by retrograde flow through the posterior interosseous artery[11,20] from the distal anastomosis with the anterior interosseous artery at the level of the wrist. It is useful for dorsal hand and first web space contractures,[21] but has also been shown to reach the proximal interphalangeal joint (**Fig. 13**).[22] The posterior cutaneous nerve of the forearm can be harvested with the flap to provide sensation.[23]

The pedicle enters the posterior compartment at the distal edge of the supinator and travels in a line marked between the lateral epicondyle and distal radioulnar joint between the extensor digitorum minimus and the extensor carpi ulnaris. Four to six cutaneous perforators vascularize the skin paddle on the middle third of the extensor surface of the forearm. Donor sites up to 6 cm in width can be closed primarily.[23] Larger flaps require skin graft closure, leaving a rather unsightly donor site. The dissection of the skin paddle begins above the fascia on the radial aspect and proceeds to the ulnar side.[21] The proximal posterior interosseous artery is then ligated, the pedicle dissected from between the extensor digitorum minimus and extensor carpi ulnaris, and the flap is rotated 180° for inset. The pedicle is dissected to the wrist level.

GROIN FLAP

The groin flap is a very reliable and versatile flap but mandates that the patients hand is positioned in the groin for 2 to 3 weeks before division and inset of the flap. The flap was based on the superficial circumflex iliac artery and vein, a branch of the femoral artery. A significant amount of tissue can be harvested with the groin flap measuring up to 10 × 30 cm with primary closure of the donor site (**Fig. 14**). The groin flap is a pedicle flap that mandates a staged procedure unless it is harvested as a free tissue transfer. Typically, the flap is elevated and inset into the hand as the thin edges heal on the hand the pedicle can be reliably transected 2 to 3 weeks after the initial surgery (**Fig. 15**). The course of the pedicle is about 2 cm below and parallel to the inguinal ligament. The pedicle travels lateral to the sartorius muscle in a more superficial plain than does its medial counterpart. This is important to remember because the flap is elevated from lateral to medial and, as the surgeons approaches the sartorius muscle, the fascia of the muscle must be elevated with the flap to preserve the integrity of the pedicle. The lateral femoral cutaneous nerve should be preserved during the elevation of the flap. Although the groin flap is a rather reliable flap, significant swelling and stiffness of the fingers can occur because of keeping the hand in the dependent position and immobilized in the patients' groin for an extended time. Consequently, the flap is used less frequently in today's age of microsurgery.

FREE FLAPS

Flap selection is based on the characteristics of the defect, including size, shape, and location, the availability of donor sites, sensory functions, and the goals of reconstruction. In scar

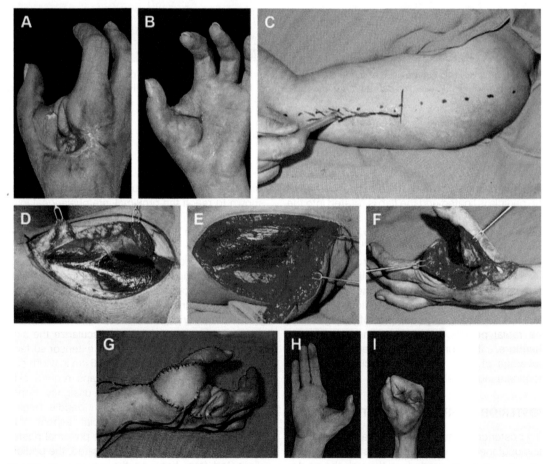

Fig. 16. The lateral arm flap is an excellent choice for first web space contractures. (*A, B*) The flap is based on the posterior radial collateral artery that is designed in the inter-muscular septum in the lateral aspect of the arm between the deltoid insertion and the lateral epicondyle. (*C, D, E*) Flaps in less than 6 cm in width can be closed primarily. Webspace release (*F*), Sutured flap (*G*), Postoperative results (*H, I*).

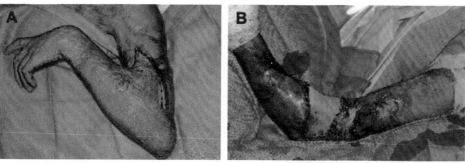

Fig. 17. (*A*) Anterior lateral thigh flap is an extremely versatile flap that offers a large amount of tissue for large contracture releases. This can be harvested as a perforator flap preserving the vastus lateralis muscle in conjunction with some muscle harvest. (*B*) The inset flap provides stable coverage of the antecubital fossa.

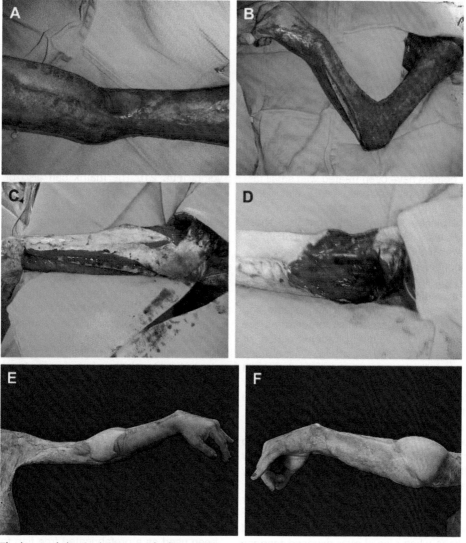

Fig. 18. The lower abdominal tissue can be harvested as a free transverse rectus abdominis myocutaneous flap or a DIEP flap or in conjunction with the skin paddle and rectus abdominis muscle. This 37 year old patient sustained a significant burn to over 40% total body surface area. She developed a contracture to the antecubital fossa and had exposed ulnar along its entire course (*A, B, C, D*). The rectus abdominis muscle along with the transverse lower abdominal tissue was harvested as a free flap to cover up both defects (*E, F*).

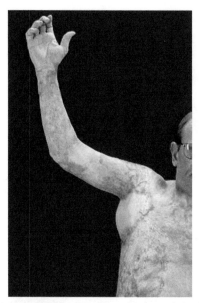

Fig. 19. Free flaps such as anterior lateral thigh flap can be rather bulky in the axilla and often require debulking procedures.

contracture, because the defect to be closed is often limited to skin, fasciocutaneous and fascial flaps are usually used.

Small defects have been treated with small fasciocutaneous flaps, such as a free first dorsal metacarpal artery from the opposite hand[24,25] or a medial plantar flap from the foot.[26,27] These small flaps were designed with the intent of replacing like with like tissue.[28–31]

Fasciocutaneous flaps are often used for reconstruction of soft tissue defect because of the similar properties the skin has to that of the lost tissue. The skin is usually soft and pliable and is easily elevated if secondary procedures are required, such as ligament reconstruction or tendon, nerve, or bone grafting. These flaps have the ability to be sensate, have improved color match, and can be taken as perforator flaps to decrease bulk and reduce donor site morbidity.[32–34] The anterior lateral thigh flap, lateral arm flap, radial forearm flap, scapular flap, and deep inferior epigastric artery perforator flap are commonly used free flaps that are used today for soft tissue reconstruction of upper extremity defects (**Figs. 16–20**).[35–38]

Fascial flaps have distinct advantage over other flaps, because they are very thin and pliable.[39,40] Numerous reports document the superiority of fascial flaps when placed over exposed tendons because of the enhanced ability of the flap to permit tendon glide without adhesions. For these reasons, fascial flaps have become ideal coverage for soft tissue defects for both the extensor and flexor surfaces of the hand. The donor site is closed primarily without tension making fascial flaps rather appealing. Examples for hand coverage include the temporal parietal fascial flap,[41,42] scapular fascia flap,[43] anterior lateral thigh fascia flap,[44,45] serratus anterior fascia flap,[46] the radial forearm fascia flap, and the lateral arm fascia flap.

Muscle flaps have also been used for coverage following contracture release. Because of their bulk, muscle flaps have somewhat limited use over flexion creases. As the hand surgeon weighs the pros and cons of each possible flap to obtain definitive soft tissue coverage, she or he must also integrate priorities of function, contour, and the need for secondary procedures.

Skin substitutes have also been used for contracture release. Acellular dermal matrices offer some advantages over flaps. The substitute is applied like a skin graft. It is technically easier, faster, and more cost-effective than regional and free flaps. A skin graft is applied to the skin substitute in 3 to 4 weeks, after the matrix is vascularized. The matrix and overlying skin graft are thin and pliable, providing stable coverage over joints (**Fig. 21**). The matrix can also be placed over small areas of exposed bone or tendon.

Integra dermal regeneration template is a bilayered construct of bovine collagen with shark glycosaminoglycan, covered with a removable silicone epidermal substitute.[47] It functions as an artificial matrix that allows migration of fibroblasts, macrophage, lymphocytes, and capillaries from wound edges. This results in rapid neodermis formation and provides additional layers of wound coverage and protection. The benefits of its use include an ideal repair of full-thickness defects by replacing like with like and recreating the dermal and epidermal components of skin.[48] Other advantages of Integra dermal substitute include simple and quick application, decreased need for flap coverage, reduced donor site morbidity, excellent cosmetic results,[49] ability to contour complex defects,[50] and less scarring of components with resultant improved function.[47]

Some technical nuances must be considered when using the skin substitute. Meticulous care must be taken to prevent contamination of the avascular product; the time needed to vascularize makes it susceptible to infection. Integra has also been used as a prefabricated free flap for coverage of a contracture of the antecubital fossa (**Fig. 20**).[51]

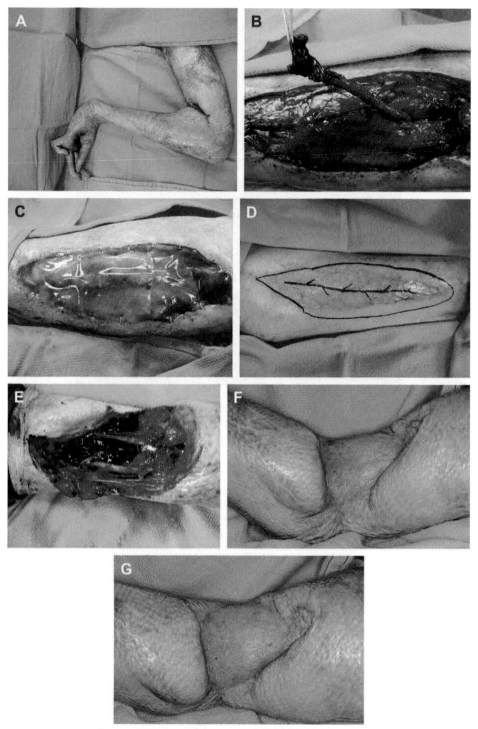

Fig. 20. Fabricated Integra® flap was used to release an antecubital fossa contracture where minimal bulk was desired yet exposed vital structures necessitated flap closure. (*A*) The minimal donor site availability in this patient precluded other flaps. The descending branch of the lateral circumflex common vessel was placed on top of the Vastus lateralis muscle. (*B*) The Integra® was then placed on top of the pedicle. (*C*) A few months later the matured skin graft on the Integra® was elevated (*D*) with the pedicle and transferred as a free tissue transfer to the ante-cubital fossa (*E*) to appropriately accomplish definitive release of the antecubital fossa contracture (*F, G*).

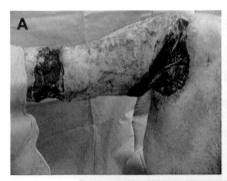
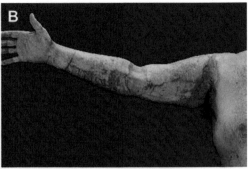
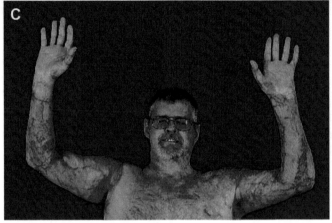

Fig. 21. Skin substitutes such as Integra® offer a readily available product that is easy to use and lower donor site morbidity (*A*). Good contour and appropriate release without further contracture are the advantages of the Integra® application (*B, C*).

POSTOPERATIVE MANAGEMENT

The principles of postoperative management follow those put in place at the time of initial injury. First, scar prevention is instituted through splinting, elevation, early motion, and scar management modalities. Each of these can be improved by adequate pain control, partnerships with hand therapists, and good patient–physician communication.

COMPLICATIONS

In addition to general surgical risks including anesthesia, bleeding, infection, and damage to surrounding tissues, one of the biggest risks is persistent scarring and contracture. Elucidation of contributing factors before surgery, optimization of risk factors, and patient compliance allows for significantly improved outcomes.

SUMMARY

The hand is essential to our sense of self and our ability to interact with our environment. It is also highly susceptible to injury. Small or partial functional deficits may compromise its function and the patient's quality of life. Scar management and revision is a common challenge for reconstructive surgeons. To appropriately treat any hand injury, the surgeon must understand all the components, and become and remain cognizant of current and emerging surgical techniques.

REFERENCES

1. Giessler G, Erdmann D, Germann G. Soft tissue coverage in devastating hand injuries. Hand Clin 2003;19:61–71.
2. Goldfarb C, Boyer M. Soft tissue and joint contracture. In: Guyuron B, Eriksson E, Persing J, editors. Plastic surgery indications and practice. Philadelphia: Saunders Elsevier; 2009. p. 1165–71.
3. Shin A, Amadio P. Stiff finger joints. In: Green D, Hotchkiss R, Pederson W, et al, editors. Green's operative hand surgery. 5th edition. Philadelphia: Elsevier; 2005. p. 417–59.
4. Kaplan FT. The stiff finger. Hand Clin 2010;26: 191–204.

5. Stern P. Fractures of the metacarpals and phalanges. In: Green D, Hotchkiss R, Pederson W, et al, editors. Green's operative hand surgery. 5th edition. Philadelphia: Elsevier; 2005. p. 277–341.

6. Bowers W, Wolf J Jr, Nehil JL, et al. The proximal interphalangeal joint volar plate. An anatomical and biochemical study. J Hand Surg 1980;5(1):79–88.

7. Neumeister MW. Examination of the hand. In: Russell RC, editor. Hand surgery. St Louis (MO): Mosby-Year Book; 2000. p. 1667–93.

8. Bunnell S, Doherty EW, Curtis RM, et al. Ischemic contracture, local, in the hand. Plast Reconstr Surg 1948;3:424–33.

9. Kwan P, Hori K, Ding J, et al. Scar and contracture: biological principles. Hand Clin 2009;25:511–28.

10. Vedder N, Hanel D. The mangled upper extremity. In: Green D, Hotchkiss R, Pederson W, et al, editors. Green's operative hand surgery. 5th edition. Philadelphia: Elsevier; 2005. p. 1587–628.

11. Browne EZ, Pederson WC. Skin grafts and skin flaps. In: Green D, Hotchkiss R, Pederson W, et al, editors. Green's operative hand surgery. 5th edition. Philadelphia: Elsevier; 2005. p. 1629.

12. Hudson D. Some thoughts on choosing a Z-plasty: the Z made simple. Plast Reconstr Surg 2000;106: 665–71.

13. Hsu V, Smartt J, Chang B. The modified V-Y dorsal metacarpal flap for repair of syndactyly without skin graft. Plast Reconstr Surg 2010;125:225–32.

14. Nathan P. Double V-Y flap for correction of proximal interphalangeal joint flexion contractures. J Hand Surg 1984;9A:48.

15. Pegahmehr M, Hafezi F, Naghibzadeh B, et al. Multiple V-Y advancement flaps: a new method for axillary burn contracture release. Plast Reconstr Surg 2008;122(1):44e–5e.

16. Omokawa S, Takaala Y, Ryu J, et al. The anatomical basis for reverse first to fifth dorsal metacarpal arterial flaps. J Hand Surg Br 2005;30:40–4.

17. Neumeister MW. Intrinsic flaps of the hand. In: Guyron B, editor. Plastic surgery, indications and practice. China: Saunders, Elsevier; 2009. p. 1001.

18. Ganchi PA, Lee WP. Fingertip reconstruction. In: Mathes SJ, editor. Plastic surgery, vol. 7. Philadelphia: Elsevier; 2006. p. 153.

19. Guimberteau JC, Goin JL, Panconi B, et al. The reverse ulnar artery forearm island flap in hand surgery: 54 cases. Plast Reconstr Surg 1988;81(6): 925–32.

20. Herndon. Surgical Reconstruction of the Upper Extremity Costa H, Soutar DS. The distally based island posterior interosseous flap. Br J Plast Surg 1988;41:221–7.

21. Zancolli EA. Posterior interosseous artery island flap for dorsal hand coverage. In: Moran S, Cooney W, editors. Soft tissue surgery. Baltimore (MD): Lippincott Williams and Wilkins; 2009. p. 179.

22. Buchler U, Frey HP. Retrograde posterior interosseous flap. J Hand Surg Am 1991;16(2):283–92.

23. Koch H, Kursumovic A, Hubmer M, et al. Defects on the dorsum of the hand—the posterior interosseous flap and its alternatives. Hand Surg 2003;8(2): 205–12.

24. Pelzer M, Sauerbier M, Germann G, et al. Free "kite" flap: a new flap for reconstruction of small hand defects. J Reconstr Microsurg 2004;20(5):367–72.

25. Takeiski M, Ishida K, Kurihara K. Free dorsal middle phalangeal finger flap. J Reconstr Microsurg 2006; 22(7):493–8 or a medial plantar flap from the foot.

26. Lee HB, Tark KC, Rah DK, et al. Pulp reconstruction of fingers with very small sensate medial plantar free flap. Plast Reconstr Surg 1998;10(4):999–1005.

27. Isik S, Sezgin M, Ozturk S, et al. Free musculofasciocutaneous medical plantar flap for reconstruction of thenar defects. Br J Plast Surg 1997;50(2): 116–20.

28. Okazaki M, Ueda K, Niu A, et al. Free lateral supramalleolar flap transfer as a small, thin flap. Ann Plast Surg 2002;49(2):133–7.

29. Hahn SB, Park JH, Kang JH, et al. Finger reconstruction with a free neurovascular wrap-around flap from the big toe. J Reconstr Microsurg 2001; 17(5):319–23.

30. Yang JW, Lee DC. Reconstruction of pulp defect using a free finger-pulp flap from an excised extra digit. Br J Plast Surg 2000;53(8):703–4.

31. Ninkovic MM, Schwabegger AH, Wechselberger G, et al. Reconstruction of large palmar defects of the hand using free flaps. J Hand Surg Br 1997;22(5): 623–30.

32. Pan CH, Chuang SS, Yang JY. Thirty-eight free fasciocutaneous flap transfers in acute burned-hand injuries. Burns 2007;33(2):230–5.

33. Yildirim S, Taylan G, Eker G, et al. Free flap choice for soft tissue reconstruction of the severely damaged upper extremity. J Reconstr Microsurg 2006;22(8):599–609.

34. Woo SH, Seul JH. Optimizing the correction of severe postburn hand deformities by using aggressive contracture releases and fasciocutaneous free-tissue transfers. Plast Reconstr Surg 2001;107(1):1–8.

35. Fan CY, Jiang J, Zeng BF, et al. Reconstruction of thumb loss complicated by skin defects in the thumb-index web space by combined transplantation of free tissues. J Hand Surg Am 2006;31(2): 236–41.

36. Offer N, Baumeister S, Ohlbauer M, et al. Microsurgical reconstruction of the burned upper extremity. Handchir Mikrochir Plast Chir 2005;37(4):245–55.

37. Baumeister S, Koller M, Dragu A, et al. Principles of microvascular reconstruction in burn and electrical burn injuries. Burns 2005;31(1):92–8.

38. Mardini S, Tsai FC, Wei FC. The thigh as a model for free style free flaps. Clin Plast Surg 2003;30(3):473–80.

39. Flugel A, Kehrer A, Heitmann C, et al. Coverage of soft-tissue defects of the hand with free fascial flaps. Microsurgery 2005;25(1):47–53.

40. Hallock GG. The utility of both muscle and fascia flaps in severe upper extremity trauma. J Trauma 2002;53(1):61–5.

41. Rogachefsky RA, Ouellette EA, Mendietta CG, et al. Free temporoparietal fascial flap for coverage of a large palmar forearm wound after hand replantation. J Reconstr Microsurg 2001;17(6):421–3.

42. Brent B, Upton J, Acland RD, et al. Experience with the temporoparietal fascial free flap. Plast Reconstr Surg 1985;76:177.

43. Jim YT, Gao HP, Chang TS. Clinical application of the free scapular fascial flap. Ann Plast Surg 1989;23:170.

44. Yildirim S, Taylan G, Akoz T. Use of fascia component of the anteriolateral thigh flap for different reconstructive purposes. Ann Plast Surg 2005;55(5):479–84.

45. Hsieh CH, Yang CC, Kuo YR, et al. Free anteriolateral thigh adipofascial perforator flap. Plast Reconstr Surg 2004;112(4):976–82.

46. Fotopoulos P, Homer P, Leicht P, et al. Dorsal hand coverage with free serratus fascia flap. J Reconstr Microsurg 2003;19(8):555–9.

47. Moiemen NS, Vlachou E, Staiano JJ, et al. Reconstructive surgery with Integra dermal regeneration template: histologic study, clinical evaluation and current practice. Plast Reconstr Surg 2006;117(7S): 160S–74S.

48. Branski LK, Herndon DN, Pereira C, et al. Longitudinal assessment of Integra in primary burn management: a randomized pediatric clinical trial. Crit Care Med 2007;35(11):2615–23.

49. Herman CK, Hoschander AS, Strauch B, et al. New strategies in surgical reconstruction of the lower extremity. Tech Orthop 2009;24(2):123–9.

50. Jeng JC, Fidler PE, Sokolich JC, et al. Seven years experience with Integra as a reconstructive tool. J Burn Care Res 2007;28(1):120–6.

51. Houle JM, Neumeister MD. A prefabricated tissue-engineered Integra free flap. Plast Reconstr Surg 2007;120(5):1322–5.

Flexor Tendon Reconstruction

Brian M. Derby, MD[a], Bradon J. Wilhelmi, MD[b],
Elvin G. Zook, MD[a], Michael W. Neumeister, MD, FRCSC[a],*

KEYWORDS

- Flexor tendon • Tendon repair • Tendon reconstruction
- Hand surgery

Early depictions of flexor tendon repair can be found in the writings of Galen (AD 129–199), physician to the gladiators. A translation of his records states, "I found one of the gladiators called Horseman with a transverse division of the tendon on the anterior surface of the thigh, the lower part being separated from the upper, and without hesitation I brought them together with suture."[1] The principles of acute tendon repair have evolved to today's debates on repair tactics, core strand number, early mobilization techniques, and so forth. Principles of atraumatic technique, a bloodless field, asepsis, and pulley preservation in flexor tendon surgery were highlighted by Bunnell in 1918.[2] Kleinert and Kutz's 1967 presentation, entitled, "primary repair of flexor tendons in no man's land," changed the dynamics of modern tendon repair that is practiced today. Primary repair occasionally fails, however, to provide the desired outcome. Lexer reported on the first series of flexor tendon graft use in the hand in 1912.[2] Basset and Carroll first described secondary reconstruction of tendons in zone II using silicone implants in 1963. Hunter refined this technique in 1971.[3] The best results of tendon surgery often rely on the condition of the tissues, patient comorbidities and commitment to therapy, and the initial surgical technique. Undesirable range of motion (ROM) outcomes may require secondary surgery to resolve the assault of scar tissue on tendon glide or tendon rupture.

Proper patient selection should always remain at the forefront of the hand surgeon's mind before embarking on the reconstruction to restore functional ROM. Before consent documentation, a candid discussion should be had with the patient regarding the prolonged postoperative rehabilitative efforts required for optimal outcome. Regardless of the elegance or precision of reconstructive efforts, poorly motivated patients will not actualize their potential gains.

Outcomes and expectations should be discussed with patients with specific issues in mind. Patient age, tissues involved in scar, occupational/functional demands, and needs for activity of daily living may alter considerations of aggressive reconstruction. Arthrodesis or amputation may be in a patient's best interest in many cases.

There are several conditions that limit the normal flexion of fingers after flexor tendon repair and rehabilitation. Adhesions, tendon rupture, joint contracture, or soft tissue constraints limit motion. Poor outcomes after primary tendon repair are often a combination of many of these elements. Hand surgeons should address each of these conditions before surgery.[4–7] Scar-related limitations of motion mandate an aggressive therapy regimen for at least 3 months before considering procedures, such as tenolysis or joint release.[2,6] Tenolysis before this may endanger nutritional supply and increase rupture rate.[6] The healing tissues are also in an environment of inflammation. Early surgery in this environment mounts inflammation on more inflammation, often making the second surgery counterproductive. As long as gains are made through physical therapy, secondary surgery should only proceed with caution.

[a] Department of Plastic Surgery, Division of Plastic Surgery, Southern Illinois University School of Medicine, 747 North Rutledge, Third Floor, Springfield, IL 62702, USA
[b] Department of Surgery, University of Louisville School of Medicine, 550 South Jackson Street, Louisville, KY 40292, USA
* Corresponding author.
E-mail address: mneumeister@siumed.edu

Clin Plastic Surg 38 (2011) 607–619
doi:10.1016/j.cps.2011.08.006

SURGICAL TECHNIQUES
Flexor Tenolysis

The indications for flexor tenolysis include limited active ROM with greater passive ROM. Consideration must be given to capsulotomy, collateral ligament release, and checkrein ligament release if passive motion is impaired. In general, the technique involves incising scar tissue between the tendons and the phalanges or surrounding tissue. Although any type of anesthesia can be performed for a tenolysis procedure, the more awake a patient is during the surgery, the more of the true active ROM potential can be realized by both patient and surgeon. By keeping patients within an appropriate state of consciousness (or even without sedation), they can participate actively in the surgery to demonstrate the effectiveness of the adhesiolysis. Patients' direct observations of intraoperative gains after tenolysis may serve to motivate their postoperative efforts in rehabilitation.

The surgical exposure to the tendons is obtained through either Bruner zigzag incisions or by the midlateral approach supported by Strickland.[6] Midlateral incisions may provide a better bed of tissue to lie across the operative site and reduce wound tension with postoperative digital motion.[2] Adhesiolysis should proceed from the proximal unscarred tissue to the distal scarred areas, identifying and preserving the neurovascular bundles during the process. Although Verdan suggested wide sheath excision during the tenolysis, most surgeons today recommend conservation of as much of the pulley/sheath system as possible.[2] The tenolysis is performed with a small Beaver blade, elevator, fine tissue scissors, or specialized tenolysis instrumentation, such as a Meals tenolysis knife (**Fig. 1**). The flexor digitorum sublimus (FDS) tendon and the flexor digitorum profundus (FDP) tendons are separated from each other, surrounding annular pulleys, and from the dorsal osseous component of the canal. Surgeons should avoid attenuating the repair site through an overaggressive tenolysis. Strickland advocates the use of a pediatric urethral sound dilator to facilitate annular pulley expansion and tendon passage through the pulley system.[2,6] Patient participation to actively flex the involved digit ensures adequacy of release. A patient who is under general anesthesia or unable to cooperate with this request can have a proximal incision made in the palm or the wrist to provide access to the proximal tendon. Traction on the proximal tendon confirms the complete release of the distal adhesions. This "traction flexor check," originally described by Whitaker, illustrates adequate flexion of the digit and

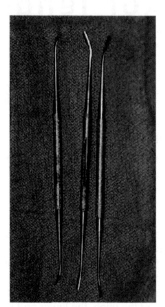

Fig. 1. Meals tenolysis knives. (*Photo courtesy of Southern Illinois University School of Medicine, Institute for Plastic Surgery.*)

signifies complete release of adhesions around the flexor tendons (**Fig. 2**).[6] An alternative to the traction test is the forearm compression test, where the flexors are compressed in the distal forearm that forces the released or unaffected digits into flexion.

An assessment of the quality of the pulley system and tendon itself should be addressed before skin closure. If greater than 30% of the involved tendon width has been lost or if tendon continuity is only maintained by a segment of scar (gap tissue), the tenolysis may be successful initially but may result in secondary tendon rupture during postoperative therapy. Efforts may be turned to staged reconstruction with a silicone implant if the quality of the tendon is too poor to risk rupture (**Fig. 3**).[6] The quality of the tendon and pulley system should be conveyed to a therapist to guide the aggressiveness of the postoperative hand therapy.

Although interpositional biologic and artificial inlays have been described for post-tenolysis adhesion reduction, none has achieved reliable results. Various inlays have included cellophane, polyethylene film, silicone sheeting, paratenon, amniotic membrane, gelatin sponge, fascia, vein, and hyaluronic acid derivatives (Seprafilm bioresorbable membrane, Genzyme, Cambridge, Massachusetts).[2,6] Corticosteroids, intended to reduce the inflammatory phase of healing by local application before wound closure, also are not universally advised because of the risk of tendon

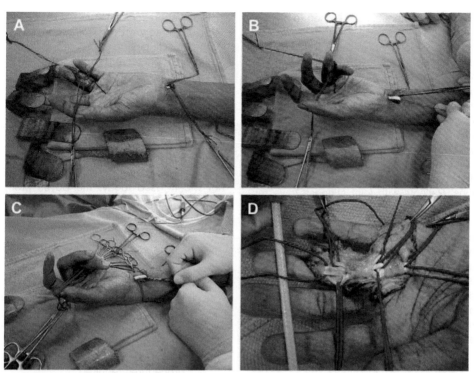

Fig. 2. Traction flexor check after adhesiolysis of zone II flexor tendon laceration repair—ring finger. A small counterincision is made across the volar wrist (*A*). Proximal tendon end is retrieved and the digit is brought through near complete ROM (*B, C*). Adhesiolysis is confirmed, with preservation of A1 and A2 pulleys (*D*). (*Photos courtesy of* Dr Michael W. Neumeister, Southern Illinois University School of Medicine, Institute for Plastic Surgery.)

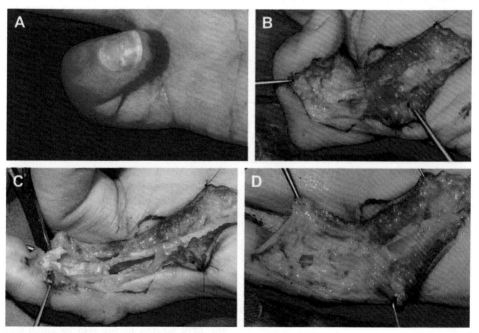

Fig. 3. Tenolysis procedure converted to staged tendon grafting. Flexion contracture deformity after zone II flexor tendon laceration repair, with passive ROM greater than active ROM on clinical examination (*A*). Intraoperative exploration demonstrates poor condition of flexor tendon and wound bed (*B, C*), requiring conversion to a staged reconstructive procedure with a silicone rod (*D*). (*Courtesy of* Southern Illinois University School of Medicine, Institute for Plastic Surgery.)

rupture and their potential contribution to delayed wound healing.

Postoperative therapy is initiated within the first week and consists of active and passive ROM, edema control, scar message, and strengthening. Therapy continues until the gains in ROM plateau in 2 to 4 months. Surgeons could consider indwelling catheters around the median and/or ulnar nerve in the wrist if pain control in the immediate postoperative period is an issue for patients during therapy.

Joint stiffness may be associated with the tendon adhesions. Patients with joint stiffness have restricted passive motion as well as restricted active motion. Capsulotomies, volar plate release, and collateral ligament release may be required at the time of tenolysis to restore active and passive motion. Unfortunately, the greater the amount of soft tissue release required to achieve motion around the proximal interphalangeal (PIP) or distal interphalangeal (DIP) joints, the worse the outcome. This is likely due to recurrent scarring and periarticular swelling.

Complications of tenolysis surgery are illustrated in **Box 1**. All complications can be devastating and may culminate in a functionless digit. Skin loss over the tendon may require flap coverage. Tendon rupture may be a consequence of infection, attenuation of the old repair site, or gap formation at the repair site. Salvage procedures of the ruptured tendon may include tendon grafts if the pulley system was intact, a two-staged silastic rod reconstruction, DIP arthrodesis, tenodesis, or amputation.

Tendon Grafting

The indications for single-stage free tendon grafting are narrow. They include[4]

1. Injuries resulting in segmental tendon loss

Box 1
Complications of tenolysis

- Infection
- Hematoma
- Volar skin necrosis
- Tendon exposure
- Injury to neurovascular structures
- Stiffness
- Contracture
- Tendon rupture
- Bowstringing

---

2. Delayed presentation greater than 3 weeks, resulting in tendon end fraying or retraction into the muscle belly
3. Delayed presentation of some FDP avulsion injuries.

The pulley system should be intact and supple motion of the digit preserved to proceed with single-stage grafting. Tendon reconstruction in zones III, IV, and V are more amenable to single-stage reconstruction due to lack of a restricted fibro-osseous canal notable in zone II. Although not widely used today, the Boyes preoperative injury classification system for tendon reconstruction provides the principles of current tendon grafting philosophy[8]:

Grade 1—minimum scar, supple joints, no trophic changes
Grade 2—scar-limiting gliding of graft
Grade 3—joint involvement with loss of passive motion
Grade 4—multiple digit involvement with tendon injury
Grade 5—devastating injury with salvage procedures required.

The most desirable preoperative condition for tendon reconstruction is a Boyes grade 1 finger, where joints are without contracture, wounds are well healed, and hand therapy efforts have maximized potential passive gains in ROM. Pulvertaft adds that circulation should be satisfactory and at least one digital nerve intact.[3,4] Contraindications to grafting include insensate, poorly vascularized fingers; patients who cannot appreciate the needs for strict adherence to postoperative hand therapy regimens (ie, children younger than age 3 years or patients who are mentally debilitated); or those patients who declare that they have minimal functional demands needs (ie, elderly).[2–4] In more significantly damaged fingers (Boyes grades 2–5), two-stage reconstruction should be pursued. If the intraoperative dissection demonstrates pulley systems in need of significant reconstruction, single-stage reconstruction should be abandoned and efforts turned to two-stage reconstruction.[2] The possibility of a two-staged reconstruction should be shared with patients during the preoperative evaluation.

Common tendon grafts include the palmaris longus tendon, the plantaris tendon, the extensor indicis proprius, the extensor digiti quinti proprius, the FDS tendon to the ring or small finger, and the long toe extensors (**Table 1**).[2,3] Tendon grafts can be intrasynovial or extrasynovial. Intrasynovial toe flexor grafts, in theory, replace like with like but the outcomes of any tendon seem similar. The

Table 1
Tendon graft selection

Tendon	Total Length (cm)
EIP	13
EDM	16
Palmaris	16
Plantaris	35
Toe extensor (second toe)	35

Abbreviations: EDM, extensor digiti minimi; EIP, extensor indicis proprius.

palmaris longus and plantaris tendons are the most frequently used tendon grafts because they are readily available, easy to harvest, and leave minimal donor morbidity. The palmaris longus and plantaris tendons are present in 85% and 80% of subjects, respectively.[2–4]

The presence of the palmaris longus tendon is confirmed preoperatively by having a patient oppose the thumb and small finger with the wrist flexed against resistance (**Fig. 4**). A 1-cm transverse incision is made at the distal wrist crease. The tendon is transected as far distally as possible, passed through a tendon stripper, and then held securely as the stripper is passed proximally with a slight twisting motion. The plantaris tendon graft is used for longer grafts that reach from the distal fingertip to the forearm.

The plantaris tendon is isolated through a vertical incision just anterior to the medial border of the Achilles tendon (**Fig. 5**). Once the plantaris is identified, it is divided as far distally as possible, and a tubular tendon stripper is passed in the proximal direction up an extended leg. Up to 12 cm to 18 cm of tendon length can be harvested. Donor site morbidity is rare but compartment syndrome after plantaris tendon harvest has been reported.[4]

Single-stage grafting

As Tubiana indicated, an intact superficialis tendon is never sacrificed.[2] If the FDS is intact on exploration, the FDP can still be grafted through the decussation. Many patients function well, however, with a well-functioning FDS alone.[3] Most of the useful motion of the maximal flexion arch provided by the profundus, sublimis, and intrinsics is maintained when the FDS is fully functional.[4] The indications for grafting through an intact FDS are narrow. Pulvertaft highlighted his discretionary pursuit of this procedure: "it should not be advised unless the patient is determined to seek perfection and the surgeon is confident of his ability to offer a reasonable expectation of success without the risk of doing harm."[2] Generally, this procedure is reserved for those patients with high occupational demands for dexterity, such as skilled technicians or musicians, generally ages 10 to 21 years.[2–4]

The dissection to the tendon sheath proceeds in a fashion similar to that of the tenolysis surgery (discussed previously).[2–4] Small windows in the cruciate regions of the sheath are used to identify the proximal and distal tendon stumps. The distal

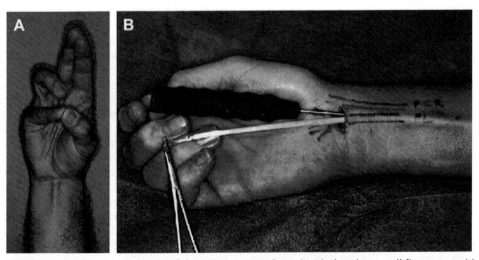

Fig. 4. Palmaris tendon harvest. Presence of the palmaris is confirmed with thumb to small finger opposition and the wrist flexed against resistance (*A*). A small transverse incision is made in the wrist crease; the tendon is isolated superficially below the skin surface, divided, and a tendon passer used to facilitate harvest (*B*). (*Photos courtesy of* Dr Michael W. Neumeister, Southern Illinois University School of Medicine, Institute for Plastic Surgery.)

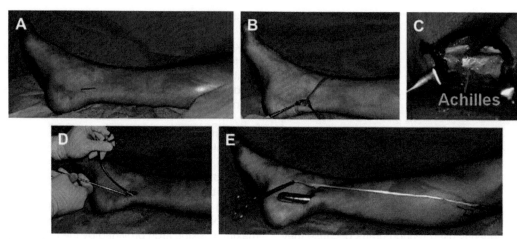

Fig. 5. Plantaris tendon harvest. Incision is made just anterior to the Achilles tendon at the level of the medial malleolus (*A*). The plantaris tendon is identified and isolated with a vessel loop (*B, C [arrow* points to the Achilles tendon]). It is divided as far distally as possible and a tubular tendon passer is passed along the tendon length, aiming laterally toward its origin (*D, E*). (*Photos courtesy of* Dr Michael W. Neumeister, Southern Illinois University School of Medicine, Institute for Plastic Surgery.)

profundus stump is identified and transected keeping 1 cm of FDP tendon attached to the distal phalanx. The proximal FDP tendon is withdrawn, along with the injured FDS tendon. The proximal FDP tendon is trimmed back to healthy tendon. Delayed presentation often results in a swollen, frayed proximal stump.[2,3] The lumbrical muscle may be resected if it is scarred. The FDS is transected and allowed to retract into the proximal forearm. Approximately 1 cm to 2 cm of distal FDS is left attached at its insertion to provide a smooth surface to support the overlying tendon graft. Theoretically, the FDS remnant in the flexor canal helps prevent hyperextension deformity at the PIP joint.

The tendon graft is passed through the intact pulley system and secured to the distal stump. Typically, a double crisscrossed monofilament suture is placed in the distal graft, as described by Bunnell.[2] The graft can be passed through or dorsal to the FDP stump. The 3.0 suture is placed around the waist of the distal phalanx or through the bone on Keith needles, secured over the nail plate distal to the germinal matrix. The graft is reinforced with another 3-0 suture to the distal FDP tendon stump. Suture anchors have also been used at the distal graft juncture.[2] Many surgeons prefer to elevate the distal FDP stump off the distal phalanx for a short distance with only the most distal portion of FDP attached to bone. The cortex of the bone is then roughened with a rongeur. The tendon is secured tightly to this area of the distal phalanx. The proximal tendon graft is commonly secured in the palm or distal forearm with a Pulvertaft weave

technique, secured with 3-0 suture.[4] If palm-to-fingertip graft is used, the proximal juncture is made just distal to the lumbrical origin. Tension on the graft is set such that the finger's position is in slightly greater flexion than its ulnar and radial neighbor.

Two-stage grafting

A two-staged flexor tendon reconstruction is preferred when the fibro-osseous canal is scarred excessively, significant joint contracture release is required, and if pulley reconstruction is needed. Scar tissue is resected, the pulley system reconstructed, a silicone rod is placed in the old tendon bed to generate a foreign body reaction pseudosheath, and therapy rehabilitation initiated early to generate a supple finger. The second-stage tendon graft insertion is performed 3 to 4 months later. Surgeon, patient, and hand therapist must be in regular communication to ensure the best outcome. Alternatives to the classic two-stage reconstruction are discussed later in this article.[9]

Currently available silicone rods (Hunter implants) have a polyester core and silicone elastomer shell, ranging in width from 2 mm to 6 mm and are typically 24.5 cm to 25 cm long (Wright Medical Technology, Arlington, TN, USA). The rod is secured distally to the FDP stump, 3-0 Prolene (**Fig. 6**). The rods are passive gliding implants with the proximal end left free in the proximal palm or forearm. If treated as an active implant, and secured proximally, the distal coaptation often breaks loose as muscle power returns to normal.

Postoperative therapy ensues to maximize passive ROM at all joints, with its time course

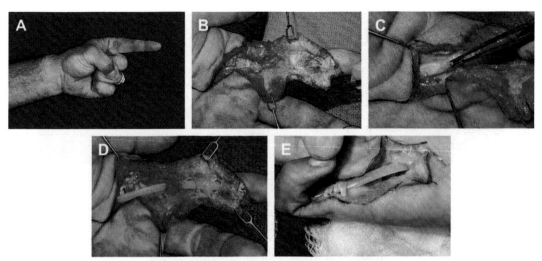

Fig. 6. Stage 1 of two-stage flexor tendon reconstruction. The stiff finger, status post flexor tendon zone II repair (*A*), is approached using Bruner incisions (*B*). Scarred sheath and poor quality tendon is excised with care to leave as much pulley system intact as possible (*C*). Silicone rod is inserted beneath the remaining pulley system and secured distally to the undersurface of the remaining FDP stump (*D*). Passive flexion of the digit is performed to ensure the silicone rod moves freely in the volar wrist without buckling (*E*). (*Photos courtesy of* Dr Elvin G. Zook, Southern Illinois University School of Medicine, Institute for Plastic Surgery.)

adjusted based on presence of associated neuro-vascular repair. It should be reiterated, however, that patients with severe neurovascular impairment or unresolved stiffness are not good candidates for staged flexor tendon reconstruction. Three months of hand therapy usually follow, before definitive grafting. Case reports of silicone rod implants removed 18 and 25 years after implantation have been published.[10]

Access to the rod and its pseudosheath is achieved through limited incisions at the proximal and distal ends of the rod (**Fig. 7**). Small chevron incisions also work well, so the intervening pseudosheath is not disrupted. The tendon graft is sutured to the proximal end of the rod. The rod is pulled out through the distal wound with the graft attached gliding easily through the pseudosheath.[11] The graft is released from the rod and secured to the distal phalanx and FDP stump through techniques (described previously).

An alternative to the standard two-stage technique of flexor tendon reconstruction was described by Viegas.[12] The graft is secured with a Pulvertaft interweave technique to either a common FDP tendon motor or single FDP tendon at the proximal site after the distal site is secure. The tension should permit the reconstructed digit to appear slightly more flexed than the normal cascade.

Paneva-Holevich[9] in 1969 described an alternative to the use of tendon grafts in the staged reconstruction. The proximal aspect of resected FDP and FDS tendons are sutured to each other in the palm in stage 1. The procedure has been modified to include insertion of a Hunter silicone rod also at this time. The FDS-FDP loop in the proximal palm is identified at the second stage and the proximal FDS in the forearm is divided and pulled out through the palm wound still attached to the FDP tendon. The FDS is secured to the rod and pulled out through the distal wound at the distal phalanx.[9,13] The proximal loop junction heals by the time the second stage is performed.

The Paneva-Holevich technique and the standard two-stage technique work well but are not without complications that may require further procedures to restore greater function in the involved finger. The need for tenolysis surgery occurs in 12% to 47% of patients after Hunter's classically described two-stage reconstruction, a rate higher than that of the Paneva-Holevich technique.[13] Other complications, however, may include joint contracture, inappropriate tendon graft length, and distal tendon rupture. Additionally, given the healing of the proximal FDP-FDS loop juncture that occurs during the 3-month interval between stages 1 and 2, proximal juncture ruptures are uncommon using the Paneva-Holevich technique. The incidence of proximal rupture in Hunter reconstructions is approximately 7%.[13]

Two-stage flexor tendon grafting in children

The presentation of flexor tendon laceration in children may be delayed, with some reports indicating a 25% late presentation rate.[3,14] To compensate for the functional loss of the involved finger,

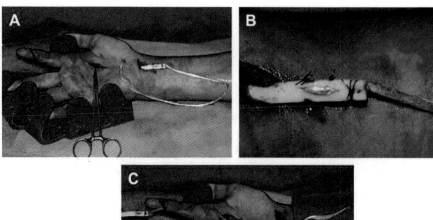

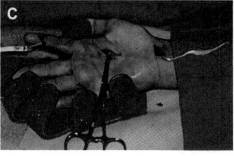

Fig. 7. Stage 2 of stage 2 flexor tendon reconstruction. Small access incisions are made on the volar digit, palm, and wrist (*A*). The graft is procured and secured to the proximal end of the silicone rod (*B*) and then brought through the pseudosheath (*C*). The graft is secured distally by one of many described methods and proximally by an interweave technique. (*Photos courtesy of* Dr Michael W. Neumeister, Southern Illinois University School of Medicine, Institute for Plastic Surgery.)

children often trap or assist the injured finger with the adjacent digit. This maneuver uses the uninvolved finger to pull the injured digit into the palm. As with any flexor tendon grafting procedure, patients must be capable of understanding and adhering to the required course of postoperative rehabilitation. Some have suggested delaying reconstruction in children until the age of 6 to 8 for best outcomes. The family is required to have an active role in the rehabilitation period.

Various investigators prefer the Paneva-Holevich procedure for staged tendon reconstruction in children.[14,15] They offer that the intrasynovial, pedicled FDS graft is anatomically stable/present, morphologically more appropriate than an extrasynovial graft, and provides for easier matching of pulleys, implant, and graft because the graft exists in the operative field during the first stage.

Pulley reconstruction

To optimize tendon excursion at the interphalangeal (IP) joints, an intricate pulley system keeps the flexor tendons closely opposed to the phalanges. Five annular pulleys (A1–A5) and three cruciate pulleys work in concert to optimize tendon position in the fibro-osseous canal. Pulleys derive from specialized thickenings of the tendon sheath, an extension of the paratenon in zone II of the hand. The odd-numbered annular

pulleys occupy positions overlying the finger joints. A2 and A4 overlie the proximal and middle phalangeal shafts, respectively. A1, A2, A3, and A4 pulleys are 11 mm, 17 mm, 5 mm, and 8 mm in width, respectively.[5] Cruciate pulleys (C1–C3) lie between their annular counterparts and are not considered critical for tendon excursion, nor are they often highlighted in pulley reconstruction discussions.

Bunnell suggested that pulley loss results in flexor tendons seeking the shortest distance between two adjacent pulleys.[4] Bowstringing reduces maximal efficiency of flexor tendon excursion and increases the muscle force required for complete composite finger flexion. Pulley reconstruction seeks to re-establish the appropriate spatial relationship between flexor tendon and bone to ultimately generate functional joint motion.

Typically, the A2 and A4 pulleys should be reconstructed to prevent bowstringing, which inhibits full flexion of the involved finger.[4,5] Reconstruction of A3 may offer even greater efficiency.[5] A1 and A5 can be considered expendable and an unnecessary focus of reconstructive efforts.

Principles of reconstruction include

1. Repairing as much of the pulley system as possible — three-pulley or even four-pulley systems should be reconstructed for optimal efficiency[4]

2. Using synovial-lined grafts to reduce resistance at the tendon-pulley interface
3. Repairing pulleys over a Hunter rod when tendon and sheath are significantly damaged
4. Tensioning the pulley appropriately to prevent bowstringing but allow for unimpeded gliding.

Options for pulley reconstruction include[5]

- Okutsu's three-loop technique
- Kleinert/Weilby's shoelace interweave technique
- Karev's belt-loop technique
- Lister's extensor retinaculum technique
- Widstrom's loop and a half technique.

Okutsu modified Bunnell's technique of using a single tendon graft looped around the phalanx, sutured to itself. The modification uses three graft loops, creating the strongest of options for pulley restoration, capable of withstanding as much load to failure as a normal pulley (**Fig. 8**).[5] Recommendations for placement of the pulley graft, in relation to the extensor apparatus, differ among

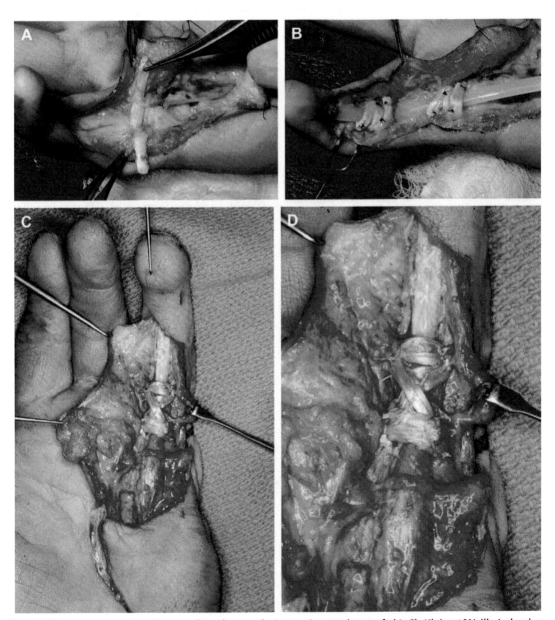

Fig. 8. Pulley reconstruction. Okutsu's three-loop technique using tendon graft (*A, B*). Kleinert/Weilby's shoelace interweave technique using tendon graft (*C, D* [magnified view of *C*]).

surgeons. Bunnell's original description placed the graft volar to the extensor apparatus at the level of the proximal phalanx for A2 reconstruction and dorsal to the extensor apparatus at the level of the middle phalanx for A4 reconstruction. Boyer and colleagues prefers placement of the graft volar to the extensor at all levels.[4]

The Kleinert/Weilby technique uses a tendon weave through the remaining fibrous rim of the pulley undergoing reconstruction (see **Fig. 8**). Typically a tail of the FDS is the source of donor tendon, but a tendon graft may be used. Karev suggested proximal and distal incisions through the volar plate, with volar displacement of the intervening "belt-loop" of tissue to provide passage for the flexor tendon dorsal to the loop. This method should only be used with concurrent flexor tendon grafting and not for reconstruction of pulleys over an intact flexor system.[5] Joint and tendon are placed in close proximity, reducing the moment arm and increasing efficiency of muscle excursion. The stiff volar plate may generate friction, potentially inhibit tendon gliding.

Lister supplemented available options with his recommendation of using extensor retinaculum for pulley reconstruction. This provides a smooth synovial surface for tendon glide. The extensor retinaculum demonstrates low load to failure, the lowest mechanical efficiency as a result of difficulties with setting, and maintaining tension on the reconstructed pulley.[5]

Widstrom and colleagues developed the loop and a half technique during his comparison of six types of pulley reconstruction.[5,16] The tendon graft is passed around the phalanx with one end passed through the substance of one limb of the graft. Tendon ends are then sutured together. Based on Widstrom's comparisons, this technique's mechanical efficiency was inferior only to Karev's method.

Finally, a tail of FDS insertion at the middle phalanx can be detached proximally, passed over a tendon implant, and sutured to the periosteum, the bone, or residual pulley on the other side.[4] This technique has been suggested as an excellent tactic for reconstruction of the A3 pulley.

POSTOPERATIVE CARE AND REHABILITATION
Flexor Tenolysis

Early active motion protocols are considered primary therapeutic modalities after flexor tenolysis.[4] Initiation of therapy should begin 2 to 3 days after the procedure. Gains in motion obtained during the first week that are maintained through the next 2 to 3 weeks usually herald maintenance of useful motion.[4] Use of continued passive motion (CPM) devices has been described. CPM has been shown to increase rupture risk, and flexion force required for passive joint flexion, and, while also resulting in less return of passive motion.[6] Compliance with the continuous wear, difficulty with the bulky apparatus, and digits slipping out of position have diminished enthusiasm for the use of the CPM.

Postoperative edema control includes hand elevation and compression with products, such as Coban (3M Company, St. Paul, Minnesota).[2,6] For those tendons judged of poor quality, a frayed tendon program is used for postoperative rehabilitation.[2] This program is pursued for 4 to 6 weeks.

Single-Stage Grafting

Traditional tactics of prolonged immobilization after tendon grafting have been supplanted by the early motion protocols used after primary tendon repairs. A dorsal blocking splint is worn at all times between therapy sessions and protects the repair for 6 weeks after surgery. The splint maintains the wrist in neutral, metacarpophalangeal (MCP) joints at 45°, and IP joints in neutral. At the postoperative days 2 to 3 visit, guided passive ROM exercises begin, followed by gentle place-and-hold exercises at 2 weeks postoperatively. Blocked flexion exercises optimize tendon gliding and may start at 4 weeks. Resistance to blocked flexion commences at weeks 6 to 8, based on the therapist's protocol. At 6 weeks the tendon and its junctures are considered sufficiently strong to tolerate a more aggressive application of motion stress.[2]

Two-Stage Grafting

Therapy starts 2 to 3 days postoperatively with passive ranging. Adjacent finger trapping can be used to assist with return of mobilization of the involved finger.

Stage 2 therapy follows the course (described previously) for single-stage grafting. Early active motion is emphasized. Joint contracture can be countered with dynamic splinting at 6 to 8 weeks.[12]

Pulley Reconstruction

Pulley reconstructions are bolstered with an external protective pulley ring, worn for 4 to 6 weeks. Close communication with a therapist should convey the need for support of the reconstructed pulleys during active and resisted rehabilitative efforts.

OUTCOMES

The goal of flexor tendon reconstruction is to restore function. This means that patients are able to flex and extend their fingers to accomplish any given activity. What defines a satisfactory gain in function is subject to the interpretation of patient, surgeon, and therapists. Ultimately, an optimum result returns patients to gainful employment and being able to perform their activities of daily living with the use of their hands. There are several classifications described to help define the ROM outcomes of tendon reconstruction and repair (**Table 2**).

Flexor Tenolysis

Azari and Meals[6] reviewed a series of reports in the literature regarding individual investigators' outcomes after flexor tenolysis. Strickland demonstrated 50% improvement in active motion through the available passive arc at the PIP and DIP joints in 64% of his tenolysed digits.[6] Comparably, Foucher identified 51% gains in active motion (135°–205° of total active motion) in 84% of his tenolysis procedures.[6] Jupiter examined total active motion (TAM) gains in replanted digits after flexor tenolysis. Significant increases in TAM were demonstrated (72°–130°).[6] The poorest outcomes were found in crush or avulsion amputations, replantation of more than two digits on the same hand, and those digits requiring capsulotomy.

Two-Stage Grafting

In Hunter and Salisbury's[11] 1970 description of their results in 19 digits undergoing two-stage reconstruction (17 fingers and 2 thumbs), 9 actively reached their passive potential—measured according to Boyes criteria of distance from fingertip to distal palmar crease after passive flexion.

COMPLICATIONS AND MANAGEMENT

Complications after tendon grafting include those shared by both single-stage and two-stage grafting procedures as well as issues specific to temporary implantation of a silicone prosthesis. The literature alludes to a 20% adhesion rate after primary tenorrhaphy. If adhesiolysis fails to improve motion to expected levels after single-stage grafting, potential management strategies include conversion to two-stage reconstruction, arthrodesis in a position of function, or, in severe cases, but not necessarily a last resort, amputation. Tendon repair rupture occurs in 3% to 9% of most reported series, with maximal risk occurring 10 to 12 days postoperatively.[7] Exploration with primary repair should be performed if early rupture is observed in the first few weeks after the initial repair. If the condition of tissues does not permit primary repair, the surgeon may opt for conversion to a two-stage procedure, DIP arthrodesis if only the FDP has ruptured, or conversion to a superficialis finger. To create a superficialis finger, the distal FDP stump is tenodesed to an intact

Table 2 Outcome assessment			
	Boyes (Tip to Distal Palmar Crease)	ASSH (TAM)	Strickland Modification Zones I and II
Excellent	0–2.5 cm	Normal (260°)	75%–100% (>131°)
Good	2.5–4 cm	>75% (>195°)	50%–74% (88°–131°)
Fair	4–6 cm	>50% (>130°)	25%–49% (44°–87°)
Poor	>6 cm	<50% (<130°)	0%–24% (<44°)
		MCP + PIP + DIP motion measured Subtract extension deficit of hyperextension	Normal = 175°

TAM = total active flexion - total extension deficit (MCP, PIP, DIP)
% = TAM of injured finger/TAM of contralateral finger

$$\text{Strickland} = \frac{(\text{Active flexion PIP} + \text{DIP}) - (\text{extension deficit PIP} + \text{DIP})}{175°} \times 100\%$$

Abbreviations: ASSH, American Society for Surgery of the Hand; MCP, metacarpophalangeal.
From Kleinert HE, Verdan C. Report of the committee on tendon injury [International Federation of Societies for Surgery of the Hand]. J Hand Surg Am 1983;8(5 Pt 2):799–8; with permission.

FDS tendon or is secured to the middle phalanx. This prevents hyperextension at the DIP joint. Superficialis fingers are fairly well tolerated.

It is essential to provide the proper length of grafts in staged reconstruction. Inappropriate tendon tension can lead to the quadrigia effect or lumbrical plus deformities. The quadrigia effect occurs with tendon grafts that are too short. This results in achievement of maximal TAM of a repaired FDP tendon before complete FDP tendon excursion of adjacent fingers. Its etiology is explained by the common FDP muscle belly that motors the FDP tendons to the long, ring, and small fingers. The index finger FDP often originates from an independent belly and is not typically subjected to the same constraints of maximum tendon advancement demonstrated by the long, ring, and small fingers. The latter 3 digits can tolerate up to 1-cm advancement before the risk of quadrigia becomes an issue.[17]

The lumbrical plus deformity can occur with an excessively long tendon graft. The lumbrical muscle contracts to extend the IP joints before the FDP tendon graft can create flexion. The result is exaggerated lumbrical effect that paradoxically extends the finger when a patient attempts to flex the digit.

Another uncommon complication of staged reconstruction is silicone synovitis, which can occur in approximately 8% of two-stage procedures.[5] Implant infection (4% incidence) often necessitates removal, débridement, antibiotic treatment, and delayed reconstruction. Flexion contractures can occur in up to 41% of cases.[5]

FUTURE OF TENDON RECONSTRUCTION—TISSUE ENGINEERING

With the knowledge that a defined quantity of autologous tendon graft may be harvested from their patients, hand surgeons have sought the creation of an unlimited, off-the-shelf source of tendon through tissue engineering. Tissue engineering reconstitutes injured tissue with constructs that assimilate the structural and functional properties of native tendon.[18] A pioneer experiment in tendon engineering was performed using a combination of polyglycolic acid fibers seeded with tenocytes.[19] It highlights two critical factors in the engineering process—scaffold (that serves for tissue in growth) and cell type (that infiltrates the scaffold).

Scaffold materials are typically classified as biologic or synthetic. Human dermis, porcine small intestinal submucosa, and type I collagen are sources of biologic material. Polyglycolic acid, silicone, and polyethylene are a few of the resorbable and nonresorbable types of synthetic scaffolds. Implantation of a scaffold that serves as a platform for cell in growth, stimulates regeneration through release of growth factors, and ultimately demonstrates the generation of a tendon that maintains the biomechanical properties of native tendon would be ideal. Use of biodegradable synthetic scaffolds, such as polyglycolic acid, poly-N-acetyl-D-glycosamine (ie, chitin), poly-ε-caprolactone, polyethylene terephthalate, and polypropylene, are being investigated as potentially ideal scaffolding materials that can be augmented with cell therapy, growth factors, and gene therapy.[18]

Unwoven polyglycolic acid fibers have been mixed with isolated tenocytes in an in vivo experimental model.[20] Results from this experimental study demonstrated that engineered tendon, after 14 weeks, displayed a typical tendon structure hardly distinguishable from that of normal tendon. In this study, engineered tendon demonstrated a breaking strength comparable to normal tendon. The need to have source tenocyte from patients, to mix with the polyglycolic acid fibers, requires additional tendon harvest from patients to obtain these cells. This necessity limits clinical applicability of these findings.

Other studies have considered acellularized tendon as the ideal scaffold.[21] Acellularized tendons address the issue of antigenicity associated with implantation of tendon allograft. The acellularization process intends to avoid graft rejection from immunogenicity. Critical to their potential use and function, acellularized constructs seem to maintain the same biomechanical properties of native tendons. Again, the reseeding of these constructs with tenocytes from additional donor tendon may limit clinical applicability.

Adipose-derived stem cells have been used to address the issue of morbidity from additional tendon harvest to obtain a cell source for scaffold seeding.[22] In vivo models demonstrate adipose-derived stem cells incorporate well into a polyglycolic acid scaffold, with the tissue engineered construct demonstrating stronger mechanical properties over time. The ideal combination of scaffold and cell source remains a topic of future research in tendon tissue engineering.

SUMMARY

The hand surgeon's familiarity with options for flexor tendon reconstruction is essential. Efforts at primary repair are not always successful nor are the conditions after injury necessarily conducive to primary coaptation of tendon ends.

Single-stage and two-stage grafting, tenolysis, and pulley reconstruction are parts of the reconstructive surgeon's armamentarium. Future interventions of tissue engineering suggest the possibility of creating a theoretically endless supply of available donor material for use in tendon reconstruction.

REFERENCES

1. Manske P. History of flexor tendon repair. Hand Clin 2005;21:123–7.
2. Strickland J. Delayed treatment of flexor tendon injuries including grafting. Hand Clin 2005;21: 219–43.
3. Freilich A, Chhabra B. Secondary flexor tendon reconstruction, a review. J Hand Surg Am 2007; 32(9):1436–42.
4. Boyer M, Taras J, Kaufmann R. Flexor tendon reconstruction. In: Green D, Hotchkiss R, Pederson W, et al, editors. Green's operative hand surgery, vol. 1. 5th edition. Philadelphia: Elsevier; 2005. p. 241–76.
5. Mehta V, Phillips C. Flexor tendon pulley reconstruction. Hand Clin 2005;21:245–51.
6. Azari K, Meals R. Flexor tenolysis. Hand Clin 2005; 21:211–7.
7. Lehfeldt M, Ray E, Sherman R. MOC-PS CME article: treatment of flexor tendon laceration. Plast Reconstr Surg 2008;121(4):1–12.
8. Boyes J, Stark H. Flexor tendon grafts in the fingers and thumb. J Bone Joint Surg Am 1971;53:1332–9.
9. Paneva-Holevich E. Two-stage tenoplasty in injury of the flexor tendons of the hand. J Bone Joint Surg Am 1969;51(1):21–32.
10. Basheer M. Removal of a silicon rod 25 years after insertion for flexor tendon reconstruction. J Hand Surg Eur Vol 2007;32(5):591–2.
11. Hunter J, Salisbury R. Use of gliding artificial implants to produce tendon sheaths. Plast Reconstr Surg 1970;45(6):564–72.
12. Viegas S. A new modification of two-stage flexor tendon reconstruction. Tech Hand Up Extrem Surg 2006;10(3):177–80.
13. Beris A, Darlis N, Korompilias A, et al. Two-stage flexor tendon reconstruction in zone II using a silicone rod and a pedicled intrasynovial graft. J Hand Surg Am 2003;28(4):652–60.
14. Darlis N, Beris A, Korompilias A, et al. Two-stage flexor tendon reconstruction in zone 2 of the hand in children. J Pediatr Orthop 2005;25(3):382–6.
15. Valenti P, Gilbert A. Two-stage flexor tendon grafting in children. Hand Clin 2000;16(4):573–8.
16. Widstrom C, Johnson G, Doyle J, et al. A mechanical study of 6 digital pulley reconstruction techniques: part 1. Mechanical effectiveness. J Hand Surg Am 1989;14:821–5.
17. Wheeless C. Wheeless' textbook of orthopaedics. Available at: http://www.wheelessonline.com/ortho/lumbrical_plus_finger. Accessed April 16, 2010.
18. DeFranco M, Derwin K, Iannotti J. New therapies in tendon reconstruction. J Am Acad Orthop Surg 2004;12:298–304.
19. Cao Y, Vacanti J, Ma X, et al. Generation of neo-tendon using synthetic polymers seeded with tenocytes. Transplant Proc 1994;26(6):3390–2.
20. Cao Y, Liu Y, Liu W, et al. Bridging tendon defects using autologous tenocyte engineered tendon in a hen model. Plast Reconstr Surg 2002;110(5):1280–9.
21. Chong A, Riboh J, Smith R, et al. Flexor tendon tissue engineering: acellularized and reseeded tendon constructs. Plast Reconstr Surg 2009;123(6):1759–66.
22. Deng D, Liu W, Yang Y, et al. OP22: repair of tendon defect with adipose derived stem cells engineered tendon in a rabbit model. Plast Reconstr Surg 2009;124(2):686–7.

Tendon Transfers for Radial, Median, and Ulnar Nerve Injuries: Current Surgical Techniques

Neil F. Jones, MD[a],*, Gustavo R. Machado, MD[b]

KEYWORDS

- Tendon transfers • Radial nerve • Median nerve
- Ulnar nerve

TENDON TRANSFERS

Tendon transfers are reconstructive techniques that restore motion or balance to the hand that has impaired or absent function of the extrinsic or intrinsic muscle-tendon units of the forearm and hand. In a typical tendon transfer, the tendon of insertion of an expendable functioning muscle is detached, mobilized, and then reattached to another tendon or bone to substitute for the action of a nonfunctioning muscle-tendon unit. Occasionally, both the tendon of origin and the tendon of insertion are detached and then reattached at different locations. Unlike a tendon graft, the transferred donor tendon remains attached to its parent muscle. A tendon transfer also differs from a microsurgical free functional muscle transfer in that the neurovascular pedicle to the muscle of the transferred tendon remains intact.

There are 3 general indications for tendon transfers in the upper extremity:

1. To restore function to a muscle paralyzed by injuries of the peripheral nerves, the brachial plexus, or the spinal cord
2. To restore function following closed tendon ruptures or open injuries to the tendons or muscles
3. To restore balance to a hand deformed by various neurologic diseases.

Tendon transfers are best conceptualized as a means to restore a lost function rather than a means of substituting for a specific muscle (ie, restoring strong pinch as opposed to restoring function of the flexor pollicis longus [FPL]). Tendon transfers are performed predominantly following peripheral nerve injuries and, therefore, the current techniques for reconstruction of radial, median, and ulnar nerve palsies are described. However, these same techniques can be used for posttraumatic reconstruction of the hand that is affected by injuries to the muscles and tendons of the forearm or hand.

General Principles

It is assumed that surgeons will already understand the general principles of tendon transfers, but these are briefly summarized:

1. All fractures should be healed or rigidly fixed by internal fixation.
2. All skin in the projected course of the transfer should be pliable and unscarred, otherwise it should be replaced by pedicle or free flap.

The authors have no conflict of interest with the article.

[a] Division of Plastic and Reconstructive Surgery and Department of Orthopaedic Surgery, University of California Irvine Medical Center, Orange, CA, USA

[b] Department of Orthopaedic Surgery, University of California Irvine Medical Center, Orange, CA, USA

* Corresponding author. 101 The City Drive South, Pavilion III, Orange, CA 92868.

E-mail address: nfjones@uci.edu

Clin Plastic Surg 38 (2011) 621–642

doi:10.1016/j.cps.2011.07.002

0094-1298/11/$ – see front matter Published by Elsevier Inc.

3. Full passive range of motion of the metacarpophalangeal (MCP) and interphalangeal joints should be achieved by therapy or splinting before any tendon transfer.
4. The muscle-tendon unit selected must be expandable so that the transfer does not create a new functional deficit. A minimum of 1 wrist extensor, 1 wrist flexor, and 1 extrinsic flexor and extensor tendon to each digit should always be retained.
5. The potential amplitude or excursion of a donor muscle-tendon unit must be sufficient to restore the specific lost function[1]:
   - Wrist extensors and flexors: 33 mm
   - Finger extensors: 50 mm
   - Finger flexors: 70 mm
   - The potential excursion of the donor muscle-tendon unit can be increased by 20 mm by the wrist tenodesis effect.
6. The tendon transfer should pass in a direct line from the origin of the donor muscle to its new insertion and should ideally only act across 1 joint.
7. The tendon transfer should perform only 1 single function, but it may perform the same function in several adjacent digits.
8. The donor muscle should be synergistic with the function of the muscle to be restored.
9. The final selection of the potential tendon transfers is done by matching the available donor muscles with the functions to be restored.

Surgical Techniques

The success of any tendon transfer depends entirely on preventing scarring or adhesions along the course of the transferred tendon. Incisions should be carefully planned before elevation of the tourniquet so that the final tendon junctures lie beneath skin flaps rather than lying immediately beneath the incisions. The donor muscle should be carefully mobilized to prevent damage to its neurovascular bundle, which usually enters in the proximal third of the muscle. The transferred tendon should glide in a tunnel through the subcutaneous tissues and should not cross bare bone or pass through small fascial windows. Tendon junctures should be performed using a Pulvertaft weave technique. The donor and recipient tendons are sutured under appropriate tension, and after 1 or 2 nonabsorbable sutures have been inserted, the tension of the transfer should be checked by observing the flexion and extension of the digit during tenodesis of the wrist. Postoperatively, the hand is immobilized for 3 to 4 weeks, at which time gentle, active range-of-motion exercises are started, usually under the supervision of a therapist,

but the hand is protected for a further 3 weeks in a light-weight plastic splint.

Timing of Tendon Transfers

Timing of tendon transfers may be classified as early, conventional, or late. A conventional tendon transfer is usually performed after reinnervation of the paralyzed muscle fails to occur by 3 months after the expected time of reinnervation, based on the rate of nerve regeneration of 1 mm per day. Brand,[2] Omer, and Burkhalter[3] have advocated early tendon transfers in certain circumstances so that a tendon transfer is performed simultaneously with the nerve repair or before the expected time of reinnervation of the paralyzed muscle. This early tendon transfer, therefore, serves as a temporary substitute for the paralyzed muscle until reinnervation occurs, by acting as an internal splint. If reinnervation is suboptimal, the early tendon transfer acts as a helper to augment the power of the partially paralyzed muscle, and if reinnervation fails to occur, it then acts as the permanent substitute.

RADIAL NERVE PALSY
Functional Deficits

The functional motor deficit in radial nerve palsy consists of the inability to extend the wrist, the inability to extend the fingers at the MCP joints, and the inability to extend and radially abduct the thumb (**Fig. 1**A). However, another significant disability is that patients are unable to stabilize their wrist so that transmission of flexor power to their fingers is impaired resulting in marked weakness of grip strength (see **Fig. 1**B). Unlike median and ulnar nerve palsies, sensory loss following radial nerve injury is not functionally disabling unless patients develop a painful neuroma.

Tendon transfers are, therefore, required to provide wrist extension, extension of the fingers at the MCP joints, and extension and radial abduction of the thumb.

Timing

Timing of tendon transfers for radial nerve palsy remains controversial. The 2 options are either to perform an early tendon transfer simultaneously with repair of the radial nerve or, more conventionally, to delay any tendon transfers until reinnervation of the most proximal muscles, brachioradialis and extensor carpi radialis longus (ECRL), fails to occur within the calculated time limit. The more proximal the nerve injury, the less likely that functional muscle reinnervation will occur.[2,3] If the nerve remains in continuity, most

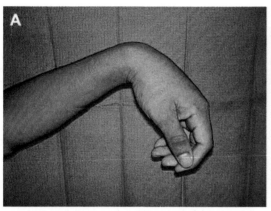 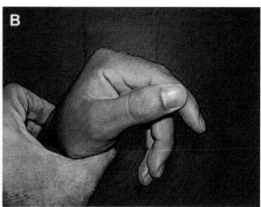

Fig. 1. (A) Typical appearance of a left radial nerve palsy with wrist drop. (B) Even with the wrist supported, the patient is still unable to actively extend their fingers and thumb at the MCP joints.

surgeons would suggest 3 months of observation are indicated to await spontaneous recovery in peripheral nerve palsies. With extensive nerve gaps or associated soft-tissue injuries or in older patients, the chances of successful reinnervation are much less predictable and, therefore, it may be more appropriate for these patients to undergo the full set of tendon transfers early.[4] In patients awaiting return of radial nerve function, it is important to maintain supple MCP joints capable of full extension and adequate radial abduction of the thumb with appropriate splinting and therapy.

Tendon Transfer Options

Franke[5] provided one of the earliest descriptions of tendon transfers for radial nerve palsy using the flexor carpi ulnaris (FCU) to extensor digitorum communis (EDC) transfer through the interosseous membrane. The flexor carpi radialis (FCR) to extensor pollicis longus (EPL) transfer has also been described. The pronator teres (PT) to ECRL and extensor carpi radialis brevis (ECRB) transfer for wrist extension was first reported in 1906 by Sir Robert Jones. Zachary[6] emphasized the importance of retaining at least one wrist flexor,

preferable the FCR to facilitate wrist control. Other authors have argued that FCU is not an expendable tendon and therefore prefer to use the FCR as the donor tendon to restore finger extension.[7] The advantage of using FCR is that it preserves the important moment of flexion and ulnar deviation of the wrist, which is so important for a power grip in working people. This factor is particularly important in patients with a posterior interosseous nerve (PIN) palsy in which ECRL function is preserved but extensor carpi ulnaris (ECU) function is lost. This condition results in radial deviation of the wrist with attempted wrist extension. Use of the FCU in this setting will only increase the radial deviation of the wrist because there would be no ulnar deviating motors of the wrist.

More than 50 modifications of tendon transfers have been reported for radial nerve palsy, but 3 patterns of transfer have evolved. The use of PT to provide wrist extension has become universally accepted, the only remaining controversy being whether to insert PT into the ECRB alone or into both the ECRL and the ECRB. The 3 patterns of tendon transfer differ, therefore, only in the technique of restoring finger extension and thumb extension and radial abduction (**Table 1**).[6,8–10]

Table 1
Tendon transfers for radial nerve palsy

	FCU Transfer	FCR Transfer	Boyes Superficialis Transfer
Wrist extension	PT to ECRB	PT to ECRB	PT to ECRB
Finger extension	FCU to EDC	FCR to EDC	FDS of ring finger to EDC long, ring, and small fingers
Thumb extension	PL to EPL	PL to EPL	FDS long finger to EIP and EPL

Abbreviations: EIP, extensor indicis proprius; FDS, flexor digitorum superficialis; PL, palmaris longus.

Standard FCU transfer

The FCU transfer is the authors' preferred technique for patients with a radial nerve palsy; the FCR transfer is preferred in patients with a PIN palsy. Through an inverted J-shaped incision over the ulnar-volar aspect of the distal forearm, the FCU tendon is transected at the wrist crease and released extensively from its fascial attachments up into the proximal third of the forearm, taking care not to damage the neurovascular pedicle, using a second incision in the proximal forearm if necessary. Through the same distal incision, the palmaris longus (PL) tendon is transected at the wrist crease and the muscle mobilized into the middle third of the forearm. An S-shaped incision is then made beginning over the volar-radial aspect of the middle third of the forearm and passing dorsally and ulnar over the radial border of the forearm, through which the tendon of the PT is elevated from the radius. The ECRB is transected at its musculotendinous junction if there is no chance of future reinnervation of the wrist extensors. The PT is then rerouted around the radial border of the forearm superficial to the brachioradialis and the ECRL tendons in a straight direction and sutured to the ECRB. The FCU tendon is passed through a subcutaneous tunnel made with a Kelly clamp from a dorsal incision around the ulnar border of the forearm into the J-shaped incision used to mobilize the FCU and sutured to the EDC tendons proximal to the extensor retinaculum. Alternatively, the FCU tendon may be passed from the palmar incision to the dorsal incision through a window in the interosseous membrane.[11] If no return of the EDC function is to be expected, the EDC tendons are transected at their musculotendinous junctions so that a more direct line of pull can be achieved. Otherwise an end-to-side juncture is performed. The EPL tendon is divided at its musculotendinous junction, removed from the third dorsal extensor tendon compartment, and passed through a subcutaneous tunnel from the base of the thumb metacarpal into the volar forearm incision and sutured to the PL. If the PL is absent, the EPL tendon is included with the EDC tendons so that the FCU provides both finger and thumb extension. To prevent a collapse flexion deformity at the carpometacarpal joint of the thumb, a tenodesis of the abductor pollicis longus (APL) may be necessary. After transection of the APL tendon in the distal forearm, it is looped around the brachioradialis proximal to the radial styloid and sutured to itself with the thumb metacarpal held in extension with the wrist in 30° of extension.

The proper tension in radial nerve tendon transfers should be tight enough to provide full extension of the wrist and digits but without restricting the flexion of the digits when the wrist is fully extended. The PT at resting tension is woven through the ECRB tendon with the wrist in 45° of extension. The distal ends of the 4 EDC tendons to the index, long, ring, and small fingers are sutured to the FCU tendon proximal to the extensor retinaculum. The extensor digiti minimi is not usually included unless there is still an extensor lag when proximal traction is applied to the EDC tendon to the small finger. With the wrist in neutral and the FCU under resting tension, each individual EDC tendon is sutured to provide full extension at the MCP joint, starting with the index finger and finishing with the small finger. Appropriate tension is then evaluated by checking that all 4 digits extend synchronously when the wrist is palmar flexed and, most importantly, that all 4 digits can be passively flexed into a fist when the wrist is extended. Finally, the PL and the EPL are interwoven over the radio-volar aspect of the wrist, with the PL at resting tension and the EPL at maximal tension with the wrist in neutral. The wrist is immobilized in 45° of extension in a volar splint, with the MCP joints positioned in slight flexion and the thumb in full extension and abduction.

Active flexion and extension of the fingers and thumb are started at 3.5 to 4.0 weeks and active exercises of the wrist are started at 5 weeks. Protective splinting is continued until 6 to 8 weeks postoperatively.

FCR transfer

The PT is transferred to the ECRB and the PL is transferred to the EPL exactly as described in the standard FCU transfer (**Fig. 2**A, B). The FCR is divided at the wrist crease and mobilized to the level of the midforearm and then rerouted around the radial border of the forearm or passed through a window in the interosseous membrane (see **Fig. 2**C). The 4 EDC tendons, and if necessary, the EDM may be woven through the donor FCR tendon proximal to the extensor retinaculum, but more usually the extensor tendons need to be rerouted superficial to the extensor retinaculum to obtain a straighter line of pull. To prevent a bulky tendon juncture, the small finger EDC and EDM may be sutured side to side to the ring finger EDC and the index finger EDC sutured side to side to the long finger EDC under appropriate tension. Then only the 2 EDC tendons to the long and ring fingers require weaving through the FCR tendon. As with the standard FCU transfer, these tendon junctures are performed with the wrist in neutral and the MCP joints in full extension with the FCR tendon under resting tension (see

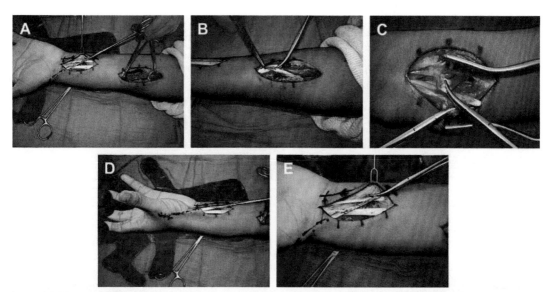

Fig. 2. (*A*) Through a volar incision in the distal third of the forearm, the palmaris longus and flexor carpi radialis are isolated and the transected extensor pollicis longus tendon rerouted into this incision. Through a separate incision over the radial aspect of the middle third of the forearm, the pronator teres is detached from the radius and the extensor carpi radialis brevis is transected at its musculotendinous junction. (*B*) The pronator teres is first sutured to the extensor carpi radialis brevis with the wrist in full extension and the pronator teres at its resting tension. (*C*) The flexor carpi radialis is passed to the radial aspect of the flexor tendons and median nerve through a window in the interosseous membrane and sutured at resting tension to the extensor digitorum communis tendons with the fingers in full extension at the MCP joints. (*D*, *E*) With the thumb in full radial abduction and extension, the rerouted extensor pollicis longus tendon is sutured to the palmaris longus tendon at its resting tension.

Fig. 2D, E). Postoperative management is similar to that for the FCU transfer (**Fig. 3**).

Boyes superficialis transfer

Boyes[8] was the first to argue that neither FCU nor FCR have sufficient amplitude (30 mm) to produce full excursion of the digital extensor tendons (50 mm) without incorporating the potential increase in amplitude obtained through the tenodesis effect of wrist flexion. He, therefore, advocated using the superficialis tendons to the long and ring fingers, which have an amplitude of 70 mm, to act as the donor tendons to restore finger extension.[8,9] The advantages of the Boyes transfer are that this transfer will potentially allow simultaneous wrist and finger extension, it may allow independent thumb and index finger extension, and it does not weaken wrist flexion. However, the long and ring fingers are deprived of superficialis function and this may result in weak grip. Harvesting of the superficialis tendons may also lead to the subsequent development of either a swan-neck deformity or a flexion contracture at the proximal interphalangeal (PIP) joint of the donor finger.

In Boyes' original description, PT was sutured to both the ECRL and the ECRB,[8] but to prevent excessive radial deviation, PT should only be woven end to end into the ECRB with the wrist in 30° of extension. The long finger superficialis is then passed to the radial side of the profundus muscles and the ring finger superficialis to the ulnar side through an interosseous window into a dorsal incision. After transection of the EPL and EIP tendons, they are woven end to end into the long finger superficialis tendon. Similarly, the transected EDC tendons to the index, long, ring, and small fingers are woven end to end into the ring finger superficialis tendon, although this arrangement can be reversed. The tendon junctures are performed proximal to the extensor retinaculum with the donor superficialis tendons at resting tension and traction on the extensor tendons to produce full extension at the MCP joints.

LOW MEDIAN NERVE PALSY
Functional Deficits

The functional deficit following injury to the median nerve distal to the innervation of the extrinsic forearm flexor muscles consists primarily of loss of opposition of the thumb and absent sensation over the thumb, index, long, and radial half of the ring finger (**Fig. 4**A).

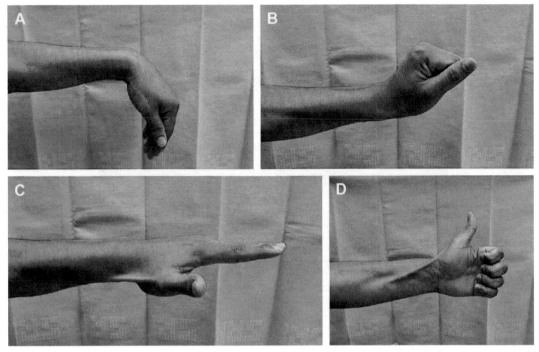

Fig. 3. (*A, B*) Two years postoperatively, the patient has excellent wrist extension. (*C*) Full finger extension with the wrist in neutral. (*D*) Full thumb extension and radial abduction.

Opposition is a composite motion that occurs at all 3 joints to position the thumb pad opposite the distal phalanx of the partially flexed long finger. Abduction, pronation, and flexion occur at the carpometacarpal joint, abduction and flexion at the metacarpophalangeal joint, and either flexion or extension at the interphalangeal joint. From a starting position of full extension and adduction, the thumb pronates approximately 90° during opposition to the long finger. Of the 3 intrinsic thenar muscles, the flexor pollicis brevis (FPB) muscle typically, although not always, receives a dual innervation from both the median and ulnar nerves.

Because the FPB may remain innervated by the ulnar nerve in approximately 70% of median nerve injuries, patients may not notice any significant functional loss, but careful testing will reveal decreased strength of the abductor pollicis brevis (APB) and lack of pronation.

Before any opposition tendon transfer, patients with median nerve injuries should be instructed to prevent the development of an adduction or supination contracture of the thumb by a program of passive abduction exercises. A static thumb–index finger web space splint may be used at night, but care should be taken to insure that

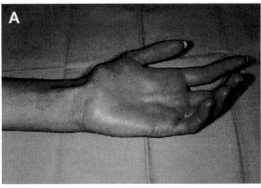
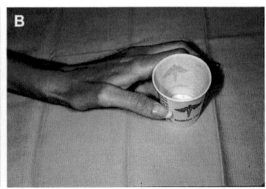

Fig. 4. (*A*) Typical spaghetti wrist with atrophy of the thenar muscles. (*B*) The patient is only able to grasp a large object by radial abduction of the thumb using the abductor pollicis longus with the forearm in pronation, which is an indication for an early opposition tendon transfer.

such splints abduct the thumb metacarpal rather than the proximal phalanx, otherwise the median nerve palsy will be compounded by attenuation of the ulnar collateral ligament of the MCP joint.

Bunnell[12] first emphasized that the pull of an opposition tendon transfer should be in an oblique direction from the thumb metacarpophalangeal joint to the region of the pisiform, and secondly that to produce pronation, the transfer should be inserted into the dorsal-ulnar base of the proximal phalanx.[13,14] Opposition transfers that are directed along the radial aspect of the palm will only produce a component of palmar abduction, whereas transfers that pass from the area of the pisiform will produce both abduction and pronation. The more distal the transfer passes across the palm, the greater the power of thumb flexion. Several sites of insertion of opposition transfers have been advocated;[15,16] however, a biomechanical study has shown that opposition tendon transfers inserted into the APB tendon alone will produce full abduction and pronation.[17]

Timing

Conventional timing of an opposition tendon transfer may be required for those patients who fail to demonstrate signs of reinnervation of the thenar muscles within the usual calculated time interval. Careful observation of thumb function following either a low or high median nerve palsy will reveal whether an early tendon transfer is necessary to restore thumb opposition. Because the FPB remains innervated by the ulnar nerve in approximately 70% of median nerve injuries, thumb function may not be significantly compromised, and, consequently, an early opposition transfer may not be necessary. Other patients, however, will adapt to their loss of opposition and abduction by substitution of the APL to provide thumb abduction, but this can only be achieved with the hand positioned in pronation. Therefore, if the surgeon or therapist observes patients attempting to grasp objects by radial abduction of the thumb with the forearm in pronation, an early opposition tendon transfer should be strongly considered (see **Fig. 4**B). If, however, patients are able to grasp an object with the forearm in neutral or with the forearm in supination, it is likely that the FPB remains innervated by the ulnar nerve and, consequently, the decision to perform an early opposition tendon transfer can be delayed.

Tendon Transfer Options

Several techniques have been described to restore opposition of the thumb using various muscles innervated by the radial or ulnar nerves, including the extensor indicis proprius (EIP), the ring finger flexor digitorum superficialis (FDS) transfer (not available in a high median nerve palsy), the PL, the abductor digiti minimi,[18–20] the extensor pollicis brevis (EPB), the ECU, and the extensor digiti minimi.[21] **Table 2** summarizes the options for opposition tendon transfers.

Burkhalter extensor indicis proprius transfer

The EIP transfer[22] is the authors' preferred technique, except in elderly patients with thenar atrophy secondary to severe carpal tunnel syndrome (**Fig. 5**). The EIP tendon is transected through a small transverse incision just proximal to the MCP joint of the index finger. The distal stump of the EIP tendon is then repaired to the EDC tendon of the index finger to prevent extensor lag at the metacarpophalangeal joint. The EIP tendon is mobilized through 2 small transverse incisions, 1 proximal and 1 distal to the extensor retinaculum, and the muscle belly mobilized through a longitudinal incision over the ulnar aspect of the dorsal distal forearm (**Fig. 6**A). A transverse incision is made just proximal to the pisiform bone and a subcutaneous tunnel developed to connect this incision to the dorsal forearm incision. The EIP tendon is then passed subcutaneously around the ulnar border of the distal forearm superficial to the ECU tendon into the pisiform incision. The insertion of the APB tendon is identified through a small incision over the radial aspect of the MCP joint of the thumb and a subcutaneous tunnel is made connecting this incision with the pisiform incision. The EIP tendon transfer is passed obliquely across the palm (see **Fig. 6**B) and woven into the tendon of the APB under maximum tension, with the wrist in neutral position and the thumb in maximal palmar abduction (see **Fig. 6**C). The tension of the transfer is then tested by the wrist tenodesis effect. Wrist extension should produce thumb abduction, and wrist

Table 2 Opposition tendon transfers	
	Donor Tendon
Burkhalter	EIP
Bunnell	FDS ring finger through a pulley of a distal-based slip of FCU
Camitz	PL extended with a rolled up strip of palmar fascia
Huber	Abductor digiti minimi
Phalen and Miller	ECU sutured to a distal-based slip of EPB
Schneider	Extensor digit minimi

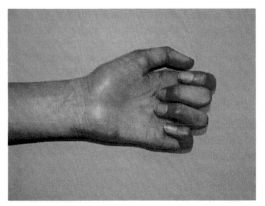

Fig. 5. A patient with a median nerve palsy about to undergo a Burkhalter opposition tendon transfer.

flexion should allow the thumb to be passively adducted. If wrist extension produces excessive flexion or extension of the thumb at the metacarpophalangeal joint, this indicates that the transfer has been inserted either too far volar or too far dorsally and should be adjusted accordingly. The thumb is immobilized in full abduction with the wrist in slight palmar flexion for 4 weeks, at which time active abduction and opposition movements are begun with protective splinting for a further 3 to 4 weeks. The only potential disadvantage with

this tendon transfer is that the EIP tendon is only just long enough to reach the APB tendon. Postoperative results have been predictable (**Fig. 7**).

Bunnell ring finger flexor digitorum superficialis transfer

In the flexor superficialis transfer originally described by Bunnell,[13] the ring finger superficialis tendon is isolated through a small transverse incision just distal to the distal palmar crease. The tendon is transected between the A1 and A2 pulleys and delivered into a proximal incision over the palmar aspect of the distal forearm. The FCU tendon is split longitudinally to create a distal-based strip of the radial half of the tendon. This strip is then passed through a slit in the FCU tendon just proximal to the pisiform and sutured to itself to create a pulley. The distal end of the ring finger superficialis tendon is passed through the pulley and through a subcutaneous tunnel obliquely across the palm to exit in an incision over the radial aspect of the MCP joint of the thumb. All the other incisions are closed and the FDS is sutured to the APB tendon with the tension adjusted as described previously.

Simple looping of the ring finger superficialis around the FCU tendon rather than creating a fixed pulley rapidly becomes ineffective and the transfer

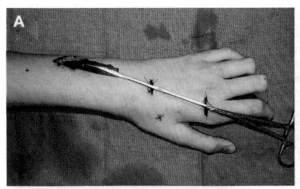
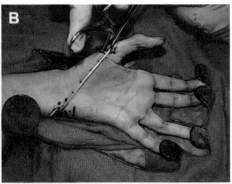
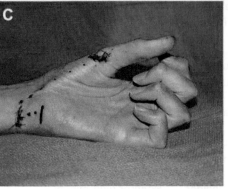

Fig. 6. (A) The extensor indicis proprius tendon is transected at the MCP joint of the index finger and mobilized through a dorsal-ulnar incision in the distal third of the forearm. (B) The extensor indicis proprius is routed around the ulnar border of the forearm as far distally as possible and then passed through a subcutaneous tunnel obliquely across the hand from the pisiform to the MCP joint of the thumb using a tendon passer. (C) Immediate intraoperative photography of the Burkhalter opposition tendon transfer.

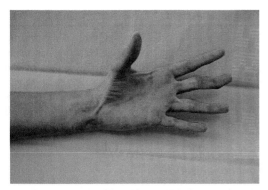

Fig. 7. Four years after the Burkhalter opposition tendon transfer, the patient has excellent palmar abduction and opposition of the left thumb.

becomes converted to a flexor of the thumb MCP joint rather than a true opposition transfer. Alternative pulleys for the ring finger superficialis transfer include passing the tendon through the Guyon canal or through a window in the transverse carpal ligament.

Compared with the EIP transfer, the ring finger superficialis is stronger and has greater length. However, the ring finger superficialis is not available as a donor tendon in a high median nerve palsy or in low median nerve injuries with associated injuries to the flexor tendons. The ring finger

superficialis transfer should also not be selected in combined low median and high ulnar nerve palsies because the ring finger superficialis is the only remaining flexor tendon in the ring finger. In low median–low ulnar nerve palsies, the ring finger superficialis may be required for correction of clawing. In addition, harvesting of the superficialis tendon may result in either a flexion contracture or a swan-neck deformity of the PIP joint of the donor finger.

Camitz palmaris longus transfer

The Camitz PL tendon transfer[23–26] is a simple transfer that will provide abduction of the thumb but little pronation or flexion and is particularly indicated in elderly patients with thenar atrophy caused by long-standing carpal tunnel syndrome (**Fig. 8**A). A strip of palmar fascia is dissected in continuity with the distal PL tendon through a standard carpal tunnel incision in the palm extending proximally into the distal forearm. A subcutaneous tunnel is developed from the radial aspect of the distal forearm incision along the thenar eminence into a midaxial incision on the radial aspect of the MCP joint of the thumb (see **Fig. 8**B). The fascial extension of the PL tendon is passed through the subcutaneous tunnel and sutured to the APB tendon under maximal tension with the wrist in neutral position (see **Fig. 8**C).

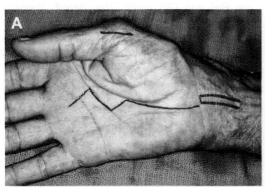

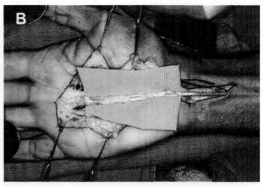

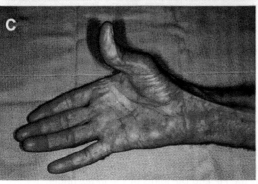

Fig. 8. (*A*) A patient with severe right carpal tunnel syndrome and thenar atrophy about to undergo a Camitz tendon transfer. (*B*) The palmaris longus tendon is extended with a rolled up sheet of palmar fascia and transferred subcutaneously to the insertion of the abductor pollicis brevis tendon at the MCP joint of the thumb. (*C*) One year postoperatively, the patient demonstrates excellent palmar abduction of the right thumb. Because the transfer does not originate from the region of the pisiform, the Camitz transfer does not provide pronation of the thumb.

HIGH MEDIAN NERVE PALSY
Functional Deficits

The functional deficit following injury to the median nerve proximal to its innervation of the extrinsic forearm flexor muscles consists of the inability to flex the index finger at the PIP and distal interphalangeal (DIP) joints and the thumb at the interphalangeal joint in addition to the loss of opposition (**Fig. 9**). This deficit is due to the paralysis of all 4 FDS muscles, the flexor digitorum profundus (FDP) tendons to the index and long fingers and the FPL muscle as well as the 3 thenar muscles. Patients are often still able to flex the long finger because of the interconnections between the profundus tendons to the long, ring, and small fingers in the distal forearm and wrist. Therefore, the 3 functions that need to be restored in patients with a high median nerve palsy are flexion at the interphalangeal joint of the thumb and flexion of the PIP and DIP joints of the index and long fingers, together with a conventional opposition tendon transfer.

Timing

Timing of tendon transfers in a high median nerve palsy remains controversial.[3] If a good primary or delayed primary median nerve repair can be performed, there is a reasonable chance of reinnervation of the extrinsic flexor muscles in young patients. Consequently, early brachioradialis to the FPL or side-to-side repair of the index and long finger profundus tendons to the ring and small finger profundus tendons is not advocated. However, if patients are seen late and require secondary nerve grafting of the median nerve, tendon transfers for restoration of thumb flexion and index and long finger flexion should be performed simultaneously with the nerve graft.

Tendon Transfers

Flexion of the interphalangeal joint of the thumb may be restored by the transfer of brachioradialis to the FPL and flexion of the DIP joints of the index and middle fingers by side-to-side tenorrhaphy of the index and long finger FDP tendons to the ring and small finger FDP tendons (**Figs. 10 and 11**).

LOW ULNAR NERVE PALSY
Functional Deficits

Injury to the ulnar nerve distal to the innervation of the ring and small finger FDP and FCU muscles produces a functional deficit consisting of the paralysis of all 7 interossei, the ulnar 2 lumbricales, the 3 hypothenar muscles, the adductor pollicis, and the deep head of FPB muscle. This deficit results in an imbalance of the flexor and extensor forces at the MCP, PIP, and DIP joints of the fingers. Because the interossei are the main flexors at the MCP joints, extension of the proximal phalanges at the MCP joints by the extrinsic extensor tendons is unopposed and the MCP joint hyperextension occurs to the extent allowed by the volar plates. Because the extrinsic extensor tendons concentrate their extension at the MCP joints and the interossei are unable to actively extend at the PIP and DIP joints, increased tension in the flexor tendons, which occurs as the MCP joints begin to hyperextend, will be unopposed at the PIP and DIP joints. This deficit, therefore, results in the typical claw hand with hyperextension at the MCP joints and reciprocal flexion at the PIP and DIP joints (Duchenne sign). Imbalance between the extrinsic extensor and flexor tendons leads to the asynchronous flexion of the fingers and weak grip strength (**Fig. 12**). The MCP joints do not flex until after the interphalangeal joints

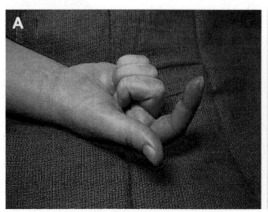
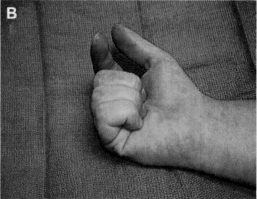

Fig. 9. (*A, B*) Typical posture of a high median nerve palsy affecting the right hand with loss of flexion at the interphalangeal joint of the thumb and loss of flexion at the PIP and DIP joints of the index finger.

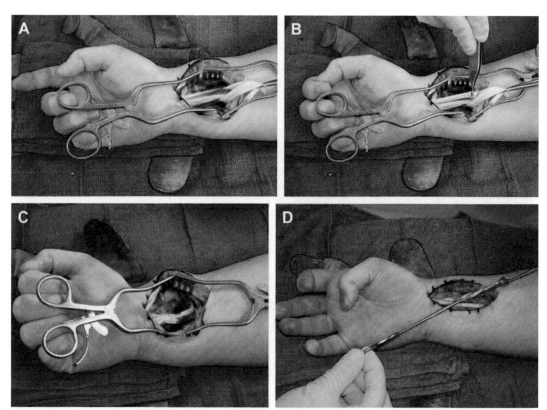

Fig. 10. (*A*) Through a palmar incision in the distal third of the forearm, the flexor digitorum profundus tendons can be isolated. (*B*) The flexor digitorum profundus tendons to the index and long fingers can be retracted proximally so that all 4 fingers have a symmetric cascade. The flexor digitorum profundus tendons to the index and long fingers are sutured to the flexor digitorum profundus tendons to the ring and small fingers, which are still innervated by the ulnar nerve. (*C, D*) The flexor pollicis longus tendon is sutured to the brachioradialis tendon to restore flexion at the interphalangeal joint of the thumb.

have become completely flexed, resulting in the curling of the tips of the fingers into the palm with the loss of the ability to grasp large objects. In a low ulnar nerve palsy, the clawing and loss of integrated MCP and interphalangeal joint flexion are confined to the ring and small fingers and, to a lesser extent, the long finger because the lumbricales to the index and long fingers remain innervated by the median nerve. However, with a combined median and ulnar nerve palsy, all 4 fingers are affected.

The other significant impairment in patients with low ulnar nerve palsy is weak thumb–index finger pinch, which may be only 20% to 25% of normal because of the paralysis of the adductor pollicis, one-half of the FPB, and the first dorsal interosseous muscles. Loss of key pinch is usually manifest by compensatory activation of the FPL producing excessive flexion at the interphalangeal joint (Froment sign) and occasionally hyperextension at the MCP joint (Jeanne's sign) as patients attempt a forceful pinch. In such patients with

weak a pinch, tendon transfers will be required to restore adduction of the thumb and abduction of the index finger.

Patients may also develop an irritating ulnar deviation of the small finger in addition to clawing at the MCP joint of the small finger (Wartenberg sign) caused by the unopposed action of the extensor digiti minimi tendon because of the paralysis of the third palmar interosseous muscle. Occasionally, a tendon transfer may be required to correct this ulnar deviation of the small finger.

Therefore, tendon transfers may be indicated in an ulnar nerve palsy to correct (1) clawing and asynchronous flexion of the fingers, (2) weak thumb–index finger pinch, (3) ulnar deviation deformity of the small finger, and (4) weak FDP flexion at the DIP joints of the ring and small fingers.

Timing

Timing of tendon transfers for ulnar nerve palsy is primarily dependent on 2 factors: the probability

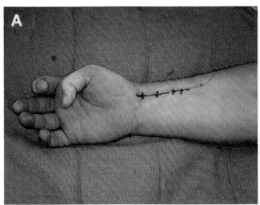

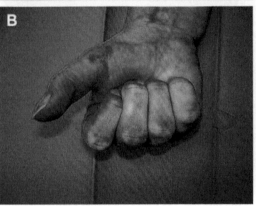

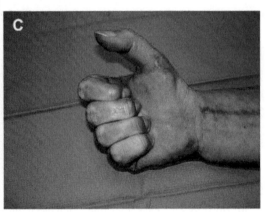

Fig. 11. (*A*) Immediate postoperative posture of the hand showing increased flexion at the PIP and DIP joints of the index finger and flexion at the interphalangeal joint of the thumb. (*B, C*) Two years postoperatively, the patient has excellent flexion at the PIP and DIP joints of the index finger and at the interphalangeal joint of the thumb. She has also undergone a Burkhalter opposition tendon transfer to restore palmar abduction and opposition of the thumb.

of motor recovery after nerve repair and the severity of the functional deficit. Although clawing should be treated proactively using a lumbrical block splint, some patients may benefit from early static procedures or tendon transfers to prevent hyperextension of the MCP joints leading to a debilitating claw deformity.

Fig. 12. A patient with a combined low median–low ulnar nerve palsy, demonstrating the asynchronous flexion of the fingers with flexion at the PIP and DIP joints occurring before flexion at the MCP joints.

Static procedures to prevent hyperextension of the proximal phalanges at their MCP joints include A1 pulley release, fasciodermadesis at the MCP joint level, Zancolli capsulodesis,[27] and various tenodeses.

Tendon Transfer Options to Correct Clawing

All of the following donor muscle-tendon transfers have been described to correct asynchronous finger flexion and clawing in ulnar nerve palsy:

1. Flexor digitorum superficialis (modified Stiles-Bunnell)
2. Extensor carpi radialis brevis
3. Extensor indicis proprius and extensor digiti minimi
4. Flexor carpi radialis
5. Extensor carpi radialis longus
6. Palmaris longus.

The various dynamic tendon transfers that have been described to correct clawing differ primarily as to whether they provide only MCP joint flexion or whether they provide both MP joint flexion and interphalangeal joint extension (**Table 3**). The hand surgeon can determine which general type

Table 3
Tendon transfers for ulnar nerve palsy

Function to be Restored	Preferred Tendon Transfer
Clawing of the ring and small fingers	2 slips of the ring finger or long finger FDS to the radial lateral bands; proximal phalanges; or A1 or A2 pulleys of the ring and small fingers
Clawing of all 4 fingers	EF4T or PL4T transfers to the radial lateral bands of the long, ring, and small fingers and the ulnar lateral band of the index finger; or to the combined interosseous tendon insertions
Thumb adduction	ECRB + tendon graft to adductor pollicis
Index finger abduction	Accessory APL to first dorsal interosseous
Severe thumb MCP joint hyperextension	MCP joint arthrodesis
Fixed thumb IP joint flexion contracture	IP joint arthrodesis
Weak DIP joint flexion ring and small fingers	Side-to-side tenorrhaphy of the ring and small finger FDP tendons to the long finger FDP tendon

Abbreviations: EF4T, extensor tendon flexor route 4-tailed graft; IP, interphalangeal; PL4T, palmaris 4-tail tendon graft.

of transfer is most appropriate by preoperative testing of PIP and DIP joint extension with the MCP joints held passively flexed: the Bouvier maneuver (**Fig. 13**). If, with the MCP joints flexed, the extrinsic extensor tendons can produce full extension at the PIP and DIP joints, the transfer only needs to produce strong MCP joint flexion by insertion of the transfer either into the A1 pulley (Zancolli[28]), the A2 pulley (Brooks-Jones[29]), the A1 and proximal half of the A2 pulley (Anderson[30]), or through a drill hole in the proximal phalanx (Burkhalter[31]). However, with long-standing flexion deformities of the PIP joints, the central slip of the extensor mechanism may become attenuated. Consequently, even with passive flexion of the MCP joints in the Bouvier maneuver, patients

cannot actively extend the PIP joints using their extrinsic extensor tendons. In these circumstances, the transfer has to be inserted into one of the lateral bands, into the dorsal base of the middle phalanx, or into the combined interosseous tendons (which Zancolli termed "direct interosseous activation,"[28,32]) so that both the MCP joint flexion and the PIP joint extension can potentially be restored.

If one of the superficialis tendons is used as a donor tendon to produce either MCP joint flexion alone or both MCP joint flexion and interphalangeal joint extension, it does not produce any increase in power grip, whereas adding an extra muscle-tendon unit from outside the hand to activate these transfers, such as a wrist flexor (FCR) or a wrist extensor (ECRL or ECRB), will potentially lead to increased grip strength.

Modified Stiles-Bunnell transfer

In the modified Stiles-Bunnell transfer[33] for patients with an isolated low ulnar nerve palsy, the ring finger superficialis tendon is divided just proximal to the PIP joint, withdrawn through a transverse distal palmar crease incision, and split longitudinally into 2 slips. The radial lateral bands of the ring and small fingers are exposed through radial midaxial incisions, and each slip of the superficialis tendon is passed down the lumbrical canals of the ring and small fingers. With the wrist in neutral, each slip is sutured under adequate tension to the radial lateral bands with the MCP joints in 45° to 55° of flexion and the interphalangeal joints fully extended. Tension is tested using the wrist tenodesis effect; with wrist extension, the fingers should assume the intrinsic-plus position. The hand is immobilized in a dorsal block splint with the wrist in slight flexion and the MP joints flexed 70° for 3.5 to 4.0 weeks.

One of the disadvantages of the modified Stiles-Bunnell transfer is that the ring finger superficialis is not expendable in a high ulnar nerve palsy or in a combined high median–high ulnar nerve palsy. The superficialis tendon is the only extrinsic flexor tendon in the ring finger in a high ulnar nerve palsy and, therefore, the long finger FDS tendon has to be used. Secondly, the transfer may result in progressive overcorrection of the claw deformity, eventually resulting in a swan-neck hyperextension deformity at the PIP joints. This swan-neck hyperextension deformity can be prevented by suturing one of the distal slips of the FDS across the PIP joint as a tenodesis. Thirdly, the donor long or ring finger may develop a PIP joint flexion contracture or loss of extension at the DIP joint. The modified Stiles-Bunnell transfer should, therefore, only be used in patients with mild PIP joint

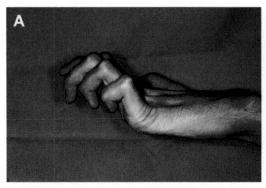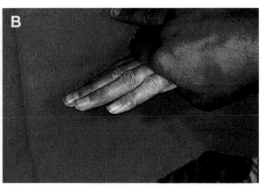

Fig. 13. (*A*) Typical claw deformity of all 4 fingers seen in a low ulnar nerve palsy with hyperextension at the MCP joints and flexion at the PIP and DIP joints. (*B*) The Bouvier maneuver. By blocking the hyperextension at the MCP joints with the surgeon's hand, the patient is able to actively extend all 4 fingers at the PIP and DIP joints through the extrinsic extensor tendons. The ability to perform this task indicates that any tendon transfer to prevent clawing only has to produce flexion at the MCP joints by insertion of the tendon transfers either into the A1 or A2 pulleys or into the proximal phalanges, rather than needing to be inserted into the lateral bands.

flexion contractures or stable fingers without passive hyperextension at the PIP joints.

Brand EE4T transfer extensor tendon, extensor route, 4-tailed graft

Because of his extensive experience with tendon transfers in patients with leprosy, Brand[1,34] originally described the transfer of the ECRB, extended with 4 tendon grafts, passed from dorsal to palmar through the intermetacarpal spaces and then down the lumbrical canals to be attached to the radial lateral bands of the long, ring, and small fingers and to the ulnar lateral band of the index finger. This extensor tendon, extensor route, 4-tailed graft transfer will only produce MCP joint flexion when the wrist is flexed, but it is an alternative transfer for a combined high median–high ulnar nerve palsy when the modified Stiles-Bunnell FDS transfer is not available.

Brand EF4T transfer extensor tendon, flexor route, 4-tailed graft

Brand[34] modified his original dorsal ECRB transfer by using ECRL extended with a 4-tailed tendon graft or fascia lata graft, which is passed through the carpal tunnel to the radial lateral bands of the long, ring, and small fingers and the ulnar lateral band of the index finger (extensor tendon, flexor route, 4-tailed graft [EF4T]) (**Fig. 14, Fig. 15**). In an isolated ulnar nerve palsy, this EF4T transfer only needs to be attached to the radial lateral bands of the ring and small fingers.

Fritschi PF4T transfer palmaris, flexor route, 4-tailed graft

Fritschi[35] described the PL as an alternative donor muscle for the Brand EF4T transfer. In the Lennox-

Fritschi palmaris 4-tail tendon graft transfer, the PL tendon is lengthened with tendon grafts or a fascia lata graft, which is then passed through the carpal tunnel to the lateral bands in a similar route to the Brand EF4T procedure. However, PL is obviously a much weaker donor muscle than the ECRL.

Tendon Transfer Options to Provide Adduction of the Thumb

The most successful tendon transfers to restore adduction of the thumb and lateral pinch have a transverse direction of pull across the palm deep to the flexor tendons to insert into the tendon of the adductor pollicis. Several techniques have been described; the most commonly performed techniques are the ECRB and FDS transfers. Other tendon transfers to restore adduction of the thumb include either the brachioradialis[36] or the ECRL[37] elongated with a tendon graft and passed through the third intermetacarpal space to the ulnar aspect of the thumb MCP joint and the EIP passed through the second intermetacarpal space.[38] Combined transfers to provide both thumb adduction and index finger abduction have been described by splitting the EIP or extensor digiti minimi tendons.[39]

Arthrodesis of the MCP joint may be necessary if there is a severe collapse deformity of the thumb with hyperextension at the MCP joint and flexion at the interphalangeal (IP) joint or an exaggerated Jeanne's sign when attempting to pinch.[33,40,41]

Littler ring finger flexor digitorum superficialis transfer

The ring finger FDS tendon is transected between the A1 and A2 pulleys through a short incision at the base of the ring finger.[33] Through a short

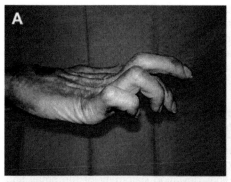

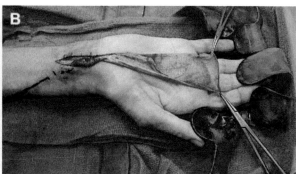

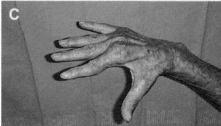

Fig. 14. (*A*) A patient with clawing of all 4 fingers caused by an ulnar nerve palsy. (*B*) The Brand EF4T transfer to prevent clawing. A triangular-shaped fascia lata graft has been sutured to the extensor carpi radialis longus tendon, which has been transected at the base of the index finger metacarpal and transposed around the radial border of the forearm into an incision just proximal to the wrist crease. The fascia lata graft is then passed through the carpal tunnel deep to the flexor tendons into a palmar incision. The graft is split into 4 slips, and each slip is passed down the lumbrical canals and sutured into the radial lateral bands of the long, ring, and small fingers and the ulnar lateral band of the index finger. (*C*) Two years postoperatively, the patient has excellent correction of the clawing of her fingers with full extension at the PIP and DIP joints of all 4 fingers and no hyperextension at the MCP joints.

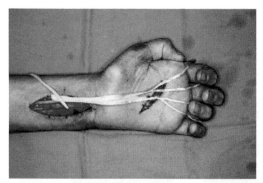

Fig. 15. In a similar Brand EF4T transfer to correct clawing of the fingers in a combined low median nerve–ulnar nerve palsy, the extensor carpi radialis longus tendon is similarly transposed around the radial border of the forearm into the palmar incision over the distal third of the forearm. This tendon is then sutured to a looped toe extensor tendon that will be subsequently passed through the carpal tunnel deep to the flexor tendons, and then each of the 2 loops is split further into 2 slips to provide 4 slips to be passed down the lumbrical canals to the radial lateral bands of the long, ring, and small fingers and the ulnar lateral band of the ring finger.

incision just to the ulnar side of the thenar crease, the superficialis tendon is then passed transversely across the palm deep to the index and long finger flexor tendons to the ulnar aspect of the thumb MCP joint. The transfer is either sutured into the adductor pollicis tendon or passed through a drill hole in the proximal phalanx just distal to the adductor insertion and tied over a button. Tension is set with the wrist in neutral and the thumb adducted against the index finger with the superficialis tendon at its resting length. Appropriate tension is confirmed by tenodesis of the wrist: with wrist flexion, the thumb should be able to be passively abducted, and with wrist extension, the thumb should adduct against the index finger. Obviously, the ring finger superficialis cannot be used as an adductor transfer in patients with a high ulnar nerve palsy because this would deprive the ring finger of its only remaining flexor tendon.

Smith extensor carpi radialis brevis transfer

ECRB is transected through a short transverse incision over the second dorsal extensor compartment just distal to the extensor retinaculum and withdrawn through a second transverse incision just proximal to the extensor retinaculum.[42] A small flap is then elevated over the ulnar aspect of the MCP joint of the thumb and a palmaris or plantaris tendon graft is sutured to the adductor pollicis tendon. Through a short transverse incision overlying the proximal third of the second intermetacarpal space, a tendon passer is used to tunnel the tendon graft deep to the flexor tendons but superficial to the adductor pollicis, withdrawing it dorsally through the second intermetacarpal space. After passing the tendon graft subcutaneously to the most proximal incision, it is woven into the ECRB tendon with the wrist in neutral and the thumb adducted. Tension is then checked by wrist tenodesis: with wrist flexion, the thumb should become strongly adducted, whereas wrist extension should allow easy passive abduction of the thumb. Postoperatively, the thumb is immobilized for 3 weeks midway between full abduction and full adduction with the wrist in 20° of extension.

Tendon Transfer Options to Provide Index Finger Abduction

Restoration of strong abduction of the index finger is the second component required for a powerful key pinch. Bunnell[43] described the transfer of the EIP extended with a short tendon graft and inserted into the first dorsal interosseous tendon. Neviaser and colleagues[44] described an accessory APL tendon elongated with a palmaris or plantaris tendon graft transferred to the insertion of the first dorsal interosseous tendon. Other tendon transfers[45–47] that have been described include EPB[46] and a PL tendon[47] lengthened with a strip of palmar fascia inserted into the first dorsal interosseous tendon.

Tendon Transfer to Correct Ulnar Deviation of the Small Finger

A variant of the Fowler transfer has been advocated by Blacker and colleagues[48] to correct the ulnar deviation deformity of the small finger (Wartenberg sign) (**Fig. 16**A). The ulnar half of the extensor digiti minimi is detached, passed volar to the deep transverse intermetacarpal ligament, and sutured into the insertion of the radial collateral ligament of the MCP joint at the base of the proximal phalanx (see **Fig. 16**B), or if there is associated clawing of the small finger, it is looped under the A2 pulley and sutured back to itself (Brooks insertion; see **Fig. 16**C). Chung and colleagues[49] have recently described transferring EIP to the distal radial aspect of the extensor hood of the small finger as an alternative transfer to correct the persistent abduction deformity of the small finger in an ulnar nerve palsy.

HIGH ULNAR NERVE PALSY
Functional Deficits

Many surgeons fail to realize the significant functional deficit associated with paralysis of the FCU

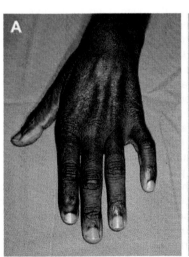
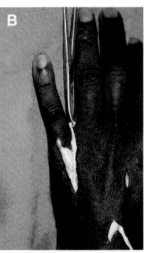
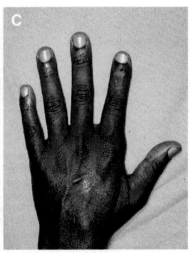

Fig. 16. (A) Typical Wartenberg sign in a patient with a left ulnar nerve palsy with an ulnar deviation deformity of the small finger caused by the unopposed action of the extensor digiti minimi tendon caused by paralysis of the third palmar interosseous muscle. (B) Half of the extensor digiti minimi tendon is rerouted around the radial collateral ligament of the MCP joint of the left small finger. (C) One year postoperatively, the patient has satisfactory axial alignment of the small finger with the ring finger and correction of the Wartenberg deformity.

and profundus tendons to the ring and small fingers in a high ulnar nerve palsy. The only remaining tendons on the ulnar side of the hand are the superficialis tendon to the ring finger and the usually diminutive superficialis tendon to the small finger. However, paralysis of the profundus tendons to the ring and small fingers will often be masked by interconnections between these 2 tendons and the long finger profundus tendon at the wrist still innervated by the median nerve.

Tendon Transfers

If there is significant weakness of the DIP joint flexion of the ring and small fingers (Pollock sign), power grip can be restored by side-to-side tenorrhaphy of the ring and small finger FDP tendons to the median-innervated long finger FDP tendon.[50] This procedure should be performed before tendon transfers to correct clawing are performed, but patients should be warned that this will temporarily exaggerate their clawing and that they should then use a lumbrical block splint. To restore independent flexion of the ring and small fingers, the FDS tendon of the long finger may be used as a donor tendon to activate the FDP tendons of the ring and small fingers. Patients requiring strong ulnar deviation and flexion of the wrist may occasionally need to be considered for transfer of the FCR tendon to the FCU.[50]

TENDON TRANSFERS FOR COMBINED NERVE INJURIES

It is much more difficult to reconstruct patients with combined nerve injuries and unwise to adopt a cookbook approach (see **Fig. 12**). Most of these patients require multiple tendon transfers, which should be individualized to address the patients' specific functional needs. In addition, the number of donor tendons is limited, there is a more profound sensory loss, and the soft tissues may be more scarred in these patients (see **Fig. 15**); so, the results of tendon transfers for combined nerve injuries are inferior to those for a single nerve injury.[51]

Tables 4 and **5** summarize the tendon transfer options for a combined low median–low ulnar palsy and a high median–high ulnar palsy.

TENDON TRANSFERS FOR RECONSTRUCTION AFTER TRAUMA

Tendon transfers are an excellent technique for restoring function to the hand and wrist following traumatic injuries of the muscles and tendons of the forearm, wrist, and hand. Simplistically, there are 4 situations in which tendon transfers can be

Table 4 Tendon transfers for combined low median–low ulnar nerve palsy	
Function to be Restored	Preferred Tendon Transfer
Thumb opposition	EIP to APB
Clawing of all 4 fingers	EF4T or PL4T transfers to the radial lateral bands of the long, ring, and small fingers and the ulnar lateral band of the index finger; or to the combined interosseous tendon insertions
Thumb adduction	ECRB + tendon graft to adductor pollicis
Index finger abduction	Accessory APL to first dorsal interosseous
Severe thumb MCP joint hyperextension	MCP joint arthrodesis
Improve palmar hand sensation	Nerve transfer of superficial radial nerve to distal median nerve

considered for posttraumatic reconstruction of the wrist and hand:

1. Restoration of thumb extension
2. Restoration of thumb flexion
3. Restoration of finger extension
4. Restoration of finger flexion.

Tendon Transfer to Restore Thumb Extension

Rupture of the EPL tendon occurs in approximately 1 in 200 distal radius fractures, classically at the Lister tubercle and approximately 6 weeks after the fracture. Paradoxically, rupture of EPL is associated with nondisplaced or minimally displaced distal radius fractures. Ischemia of the tendon caused by swelling or attrition over the roughened dorsal cortex has been postulated as the etiologic mechanism.[52–54] Patients present with painless loss of extension at the interphalangeal joint or paradoxically with incomplete extension at the MP joint as well as the loss of retropulsion of the thumb above the plane of the hand.

Although the deficit can be reconstructed with a tendon graft, the optimal choice for restoration of thumb extension is the EIP to EPL transfer, which can even be performed under local anesthesia.[55] The EIP tendon is harvested through

Table 5 Tendon transfers for combined high median–high ulnar nerve palsy	
Function to be Restored	Preferred Tendon Transfer
Thumb opposition	EIP to APB
Finger flexion	ECRL to the 4 FDPs, can be combined with tenodeses of the DIP joints of the ulnar 3 digits
Thumb flexion	Brachioradialis to FPL
Clawing of all 4 fingers	Static tenodeses, Zancolli capsulodesis, or PIP joint arthrodeses
Thumb adduction	ECRB + tendon graft to adductor pollicis
Index finger abduction	Accessory APL to first dorsal interosseous
Severe thumb MCP joint hyperextension	MCP joint arthrodesis
Improve palmar hand sensation	Fillet flap of the index finger; or first dorsal metacarpal artery flap to resurface the thumb–long finger web space; or nerve transfer of superficial radial nerve to distal median nerve

a short transverse incision just proximal to the index finger MP joint and its distal stump is then sutured end-to-side to the EDC tendon of the index finger to prevent extensor lag of this finger. The EIP is retrieved through a second transverse incision just distal to the extensor retinaculum. A third incision is made over the distal third of the thumb metacarpal and the EIP is tunneled subcutaneously to this incision (**Fig. 17**). The EIP tendon is sutured to the distal end of the EPL tendon with the wrist held in neutral and the thumb fully extended and parallel or just volar to the plane of the palm.[56] The tension of the transfer can be checked by tenodesis of the wrist. With wrist flexion, the thumb should move dorsal to the plane of the palm. Under local anesthesia, patients are even able to use the tendon transfer and extend the thumb on the operating table. Postoperatively, the wrist is immobilized in 40° of extension with the thumb in abduction and extension for 3 to 4 weeks. A removable splint is used for an additional 3 to 4 weeks, and there is usually no need for retraining in hand therapy (**Fig. 18**).

Tendon transfer to restore thumb flexion

Acute lacerations or ruptures of the flexor FPL tendon can be treated by primary or delayed primary repair or tendon grafting. However, with a missed diagnosis, it is preferable to restore thumb flexion using a tendon transfer, usually the FDS of the ring finger.[57] The ring finger superficialis is harvested through a transverse incision at the

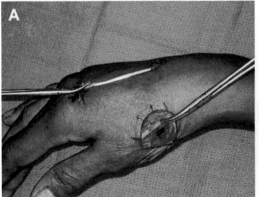
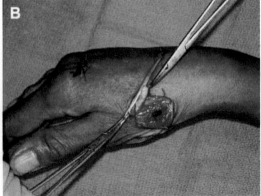

Fig. 17. (*A*) A patient with a rupture of the right extensor pollicis longus tendon caused by a minimally displaced Colles fracture. The extensor indicis proprius tendon is transected at the MCP joint of the index finger and mobilized proximally just distal to the extensor retinaculum. (*B*) The extensor indicis proprius tendon is then passed subcutaneously and sutured to the ruptured distal end of the extensor pollicis longus tendon. Tension can be adjusted with the patient awake under local anesthesia.

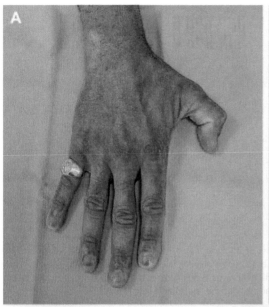
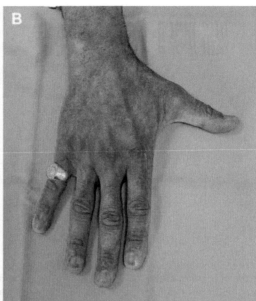
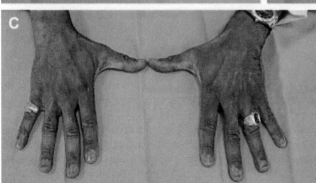

Fig. 18. (A–C) Four years postoperatively, the patient demonstrates excellent flexion and extension of the interphalangeal joint of the right thumb and symmetric extension of the right thumb with the contralateral normal left thumb.

base of the proximal phalanx and retrieved through a second incision just proximal to the wrist crease. The ring finger FDS-to-FPL tendon transfer can be performed in 1 stage by passing the FDS tendon through the FPL sheath to the base of the distal phalanx through an open incision or attaching it to a fine rubber catheter or feeding tube and withdrawing it distally through the sheath. If the bed is scarred, the transfer is performed in 2 stages with initial placement of a Silastic tendon rod.[57] If necessary, a pulley can be reconstructed using the old FPL tendon remnant or with a PL graft.[58] The FDS tendon is sutured to the distal phalanx of the thumb using a pullout suture fixed over a button. The tension of the transfer can be checked by the wrist tenodesis effect: with wrist flexion, the thumb IP joint should extend completely, and with wrist extension, the thumb should flex to touch the ring finger MP joint.

Tendon transfers to restore finger extension

Restoration of extension to one or more fingers after trauma can be accomplished by tendon transfers similar to those described for radial nerve palsy, including the transfer of either of the wrist flexors FCU or FCR to the EDC or the Boyes transfer of the FDS of the long and ring fingers to the EDC.

Tendon transfers to restore finger flexion

Occasionally, patients may present with severe crushing or avulsion injuries involving the forearm flexor muscles with loss of finger and thumb flexion (**Fig. 19**A). The 2 options for secondary reconstruction of finger flexion are either a tendon transfer of the ECRL to all 4 FDP tendons or a free gracilis functioning muscle transfer. ECRL is transected at the base of the index finger metacarpal and mobilized through a longitudinal incision on

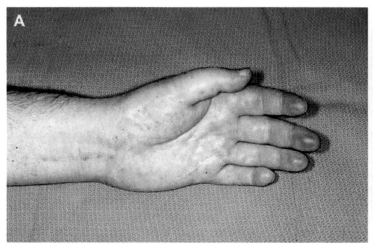
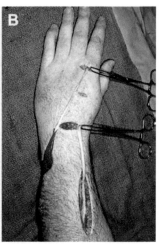

Fig. 19. (*A*) This 11-year-old boy sustained segmental loss of all the forearm flexor muscles as well as the median nerve and is unable to flex any of his fingers or his thumb. (*B*) The extensor indicis proprius tendon is mobilized to restore opposition of the thumb. The extensor carpi radialis longus tendon is mobilized to restore finger flexion. Through the same distal forearm incision, the brachioradialis can be mobilized into the middle third of the forearm to restore thumb flexion.

the dorsum of the distal forearm (see **Fig. 19**B). It is then tunneled subcutaneously around the radial border of the forearm to a palmar incision over the distal forearm. Adjusting the tension when suturing the ECRL to all 4 FDP tendons is crucial because the ECRL only has 30 mm amplitude, whereas the FDP tendons require 70 mm of excursion for full finger flexion. Inserting the transfer too tightly will prevent full finger extension. The wrist tenodesis effect is vitally important in this transfer: wrist extension should cause the fingers to flex down into the palm, whereas wrist flexion should allow the fingers to come out into full extension (**Fig. 20**).

If the FPL is also nonfunctioning, thumb flexion can be restored by transferring brachioradialis to FPL through the same palmar incision, similar to the transfer for a high median nerve palsy.

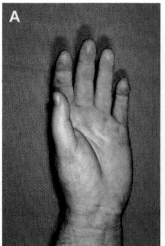
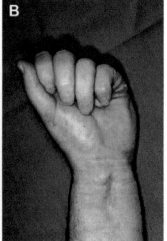

Fig. 20. (*A, B*) Preoperative and 1-year postoperative photographs demonstrating restoration of finger flexion by transfer of the extensor carpi radialis longus to the flexor digitorum profundus tendons of all 4 fingers; restoration of flexion at the interphalangeal joint of the thumb by transfer of the brachioradialis to the flexor pollicis longus and restoration of thumb opposition using the extensor indicis proprius Burkhalter transfer.

SUMMARY

Tendon transfers, if carefully selected and performed meticulously, will provide a gratifying functional improvement to the hand affected by radial, median, ulnar, or combined nerve palsies as well as severe trauma affecting the extrinsic flexor and extensor muscles and tendons. Surgeons and patients are gratified by the significant benefits derived from these tendon transfers. Comparative studies must be designed in the future to document the effectiveness of the various transfers and their ultimate impact on hand function and return to work.

REFERENCES

1. Brand PW. Clinical mechanics of the hand. St Louis (MO): CV Mosby Co; 1985.
2. Brand PW, Beach RB, Thompson DE. Relative tension and potential excursion of muscles in the forearm and hand. J Hand Surg Am 1981;6:209–19.
3. Burkhalter WE. Early tendon transfer in upper extremity peripheral nerve injury. Clin Orthop 1974;0: 68–79.
4. Bevin AG. Early tendon transfer for radial nerve transection. Hand 1976;8:134–6.
5. Ueber Sehnenüberpflanzung FF. Arch Klin Chir 1896;52:87–91.
6. Zachary RB. Tendon transplantation for radial paralysis. Br J Surg 1946;23:350.
7. Starr CL. Army experiences with tendon transference. J Bone Joint Surg 1922;4:3.
8. Boyes JH. Tendon transfers for radial palsy. Bull Hosp Joint Dis 1960;21:97.
9. Chuinard RG, Boyes JH, Stark HH, et al. Tendon transfers for radial nerve palsy: use of superficialis tendons for digital extension. J Hand Surg Am 1978;3:560–70.
10. Tsuge K, Adachi N. Tendon transfer for extensor palsy of forearm. Hiroshima J Med Sci 1969;18: 219–32.
11. Chandraprakasam T, Gavaskar AS, Prabhakaran T. Modified Jones transfer for radial nerve palsy using a single incision: surgical technique. Tech Hand Up Extrem Surg 2009;13:16–8.
12. Bunnell S. Opposition of the thumb. J Bone Joint Surg 1938;20:269.
13. Royle ND. An operation for paralysis of the intrinsic muscles of the thumb. JAMA 1938;111:612.
14. Thompson TC. A modified operation for opponens paralysis. J Bone Joint Surg 1942;24:632.
15. Edgerton MT, Brand PW. Restoration of abduction and adduction to the unstable thumb in median and ulnar paralysis. Plast Reconstr Surg 1965;36:150.
16. Phalen GS, Miller RC. The transfer of wrist extensor muscles to restore or reinforce flexion power of the fingers and opposition of the thumb. J Bone Joint Surg 1947;29:993.
17. Cooney WP, Linscheid RL, An KN. Opposition of the thumb: an anatomic and biomechanical study of tendon transfers. J Hand Surg Am 1984;9:777–86.
18. Huber E. Hilfsoperation bei medianus slahmung. Dtsch Z Chir 1921;126:271.
19. Nicolaysen J. Transplantation des M. abductor dig. V bei fehlender Oppositionsfahigkeit des Daumens. Dtsch Z Chir 1922;168:133.
20. Cawrse NH, Sammut D. A modification in technique of abductor digiti minimi (Huber) opponensplasty. J Hand Surg Br 2003;28:233–7.
21. Schneider LH. Opponensplasty using the extensor digiti minimi. J Bone Joint Surg Am 1969;51: 1297–302.
22. Burkhalter W, Christensen RC, Brown P. Extensor indicis proprius opponensplasty. J Bone Joint Surg Am 1973;55:725–32.
23. Camitz H. Ueber die Behandlung der Opposition-Slahmung. Acta Chir Scand 1929;65:77.
24. Littler JW, Li CS. Primary restoration of thumb opposition with median nerve decompression. Plast Reconstr Surg 1967;39:74–5.
25. Braun RM. Palmaris longus tendon transfer for augmentation of the thenar musculature in low median palsy. J Hand Surg Am 1978;3:488–91.
26. Foucher G, Malizos C, Sammut D, et al. Primary palmaris longus transfer as an opponensplasty in carpal tunnel release. A series of 73 cases. J Hand Surg Br 1991;16:56–60.
27. Zancolli EA. Claw hand caused by paralysis of the intrinsic muscles. A simple surgical procedure for its correction. J Bone Joint Surg 1957;39A: 1076–80.
28. Zancolli EA. Intrinsic paralysis of the ulnar nerve—physiopathology of the claw hand. In: Structural and dynamic bases of hand surgery. 2nd edition. Philadelphia: JB Lippincott; 1979. p. 159–206.
29. Brooks AL, Jones DS. A new intrinsic tendon transfer for the paralytic hand. J Bone Joint Surg 1975;57:730.
30. Anderson GA. Analysis of paralytic claw finger correction using flexor motors into different insertion sites [master's thesis]. Liverpool (UK): University of Liverpool; 1988.
31. Burkhalter WE, Strait JL. Metacarpophalangeal flexor replacement for intrinsic-muscle paralysis. J Bone Joint Surg Am 1973;55:1667–76.
32. Palande DD. Correction of intrinsic minus hands with reversal of transverse metacarpal arch. J Bone Joint Surg Am 1983;65:514–52.
33. Littler JW. Tendon transfers and arthrodeses in combined median and ulnar nerve paralysis. J Bone Joint Surg 1949;31A:225–34.
34. Brand PW. Tendon grafting illustrated by a new operation for intrinsic paralysis of the fingers. J Bone Joint Surg 1961;43B:444–53.

35. Fritschi EP. Nerve involvement in leprosy; the examination of the hand; the restoration of finger function. In: Reconstructive surgery in leprosy. Bristol (UK): John Wright & Sons; 1971. p. 11–27, 28–41, 42–65.

36. Boyes JH. Bunnell's surgery of the hand. 4th edition. Philadelphia: JB Lippincott; 1964. p. 514.

37. Omer GE Jr. Reconstruction of a balanced thumb through tendon transfers. Clin Orthop 1985;195: 104–16.

38. Brown PW. Reconstruction for pinch in ulnar intrinsic palsy. Orthop Clin North Am 1974;5:323–42.

39. Robinson D, Aghasi MK, Halperin N. Restoration of pinch in ulnar nerve palsy by transfer of split extensor digiti minimi and extensor indicis. J Hand Surg Br 1992;17:622–4.

40. Mannerfelt L. Studies on the hand in ulnar nerve paralysis. A clinical-experience investigation in normal and anomalous innervation. Acta Orthop Scand 1966;(Suppl 87):1+.

41. Tubiana R. Palliative treatment of paralytic deformities of the thumb. Orthop Clin North Am 1973;4: 1141–60.

42. Smith RJ. Extensor carpi radialis brevis tendon transfer for thumb adduction–a study of power pinch. J Hand Surg Am 1983;8:4–15.

43. Bunnell S. Surgery of the intrinsic muscles of the hand other than those producing opposition of the thumb. J Bone Joint Surg 1942;24:1.

44. Neviaser RJ, Wilson JN, Gardner MM. Abductor pollicis longus transfer for replacement of first dorsal interosseous. J Hand Surg Am 1980;5:53–7.

45. Graham WC, Riordan D. Sublimis transplant to restore abduction of index finger. Plast Reconstr Surg 1947;2:459–62.

46. Bruner JM. Tendon transfer to restore abduction of the index finger using the extensor pollicis brevis. Plast Reconstr Surg 1948;3:197–201.

47. Hirayama T, Atsuta Y, Takemitsu Y. Palmaris longus transfer for replacement of the first dorsal interosseous. J Hand Surg Br 1986;11:31–4.

48. Blacker GJ, Lister GD, Kleinert HE. The abducted little finger in low ulnar nerve palsy. J Hand Surg Am 1976;1:190–6.

49. Chung MS, Baek GH, Oh JH, et al. Extensor indicis proprius transfer for the abducted small finger. J Hand Surg Am 2008;33:392–7.

50. Omer GE Jr. Evaluation and reconstruction of the forearm and hand after acute traumatic peripheral nerve injuries. J Bone Joint Surg Am 1968;50: 1454–78.

51. Omer GE Jr. Tendon transfers in combined nerve lesions. Orthop Clin North Am 1974;5:377–87.

52. Christophe K. Rupture of the extensor pollicis longus tendon following Coles' fracture. J Bone Joint Surg 1953;35:1003.

53. Duplay S. Rupture sous-cutanee du tendon du long extenseur du pouce au niveau dala tabatiere anatomique. Bull Mem Soc Chir 1876;2:788.

54. Schneider LH, Rosenstein RG. Restoration of extensor pollicis longus function by tendon transfer. Plast Reconstr Surg 1983;71:533–7.

55. Bezuhly M, Sparkes GL, Higgins A, et al. Immediate thumb extension following extensor indicis proprius-to-extensor pollicis longus tendon transfer using the wide-awake approach. Plast Reconstr Surg 2007; 119(5):1507–12.

56. Low CK, Pereira BP, Chao VT. Optimum tensioning position for extensor indicis to extensor pollicis longus transfer. Clin Orthop 2001;388:225–32.

57. Posner MA. Flexor superficialis tendon transfers to the thumb–an alternative to the free tendon graft for treatment of chronic injuries within the digital sheath. J Hand Surg Am 1983;8:876–81.

58. Brand PW. Tendon transfers for median and ulnar nerve paralysis. Orthop Clin North Am 1970;1:447–54.

Nerve Reconstruction in the Hand and Upper Extremity

Kirsty U. Boyd, MD, FRCS(C)[a],
André S. Nimigan, MD, FRCS(C)[b],
Susan E. Mackinnon, MD, FRCS(C)[c],*

KEYWORDS

- Nerve reconstruction • Hand • Upper extremity
- Surgical management

Peripheral nerve reconstruction continues to evolve and expand with the ongoing improvement in our understanding of internal nerve topography, advances in microsurgical technique, and current basic science and clinical research pertaining to nerve injury and repair.[1]

An understanding of the classification of nerve injury, as well as the numerous factors that influence recovery, is critical in the management of traumatic peripheral nerve injuries (Table 1).[1] Multiple factors influence nerve recovery, including patient age, time elapsed since injury, proximity of nerve injury, presence of a nerve gap, associated vascular or soft tissue injuries, and mechanism of injury.[1–4] The severity or degree of injury dictates the decision making between surgical management (fourth-degree and fifth-degree injuries) versus conservative management and serial examination (first-degree, second-degree, and third-degree).[1]

This review explores some of the recent literature as it relates to current techniques, debates, and advances in nerve reconstruction of the hand and upper extremity. Specifically addressed are the recent basic science advances in end-to-side and reverse end-to-side recovery, Schwann cell migration, and neuropathic pain. The management of nerve gaps, including the use of nerve conduits and acellularized nerve allografts, is examined.

Current commonly performed nerve transfers are detailed with focus on both motor and sensory nerve transfers, their indications, and a basic overview of selected surgical techniques.

MANAGEMENT OF NERVE GAPS

The optimal method of nerve reconstruction is prompt, tension-free, primary anatomic end-to-end neurorrhaphy.[1,4] Animal studies have shown that across every coaptation site a percentage of nerve fibers are lost, resulting in fewer nerve axons reaching the target organ.[5,6] It is also important to consider that excessive tension has been shown to significantly impair regeneration across a nerve repair by causing a reduction in microvascular flow and an increase in scarring.[7,8] If a truly tension-free repair is not possible, another method must be used to bridge the gap (Table 2).

Autogenous Nerve Grafts

Nerve autografting is the current gold standard for addressing a nerve gap in peripheral nerve reconstruction. In addition to providing immunogenically inert scaffolds, autogenous grafts contain a viable source of Schwann cells required for axonal regeneration.[1,9,10] However, several disadvantages are associated with this technique. Harvesting

[a] Division of Plastic and Reconstructive Surgery, Department of Surgery, University of Ottawa, 1053 Carling Avenue, Ottawa, ON K1Y 4E9, Canada
[b] The Medical Centre, 707 Charlotte Street, PO Box 4200, Peterborough, ON K9J 7B3, USA
[c] Division of Plastic and Reconstructive Surgery, Department of Surgery, School of Medicine, Washington University, Campus Box 8238, 600 South Euclid Avenue, St Louis, MO 63110, USA
* Corresponding author.
E-mail address: mackinnons@wustl.edu

Clin Plastic Surg 38 (2011) 643–660
doi:10.1016/j.cps.2011.07.008
0094-1298/11/$ – see front matter © 2011 Elsevier Inc. All rights reserved.

Table 1
Classification of nerve injuries

Degree of Injury		Tinel Sign Present	Recovery	Rate of Recovery	Surgical Procedure
I	Neurapraxia	No	Complete	Up to 12 wk	None
II	Axonotmesis	Yes	Complete	2.5 cm (1 inch) per mo	None
III		Yes	Varies[a]	2.5 cm (1 inch) per mo	None or neurolysis
IV	Neuroma in continuity	Yes, but no advancement	None	None	Nerve repair, graft, or transfer
V	Neurotmesis	Yes, but no advancement	None	None	Nerve repair, graft, or transfer
VI	Mixed injury (I to V)	Some fascicles (II, III)	Some fascicles (II, III)	Depends on degree of injury (I–V)	Neurolysis, nerve repair, graft, or transfer

[a] Recovery can vary from excellent to poor depending on the amount of scarring and the sensory versus motor axon misdirection to target receptors.

donor autograft requires a second operative site and results in donor sensory loss.

Regardless of the disadvantages, when faced with the need for motor reconstruction, critical sensory reconstruction, and any large-diameter nerve reconstruction, autologous grafting or nerve transfer is our preference. A branch of the medial antebrachial cutaneous nerve is an excellent option to consider for upper extremity grafting needs, and is overlooked by many hand surgeons in favor of the more commonly used sural nerve. When autogenous nerve grafts are undesirable, alternate options must be explored.

Nerve Conduits

One alternative option for addressing the nerve gap is the use of a synthetic or biologic nerve conduit (**Fig. 1**). Originally the use of autologous material was described, with several biologic options including vein, bone, artery, collagen, small intestine submucosa, and muscle.[11–15] Several synthetic conduits have also been developed. Although nonbiodegradable conduits have since fallen out of favor, conduits made from polyglycolic acid and purified bovine type I collagen remain in use.[1,4,16] Bioresorbable conduits have been associated with both improved axonal sprouting and reduced axonal compression.[16–18]

The use of nerve conduits has been studied in rodents, primates, and humans with varying levels of success.[4,19–21] In a prospective, randomized controlled trial, Weber and colleagues[19] reported improved 2-point discrimination after digital nerve repair with conduits compared with end-to-end repair with nerve grafts. These investigators postulated that the improved sensation associated with conduits in gaps of less than 4 mm (and for >8 mm)

may come about because conduits permit regenerating axons to better align themselves as a result of guided neurotropism. Agnew and Dumanian[18] report restoration of good or excellent sensory function, and functional recovery for larger mixed nerves, in 75% of patients with a 1-cm to 4-cm gap. Despite these promising results, nerve conduits are not without limitations. In addition to being costly, conduits lack both laminin scaffolding and Schwann cells, which are crucial to axonal regeneration.[1] To help circumvent the absence of Schwann cells, it is possible to mince a portion of donor nerve and place it within the conduit.[18] Also, the indications for using a conduit are specific. Moore and colleagues[22] report 4 cases of conduit failure in large-diameter nerve reconstruction, which may be related to a decreased concentration of neurotrophic factors associated with larger-diameter conduits. For these reasons, we believe the use of conduits should be limited to small-diameter, noncritical sensory nerves with a gap of less than 3 cm.[1,22,23] In our practice, when an autograft is not being used, nerve conduits have largely been replaced by acellularized nerve allografts.[4,23]

Acellularized Nerve Allografts

Cadaveric nerve allografts are a potential source of nerve grafting material with no additional donor site morbidity, abundant supply, and ready availability. However, the use of allografts requires temporary systemic immunosuppression for approximately 18 months while host axons traverse the allograft to reach host sensory and motor targets. This situation potentially leaves recipients vulnerable to opportunistic infections or neoplastic

Table 2
Management of a nerve gap

	Advantages	Disadvantages

Nerve autograft	Gold standard for reconstruction	Second operative site
		Results in donor sensory loss
		Potential for neuroma
		  formation/pain
		Sensory nerve autografts do not
		  support motor regeneration as
		  well as motor or mixed
		  sensorimotor nerves
		Limited available length

Allograft	Can potentially allow functional
	  recovery equivalent to autograft
	No donor site morbidity
		Requires patient systemic
		  immunosuppression (~18 mo)
		Patients vulnerable to
		  opportunistic infections

Conduits	Circumvents adverse effects of
	  autografts and allografts
	Guides regenerating nerve to
	  intended target
		Length limitation (<3 cm)
		Only for sensory,
		  small-diameter nerves
		No Schwann cells
		No matrix
		Expensive

Acellularized allograft	Retain scaffolding of nerve tissue
	Nonimmunogenic and inert
	Biologic substrate for nerve
	  regeneration without need for
	  immunosuppression
		Length limitation (<5 cm)
		No Schwann cells
		Only for small-diameter nerves
		Very expensive

End-to-side	No length limitation	Poor sensory results Motor requires donor neurectomy

Reverse end-to-side	Augment partial
	  motor/sensory nerve injury
		Requires knowledge of topography
		Requires expendable motor donor
		May need nerve autograft
		  or acellular allograft

Nerve transfer	Earlier motor/sensory
	  target recovery
		Requires expendable donor
		Requires motor (sensory)
		  reeducation
		Requires knowledge
		  of nerve topography

processes.[24] To circumvent this obvious downside, an alternative is processed donor allograft, which is a human cadaveric nerve graft that has undergone multistep detergent treatment to render it acellular and thus nonimmunogenic.[4] This process, while removing the donor Schwann cells, allows the acellularized graft to retain its three-dimensional scaffolding and to act as a biologic substrate for nerve regeneration without the need for any systemic immunosuppression.

In 1998, Sondell and colleagues[25] investigated the regeneration of rat sciatic nerve into acellular allografts and found evidence of Schwann cell migration and axonal outgrowth. Another group showed that in the rhesus monkey ulnar nerve, acellular allogenic nerve segments implanted with mesenchymal stem cells resulted in structurally and functionally repaired nerves in 100% of animals by 6 months.[26] The use of processed allograft has also been evaluated in a rat model. For short gaps, autograft was found to be superior to processed allograft, which was, in turn, superior to conduits at 6 weeks after repair. However, that difference did not persist by 12 weeks.[4] For longer gaps conduits were found to be insufficient. On the other hand, processed allografts showed evidence of successful reinnervation of distal targets, albeit inferior when compared with autografting.[4] Acellular processed allografts likely support regeneration to 4 to 5 cm, although they have been tested only to 3 cm.[27]

The clinical use of acellularized nerve allografts is a recent development, despite the thorough study of its use in rodents and primates. However,

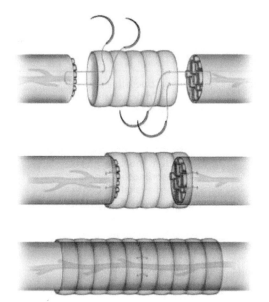

Fig. 1. The use of a nerve conduit for management of a nerve graft. The freshened edges of the nerve are telescoped into the conduit and held in place using a single horizontal mattress epineurial suture. Care is taken to ensure that all fascicles are tucked into the conduit and that the conduit is trimmed to an appropriate length to avoid either redundancy or tension.

Karabekmez and colleagues[28] reported on their experiences with this product in sensory nerve defects of the hand. Traumatic and postneuroma resection defects ranging from 0.5 to 3.0 cm were treated with acellular nerve allografts. A hand therapist blinded to the intervention evaluated functional recovery. These investigators concluded that acellular nerve allografts were capable of restoring adequate sensation with no evidence of infection or rejection.

The use of acellularized nerve grafts has largely replaced the use of conduits in our practice (**Fig. 2**). Indications for processed grafts include

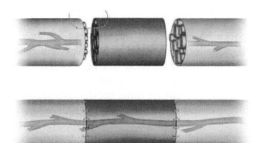

Fig. 2. The use of acellularized nerve allograft for management of a nerve gap. The allograft is coapted to the proximal and distal free nerve ends using epineurial sutures. Care is taken to avoid either redundancy or excessive tension.

small-diameter, noncritical, sensory nerve defects of less than 4 cm. In addition, processed grafts can be used as an extender to restore donor site sensation and prevent hyperalgesia, in nerve supercharging, and in an end-to-side fashion for sensory nerve transfers in the hand. These procedures are discussed later. In our opinion, contraindications for processed grafts include motor nerve reconstruction, critical sensory reconstruction, large-diameter nerve reconstruction, and sensory grafts for gaps longer than 4 cm. In these circumstances, autologous repair with either autograft or nerve transfers is always our reconstruction of choice.

As mentioned earlier, there may be an emerging role for acellularized nerve allograft in neuroma prevention. In 2008, Dorsi and colleagues[29] showed in a tibial neuroma transposition model that surrounding normal sensory nerves were found to collaterally sprout, thus causing hyperalgesia in the previously denervated territory. Acellularized nerve allograft can be used to extend the proximal nerve stump, providing a scaffold for the regenerating axon or to bridge a gap after direct neuroma excision. With this strategy, a neuroma at the site of nerve transposition is avoided, and the nerve is redirected away from the hyperalgesic response.

Further clinical investigation into the limitations and validity of processed nerve graft is indicated; however, early evidence is promising for recovery of small-diameter, noncritical sensory defects of a relatively short (<4 cm) length.

NERVE TRANSFERS

Originally reserved for otherwise unsalvageable brachial plexus injuries, the use of nerve transfers in the treatment of upper extremity nerve reconstruction has become well integrated into our practice.[30–32] Nerve transfers offer several advantages, including providing expendable donor axons close to the target end organ, minimizing time for reinnervation, the capacity to restore both sensory and motor function, restoration of multiple muscle groups with a single transfer, and the ability to operate well outside the original zone of injury.[1,30,31] Optimal muscle reinnervation requires regenerating axons to reach their target muscle in a timely fashion to avoid irreversible loss of target motor end plates by degeneration and fibrosis.[33] Given that reinnervation of denervated muscle is not possible after 12 to 18 months, and that axonal regeneration occurs at a rate of approximately 2.5 cm (1 inch) per month, nerve transfers offer a valuable alternative that can facilitate meaningful, prompt reinnervation.[34]

Indications for Nerve Transfers

The surgical indications for nerve transfer to the hand include proximal brachial plexus injuries in which grafting is not possible, proximal nerve injuries requiring long distances for reinnervation of distal targets, severely scarred regions with probability for injury to critical bony, nervous, or vascular structures, segmental nerve loss associated with major upper extremity trauma, partial nerve injuries with a functional loss, and patients with delayed presentation (**Box 1**).[1,30–32,35] As our understanding of nerve topography increases, the surgical indications for nerve transfers are expanding to include more distal and isolated nerve injuries in the forearm and hand.[31,32]

Principles of Nerve Transfers

The difficulties inherent in nerve reconstruction are exacerbated when proximal nerve stumps are either surgically inaccessible or distant from functionally important distal muscle targets.[5] This clinical scenario is common and usually occurs as a result of either surgical resection or traumatic nerve injury. If end-to-end nerve repair or autogenous nerve grafting is far removed from the target muscle, the potential for functional recovery is severely diminished because of the effects of prolonged muscle denervation (**Fig. 3**A).[36] When the proximal nerve stump is not available, conventional techniques for nerve reconstruction cannot be applied. This situation holds true not only for severe traumatic injuries such as root avulsion but also for cervical disc disease with irreparable root damage or neuritis with cell body damage.[37]

Nerve transfers require the availability of an expendable motor or sensory donor that is close

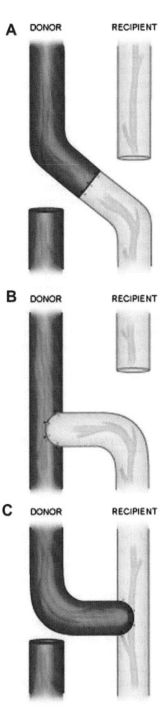

Fig. 3. Options for nerve transfer. (*A*) An end-to-end nerve transfer, where the proximal end of the donor nerve is coapted directly to the distal end of the recipient nerve. (*B*) An end-to-side nerve transfer, where the distal end of the recipient nerve is coapted to the side of the normal donor nerve. (*C*) A reverse end-to-side nerve transfer, where the proximal end of the divided donor nerve is coapted to the side of the intact injured recipient.

Box 1
Indications for nerve transfer

Indications for Nerve Transfers

Proximal brachial plexus injuries where grafting is not possible

Proximal peripheral nerve injuries requiring long distance for reinnervation of distal targets

Severely scarred areas with risk of damage to critical structures

Segmental nerve loss

Major upper extremity trauma

Partial nerve injuries with functional loss

Delayed presentation with inadequate time for reinnervation of distal targets with grafting

Sensory nerve deficits in critical regions

to the desired target. Use of a synergistic donor nerve, although not essential, is preferable, because it facilitates postoperative therapy and motor or sensory reeducation.[31] Similarly, size match between donor and recipient is optimal, although not always possible. Knowledge regarding motor and sensory axon counts in donor and recipient nerves can be helpful in planning possible transfers. Unlike with tendon transfers, amplitude, excursion, and line of pull are not considerations when selecting a donor nerve.[30] In addition, a single donor nerve can be used to power multiple muscle groups.[30,31] Nerve transfers must be conducted without tension, which should be confirmed by taking adjacent joints through a full range of motion before inset. Nerve transfers may be performed in an end-to-end, end-to-side, or reverse end-to-side manner depending on the degree of injury to the recipient nerve and the type of defect being reconstructed. Remembering to mobilize each involved nerve as much as possible, and to harvest the donor nerve distally and the recipient nerve proximally, assists in obtaining adequate length for coaptation without tension. We make use of the mantra "donor distal, recipient proximal" in surgical planning and when performing these transfers.[38]

End-to-side Transfers: Motor and Sensory

End-to-side neurorrhaphy, also known as lateroterminal neurorrhaphy, is attracting growing interest because it overcomes several limitations of both end-to-end repair and autologous nerve grafting. End-to-side neurorrhaphy involves the coaptation of the distal end of an injured recipient nerve into the lateral aspect of an intact nerve (see **Fig. 3**B). This intact nerve then serves as a donor nerve capable of providing a proximal source of either motor or sensory axons.

Historically, reports of end-to-side nerve transfer date as far back as the late 1800s.[39] However, it was not until the late 1980s that the surgical technique was published.[40–42] Since that time, the clinical use of end-to-side nerve transfer has been controversial. Although functional motor recovery after end-to-side nerve transfer has been reported, results have been conflicting, with sensory recovery typically being more successful than motor recovery.[39] The end-to-side approach has been shown to be effective through experimental work by Viterbo and colleagues as well as numerous subsequent investigators.[39,43–50] We conclude that it yields some but not excellent sensory recovery, but does not result in meaningful motor recovery without injury to the donor motor axons.[50]

Several studies show that the donor nerve in an end-to-side neurorrhaphy can sprout axons into a recipient nerve, thereby eliminating the need for a proximal nerve stump.[35,50–56] This approach has rapidly growing clinical potential for the reconstruction of peripheral nerves in the upper extremity.[57–61]

An interesting question in end-to-side neurorrhaphy is the role of donor nerve injury for enhancement of neural regeneration. In the absence of some degree of injury to the donor nerve, only sensory axons traverse an end-to-side repair in a useful manner.[49,62,63] Using this method prevents noticeable downgrading within the donor nerve territory; however, the resulting transmitted axons are expected to provide only protective sensation. As a result, we favor this technique for noncritical regions that would benefit from protective sensation, such as the dorsal cutaneous branch of the ulnar nerve, which innervates the dorsum of the hand, or to recover some sensation in the distal territory of a sensory nerve graft or transfer.

Unlike with a sensory nerve end-to-side transfer, donor nerve axonotmetic injury is a prerequisite for significant motor neuronal regeneration across end-to-side repairs.[49] The donor motor nerve must be subjected to axotomy or a compressive stimulus for significant regeneration to occur. Performing an epineurotomy in the donor nerve with inadvertent axotomy effectively induces early regenerative sprouting into the recipient nerve with robust motor end plate reinnervation. However, this result can come at the expense of a measurable donor nerve deficit because more donor nerves are injured.[50]

Reverse End-to-side Transfers

In a reverse end-to-side nerve transfer, the donor nerve is completely transected, maximizing the number of potential motor axons available. In this manner, a donor nerve can be coapted into the side of the recipient nerve, which remains in continuity (see **Fig. 3**C). The potential for recovery in the recipient nerve is maintained and viable donor motor or sensory axons are recruited to aid in distal target reinnervation in a supercharging type of arrangement. This is a new technique that we are currently investigating, but have also added clinically.[64]

Sensory nerves have been used to innervate a denervated muscle temporarily until the native motor axons are able to regenerate and reach the target motor end plates.[52] Animal studies using this technique have shown prevention of muscle atrophy and loss of muscle fibrillation potential, reduction in motor end plate and muscle spindle degeneration, as well as preservation of muscle cross-sectional area and fiber distribution.[53–57] However, although sensory protection may be useful in this manner, it lacks the benefit of donating functional motor axons that occurs with the reverse end-to-side nerve transfer of a motor nerve.

Fujiwara and colleagues[65] reported an axonal augmentation effect using the reverse end-to-side technique in the repair of sciatic nerve injuries with clinical improvement over direct repair alone. In our center the reverse end-to-side motor nerve transfer has recently been shown in the rat model to improve nerve regeneration and protect target muscles from denervation atrophy. Donor motor axons can readily regenerate through a reverse end-to-side coaptation.[64] This regenerative potential is comparable with using a direct end-to-end repair, and this knowledge opens many new possibilities in nerve reconstruction, several of which are discussed later.

Currently Preferred Motor Nerve Transfers in the Upper Extremity

Many potential nerve transfers have been described for upper extremity reconstruction, and the list continues to grow. However, with time and experience, we have revised our preferences to include several transfers that have been associated with reproducible and useful clinical outcomes.

Restoration of shoulder function

In extensive plexus injuries, the primary goal of achieving elbow flexion and shoulder function has driven surgical innovation. Although surgeons have traditionally relied on nerve grafts or muscle and tendon transfers to restore elbow flexion[66–70] and shoulder function,[71–73] nerve transfer procedures are now being used with increasing frequency and success. Our preference for restoration of shoulder stability and external rotation commences with transfer of the spinal accessory to suprascapular nerve. The transfer can be conducted with either an anterior or a posterior approach. In the posterior approach, the suprascapular nerve is located midway between the medial border of the scapula and the acromion as it runs through the suprascapular notch (**Fig. 4**). The spinal accessory nerve runs parallel to the border of the trapezius, approximately 1 cm from the distal margin on the deep surface of the muscle.[74] With respect to the surface markings, it is localized 40% of the way along a line connecting the dorsal midline to the acromion at the level of the superior border of the scapula. This technique has been described in detail by Colbert and Mackinnon.[75]

More recently, we have performed the spinal accessory to suprascapular nerve transfer through an anterior approach (**Fig. 5**).[48] An incision is designed 2 cm superior to the clavicle that extends laterally from the posterior border of the sternocleidomastoid muscle approximately 6 cm in length. The upper trunk is located between the anterior and middle scalene muscles, and the suprascapular nerve is localized as a distinct branch on the superolateral aspect. The spinal accessory nerve is located on the deep surface of the trapezius by elevating the muscle off the clavicle. Using this technique, it is possible to perform an end-to-side transfer from a direct neurotomy of one-half of the spinal accessory nerve using a short interpositional nerve graft to an end-to-end repair with the suprascapular nerve. Crushing the spinal accessory proximal to the transfer causes a second-degree nerve injury, thus encouraging axonal regeneration without a permanent loss of function to the upper trapezius muscle.

In a 2001 meta-analysis, better results for shoulder function were achieved by reinnervating both the suprascapular and axillary nerves, as opposed to targeting only a single nerve for reconstruction.[76] Transfer of either the medial pectoral nerve or the medial branch of triceps to the axillary nerve improves shoulder stability, external rotation, and abduction. Of the 2 options, the use of the medial branch of triceps is more common in our practice (**Fig. 6**). This transfer is conducted with the patient in prone position through a longitudinal incision on the posterior surface of the upper arm.[75,77] The axillary nerve is identified in the quadrangular space and dissected as far proximally as possible to include the branch to teres minor. Dissection between the long and lateral heads of the triceps muscle exposes the radial nerve as it runs along the humerus. The branch to the medial triceps is distinct from the main portion of the radial nerve, sitting superficially and medially, and can be confirmed with a nerve stimulator.[75]

If the medial pectoral nerve is selected as a donor for reinnervation of the axillary nerve, the procedure is conducted with the patient supine through an incision in the deltopectoral groove. The tendinous insertion of pectoralis major is divided to expose the pectoralis minor. The medial pectoral nerves are found on the deep surface of the pectoralis minor muscle. A nerve graft is typically required to allow adequate length to reach the axillary nerve. We preferentially use the medial antebrachial cutaneous nerve as a graft donor in this scenario.

In select cases, transfer of the thoracodorsal nerve to the long thoracic nerve further aids in

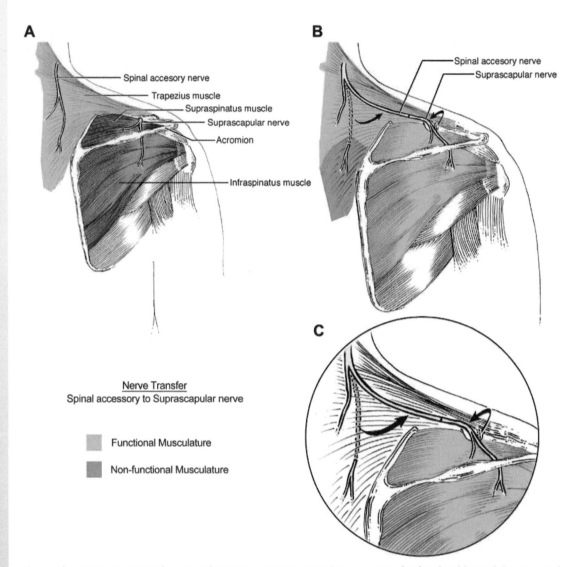

A

- Spinal accesory nerve
- Trapezius muscle
- Supraspinatus muscle
- Suprascapular nerve
- Acromion
- Infraspinatus muscle

Nerve Transfer
Spinal accessory to Suprascapular nerve

Functional Musculature

Non-functional Musculature

B

- Spinal accesory nerve
- Suprascapular nerve

C

Fig. 4. The posterior approach to spinal accessory to suprascapular nerve transfer for shoulder stabilization and external rotation (*A–C*).

shoulder function by stabilizing the scapula and assisting with scapular rotation.[78] To perform this transfer, an incision is made parallel to the infero-lateral border of the latissimus dorsi muscle. The long thoracic nerve and the thoracodorsal nerves are identified. An appropriately sized branch of the thoracodorsal nerve is selected and transferred in an end-to-end fashion to the long thoracic nerve. This transfer results in good functional recovery of the serratus anterior muscle to prevent scapular winging and preserves some branches to the latissimus dorsi muscle.[78] If the thoracodorsal nerve is not available, intercostal nerves can be used.

Restoration of elbow flexion

Our preference to restore elbow flexion is the double fascicular transfer (**Fig. 7**). This transfer involves using redundant branches of the median and ulnar nerves to reinnervate the biceps brachii branch of the musculocutaneous nerve and the brachialis branch of the musculocutaneous nerve. This strategy allows for reinnervation of both the brachialis, which is the primary muscle providing elbow flexion, and the biceps brachii, which primarily supinates the forearm but also secondarily provides elbow flexion.[79] To perform this transfer, a longitudinal incision is designed along the bicipital sulcus and the musculocutaneous

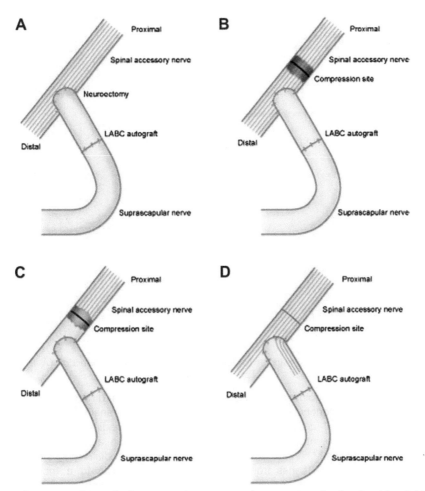

Fig. 5. The anterior approach to spinal accessory to suprascapular nerve transfer for shoulder stabilization and external rotation. This approach, performed in an end-to-side manner, preserves function to the upper trapezius muscle (*A–D*).

nerve is identified between the biceps brachii and the brachialis muscles. The biceps brachii branch arises proximally from the lateral aspect of the musculocutaneous nerve. The nerve then divides into the lateral antebrachial cutaneous nerve, which travels superficially and laterally, and the brachialis branch, which projects medially and deeper into the arm.[80] The median and ulnar nerves are identified through the same incision, and a nerve stimulator is used to identify expendable motor fascicles. The expendable donor fascicle group from the median nerve is medial and superficial, whereas the donor group from the ulnar nerve is lateral and superficial. In this way, the donor fascicles are facing each other anatomically.

Most commonly these redundant fascicles innervate the flexor carpi ulnaris, flexor carpi radialis, flexor digitorum superficialis, or palmaris longus.[80] The redundant fascicles are then coapted

end-to-end with the recipient nerve branches, generally ulnar nerve to biceps brachii, and median nerve to brachialis branch given the orientation, although either transfer is possible.[80] The double fascicular nerve transfer has been associated with Medical Research Council grade 4 to 4+ recovery in most patients, with no detectable motor or sensory deficits in the donor nerve distribution.[79,80]

Restoration of elbow extension

Triceps muscle function is necessary to achieve elbow extension and overhead and forward reach, as well as stabilization of the hand in space during many daily activities.[81–83] Loss of this capability entails significant functional restriction, and few reconstructive surgical options are described in the literature.[84] Frequently, patients compensate by using gravity for passive extension. Published results of nerve transfers to the proximal radial

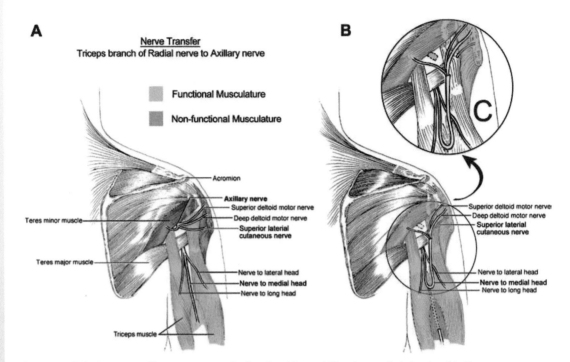

A

Nerve Transfer
Triceps branch of Radial nerve to Axillary nerve

Functional Musculature

Non-functional Musculature

Acromion

Axillary nerve
Superior deltoid motor nerve
Deep deltoid motor nerve
Superior lateral cutaneous nerve

Teres minor muscle

Teres major muscle

Nerve to lateral head
Nerve to medial head
Nerve to long head

Triceps muscle

B

C

Superior deltoid motor nerve
Deep deltoid motor nerve
Superior lateral cutaneous nerve

Nerve to lateral head
Nerve to medial head
Nerve to long head

Fig. 6. Medial triceps to axillary nerve transfer for shoulder stabilization and abduction (A, B).

nerve have been largely disappointing, and have included a wide variety of donors, including the contralateral C7 root, spinal accessory nerve, cervical plexus, phrenic nerve, intercostal nerves, and various intraplexal nerves.[83–86]

In a recently published case series from our institution we describe and show the feasibility of 3 novel nerve transfers to a triceps motor branch of the radial nerve for the restoration of elbow extension after brachial plexus injury.[87] Expendable ulnar and radial nerve fascicles, along with the thoracodorsal nerve, were used as motor donors without creating functional deficits in the donor distributions.

We have previously proposed ulnar fascicular transfer to a triceps motor branch for the restoration of elbow extension and have since documented the excellent outcome of this procedure in 2 patients.[87,88] However, most cases of triceps paralysis occur in conjunction with musculocutaneous nerve palsy when upper plexus injuries extend caudally to involve the C7 nerve root or posterior cord. Because elbow flexion is a higher priority in restoring function to the upper limb, the redundant ulnar fascicle is in these cases used for the double fascicular transfer, and thus is unavailable for triceps reinnervation.

In the case of extensive upper plexus injury, with paralysis of shoulder muscles, elbow flexors, and the triceps, we describe the use of a redundant wrist extensor fascicle from the radial nerve.

Radial intraneural dissection and selective fascicular stimulation analogous to that routinely performed in the median and ulnar nerves allows for the identification a radial nerve fascicle to the extensor carpi radialis longus muscle. Transfer of this nerve fascicle to a triceps motor branch allowed the recovery of M4 elbow extension strength without downgrading wrist extension.[87]

The thoracodorsal nerve is another intraplexal donor option that can provide abundant and readily available motor axons for nerve transfer.[89] This nerve has been successfully used to reinnervate the musculocutaneous, axillary and long thoracic nerves with no resultant functional deficit.[78,89–91] In our case series we document the use of the thoracodorsal nerve as donor to a triceps motor branch of the radial nerve.[87]

Restoration of wrist and finger extension

Although nerve transfers for restoration of radial nerve function have replaced nerve grafting in our practice, tendon transfers have a role in treating these patients when the timing does not favor nerve transfers. Our group has recently published a detailed account of our preferred nerve transfers for restoration of radial nerve function in the forearm.[27,92] This technique has evolved to consistently include coaptation of the flexor digitorum superficialis nerve to the extensor carpi radialis brevis nerve as well as the flexor carpi radialis nerve to the posterior interosseous nerve. We offer

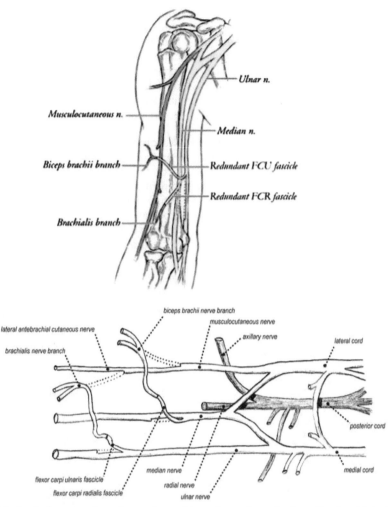

Fig. 7. The double fascicular nerve transfer performed to restore elbow flexion after brachial plexus injury. This transfer involves transfer of function from the intact median and ulnar nerves to the injured musculocutaneous nerve.

these transfers if no clinical or electrical evidence of target muscle reinnervation can be observed by 3 to 4 months after injury.[87,92]

A lazy-S type incision is used over the volar forearm and a step-lengthening of the superficial head of the pronator teres is performed to facilitate exposure of the median nerve. At the proximal end of the incision and ulnar to the radial vessels the branches of the median nerve are identified in a consistent branching pattern. Releasing the tendinous arch of the deep head of the pronator teres and the flexor digitorum superficialis allows for further exposure of the median nerve branches. The nerve to the pronator teres is found in the proximal antecubital fossa. Distal to the antecubital crease the branches to the flexor carpi radialis and the palmaris longus are identified branching medially. Moving distally, the 2 branches to the

flexor digitorum superficialis are seen, followed shortly by the main sensory branch and the anterior interosseous nerve. Once the median nerve branches are identified and mobilized, intraoperative nerve stimulation was used to verify the identification of the donor fascicles. The recipient nerves are localized by following the radial sensory branch deep to the brachioradialis, on the lateral side of the radial vessels. After the posterior interosseous nerve and extensor carpi radialis brevis branches are identified the transfers are undertaken without the use of interposition grafts. Other orientations of these transfers are occasionally used, albeit with less pleasing results and more difficult motor reeducation.[87]

In this patient group it is worth considering a concomitant pronator teres to extensor radialis brevis tendon transfer to augment the nerve transfer and provide wrist extension in the early postoperative period. The median to radial nerve transfers, when successful, allow independent finger and thumb extension, as the radially innervated muscles with their original muscle tension are being individually reinnervated.[27,92]

Restoration of pronation or anterior interosseous nerve function

Although not a transfer performed as commonly as other extremity nerve transfers, several options for restoration of pronation have been explored with success, including using flexor carpi ulnaris, flexor digitorum superficialis, flexor carpi radialis, and even extensor carpi radialis brevis as potential donors. To restore anterior interosseous nerve function, potential donors include flexor digitorum

superficialis, extensor carpi radialis brevis, supinator, and brachialis. Deciding on a donor requires knowledge of nerve internal topography, redundancy, and availability. In the setting of a devastating upper extremity injury, nerve transfers are guided by what nerves remain functional as potential donors and what are expendable donors that do not cause a downgrade in function.

Restoration of intrinsic muscle function

Proximal ulnar nerve injuries are associated with poor intrinsic motor recovery with a devastating impact on hand function. Tendon transfers are notoriously limited and are really considered salvage procedures.[27] Our preference for restoration of intrinsic muscle function is coaptation of the anterior interosseous nerve to the deep motor branch

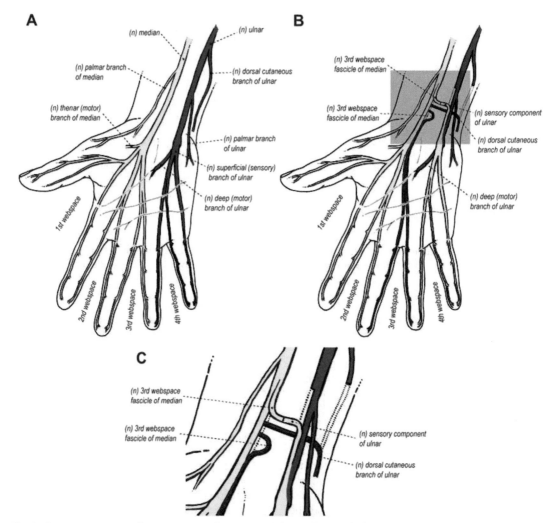

Fig. 8. Sensory nerve transfers to restore ulnar nerve deficits. This triad of transfers involves end-to-end coaptation of the third webspace to the main sensory component of the ulnar nerve, end-to-side coaptation of the dorsal cutaneous ulnar branch to the median nerve, and end-to-side coaptation of the distal third webspace to the median nerve (A–C).

of the ulnar nerve, in either an end-to-end (for complete loss of function) or reverse end-to-side (to augment or supercharge an incomplete or recovering nerve injury) manner.[32] Decompression of the ulnar nerve through the Guyon canal, paying special attention to releasing the deep motor branch as it travels under the tendinous leading edge of the hypothenar muscles and turns radially around the hamate, is performed. The anterior interosseous nerve is harvested as far distally as possible, just before or at the level of the branches at the midsubstance of the pronator quadratus. The deep ulnar motor branch is identified at the level of the distal forearm, where the coaptation can be

conducted without tension. The technical nuances of this transfer are described by Brown and colleagues.[27] This transfer has been associated with improved lateral pinch and grip strength, despite the discrepancy between the number and intelligence of motor axons in the branch to pronator quadratus (912 $\pm$ 88) and the deep motor branch of the ulnar nerve (1216 $\pm$ 108).[27,35,93]

Currently Preferred Sensory Nerve Transfers in the Upper Extremity

Sensory nerve transfers are performed to restore critical digit sensation to the contact surfaces of

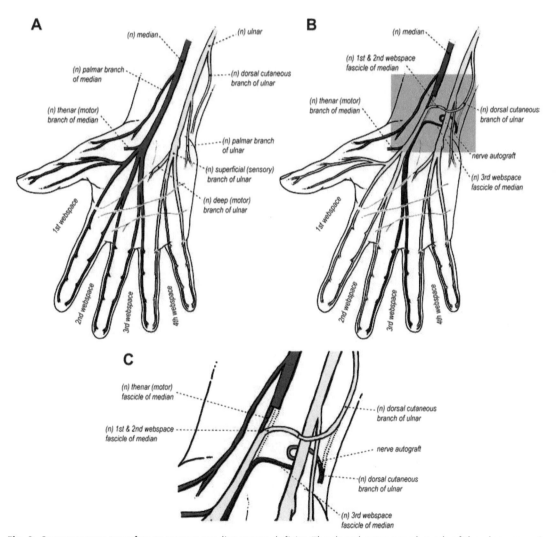

Fig. 9. Sensory nerve transfers to restore median nerve deficits. The dorsal cutaneous branch of the ulnar nerve is transferred end-to-end to the radial portion of the median nerve to restore thumb and first webspace sensation. The third webspace nerve is transferred end-to-side to the main sensory component of the ulnar nerve for restoration of third webspace protective sensation. The distal end of the transected dorsal cutaneous ulnar nerve is coapted end-to-side to the ulnar nerve to restore the donor deficit (A–C).

the thumb and fingers. Nerve branches from noncritical areas are sacrificed. Pure sensory nerves that are an approximate size match are preferred.[32] Most frequently, sensory nerve transfers are performed at the level of the distal forearm just proximal to the wrist, because transfer at a distal level results in earlier recovery of sensation.[27,32] The distal end of a transferred donor sensory nerve is coapted in an end-to-side manner to an adjacent normal sensory nerve, or to a sensory nerve that has been reinnervated proximally and to which it is assumed excellent sensation is forthcoming, to allow restoration of protective sensation in the donor nerve distribution.[32]

Restoration of sensation for ulnar nerve deficits

Our preference for restoration of sensation in an ulnar nerve deficit involves a triad of nerve transfers (**Fig. 8**). The proximal third webspace fascicle of the median nerve, which is readily identified as the ulnar most distinct fascicular group in the midforearm to distal forearm is coapted end-to-end with the main sensory component of the ulnar nerve to restore critical sensation to the small finger.[94] The distal dorsal cutaneous branch of the ulnar nerve is coapted end-to-side with the sensory portion to the median nerve to restore sensation to the ulnar aspect of the hand. The distal third webspace

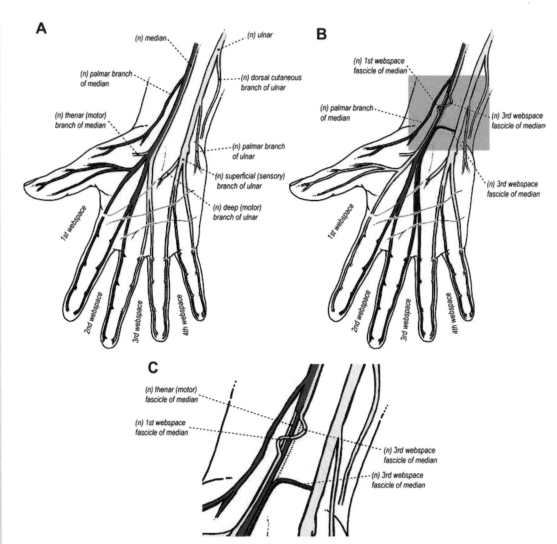

Fig. 10. Sensory nerve transfers to restore C5 to C6 sensory nerve deficit. The third webspace is transected and coapted end-to-end to the radial aspect of the median nerve to restore thumb and first webspace sensation. The distal end of the transected third webspace is coapted end-to-side to the ulnar nerve to restore protective sensation of the donor site (A–C).

fascicle is coapted in an end-to-side fashion back to the sensory portion of the median nerve to restore protective sensation in the donor nerve distribution in the hand. These transfers are described in more detail by Brown and colleagues.[27]

Restoration of sensation for median nerve deficits

Our preference for restoration of sensation in a median nerve deficit also involves a triad of nerve transfers (**Fig. 9**). The proximal portion of the dorsal cutaneous branch of the ulnar nerve is transferred end-to-end to the radial side of the median nerve to restore sensation in the thumb and first webspace. The third webspace fascicle of the median nerve is identified as described earlier, divided and coapted in an end-to-side manner to the main sensory portion of the ulnar nerve. The distal aspect of the dorsal cutaneous branch of the ulnar nerve is coapted end-to-side to the sensory portion of the ulnar nerve to restore protective sensation in the donor distribution.

Restoration of sensation in C5 to C6 nerve root injuries

In a C5 to C6 injury, the noncritical third webspace nerve remains as a viable source of sensory axons. Therefore, to restore critical sensation to the first webspace, the third webspace fascicle is divided in the distal forearm and coapted end-to-end to the radial side of the median nerve. The distal aspect of the third webspace fascicle is then coapted end-to-side to the main sensory component of the ulnar nerve to restore protective sensation in the third webspace (**Fig. 10**).

SUMMARY

The management of peripheral nerve injuries that cannot be primarily repaired involves many potential options; however, the gold standard remains nerve autografting. For noncritical, sensory, small-diameter nerve defects of less than 4 cm, we have moved away from conduits in favor of acellularized nerve allografts, which have been shown to have superior results.[4] For larger gaps, larger-diameter nerves, and motor nerves, we prefer either autografts or nerve transfers. In our practice, the indications for nerve transfers are expanding, and we have highlighted several currently preferred transfers in this article. For restoration of shoulder function a combination of spinal accessory to suprascapular nerve and medial branch of triceps to axillary nerve transfers are performed. The double fascicular nerve transfer is used to restore elbow flexion. Anterior interosseous nerve to deep motor branch of ulnar nerve transfers can be used to either augment or restore intrinsic muscle function of the hand. The

sensory nerve transfers described are more recent, and the long-term results remain unclear; however, they seem promising and are an important option in restoring critical hand sensation.

Peripheral nerve surgery continues to expand and evolve rapidly as our understanding of nerve topography and redundancy improves. With basic science and clinical research providing more knowledge about the potential role for end-to-side and reverse end-to-side transfers, even more options have become available. Nerve injuries that have traditionally been considered devastating and insurmountable now have promising options.

REFERENCES

1. Ray WZ, Mackinnon SE. Management of nerve gaps: autografts, allografts, nerve transfers, and end-to-side neurorrhaphy. Exp Neurol 2010;223(1):77–85.
2. Gilbert A, Pivato G, Kheiralla T. Long-term results of primary repair of brachial plexus lesions in children. Microsurgery 2006;26(4):334–42.
3. Hentz VR, Narakas A. The results of microneurosurgical reconstruction in complete brachial plexus palsy. Assessing outcome and predicting results. Orthop Clin North Am 1988;19(1):107–14.
4. Whitlock EL, Tuffaha SH, Luciano JP, et al. Processed allografts and type I collagen conduits for repair of peripheral nerve gaps. Muscle Nerve 2009;39(6):787–99.
5. Myckatyn TM, Mackinnon SE. A review of research endeavors to optimize peripheral nerve reconstruction. Neurol Res 2004;26(2):124–38.
6. Trumble TE, Archibald S, Allan CH. Bioengineering for nerve repair in the future. J Am Soc Surg Hand 2004;4(3):124–38.
7. Driscoll PJ, Glasby MA, Lawson GM. An in vivo study of peripheral nerves in continuity: biomechanical and physiological responses to elongation. J Orthop Res 2002;20(2):370–5.
8. Trumble TE, McCallister WV. Repair of peripheral nerve defects in the upper extremity. Hand Clin 2000;16(1):37–52.
9. Flores AJ, Lavernia CJ, Owens PW. Anatomy and physiology of peripheral nerve injury and repair. Am J Orthop (Belle Mead NJ) 2000;29(3):167–73.
10. Siemionow M, Brzezicki G. Chapter 8: current techniques and concepts in peripheral nerve repair. Int Rev Neurobiol 2009;87:141–72.
11. Chiu DT, Janecka I, Krizek TJ, et al. Autogenous vein graft as a conduit for nerve regeneration. Surgery 1982;91(2):226–33.
12. Chiu DT, Strauch B. A prospective clinical evaluation of autogenous vein grafts used as a nerve conduit for distal sensory nerve defects of 3 cm or less. Plast Reconstr Surg 1990;86(5):928–34.

13. Kim DH, Connolly SE, Zhao S, et al. Comparison of macropore, semipermeable, and nonpermeable collagen conduits in nerve repair. J Reconstr Microsurg 1993;9(6):415–20.

14. Chen LE, Seaber AV, Urbaniak JR, et al. Denatured muscle as a nerve conduit: a functional, morphologic, and electrophysiologic evaluation. J Reconstr Microsurg 1994;10(3):137–44.

15. Smith RM, Wiedl C, Chubb P, et al. Role of small intestine submucosa (SIS) as a nerve conduit: preliminary report. J Invest Surg 2004;17(6):339–44.

16. Meek MF, Coert JH. Clinical use of nerve conduits in peripheral-nerve repair: review of the literature. J Reconstr Microsurg 2002;18(2):97–109.

17. Krarup C, Archibald SJ, Madison RD. Factors that influence peripheral nerve regeneration: an electrophysiological study of the monkey median nerve. Ann Neurol 2002;51(1):69–81.

18. Agnew SP, Dumanian GA. Technical use of synthetic conduits for nerve repair. J Hand Surg Am 2010; 35(5):838–41.

19. Weber RA, Breidenbach WC, Brown RE, et al. A randomized prospective study of polyglycolic acid conduits for digital nerve reconstruction in humans. Plast Reconstr Surg 2000;106(5):1036–45 [discussion: 1046–8].

20. Dellon AL, Mackinnon SE. An alternative to the classical nerve graft for the management of the short nerve gap. Plast Reconstr Surg 1988;82(5):849–56.

21. Mackinnon SE, Dellon AL. Clinical nerve reconstruction with a bioabsorbable polyglycolic acid tube. Plast Reconstr Surg 1990;85(3):419–24.

22. Moore AM, Kasukurthi R, Magill CK, et al. Limitations of conduits in peripheral nerve repairs. Hand (N Y) 2009;4(2):180–6.

23. Mackinnon SE. Letter to the Editor Regarding: Agnew, SP and Dumanian GA. 2010. Technical use of synthetic conduits for nerve repair. J Hand Surg Am 35(5): p. 838–41. J Hand Surg Am 2011;36(1):183.

24. Mackinnon SE, Doolabh VB, Novak CB, et al. Clinical outcome following nerve allograft transplantation. Plast Reconstr Surg 2001;107(6):1419–29.

25. Sondell M, Lundborg G, Kanje M. Regeneration of the rat sciatic nerve into allografts made acellular through chemical extraction. Brain Res 1998; 795(1–2):44–54.

26. Hu J, Zhu QT, Liu XL, et al. Repair of extended peripheral nerve lesions in rhesus monkeys using acellular allogenic nerve grafts implanted with autologous mesenchymal stem cells. Exp Neurol 2007; 204(2):658–66.

27. Brown JM, Yee A, Mackinnon SE. Distal median to ulnar nerve transfers to restore ulnar motor and sensory function within the hand: technical nuances. Neurosurgery 2009;65(5):966–77 [discussion: 977–8].

28. Karabekmez FE, Duymaz A, Moran SL. Early clinical outcomes with the use of decellularized nerve allograft for repair of sensory defects within the hand. Hand (N Y) 2009;4(3):245–9.

29. Dorsi MJ, Chen L, Murinson BB, et al. The tibial neuroma transposition (TNT) model of neuroma pain and hyperalgesia. Pain 2008;134(3):320–34.

30. Weber RA, Mackinnon SE. Nerve transfers in the upper extremity. J Am Soc Surg Hand 2004;4(3):200–13.

31. Tung TH, Weber RV, Mackinnon SE. Nerve transfers for the upper and lower extremities. Operat Tech Orthop 2004;14:213–22.

32. Tung TH, Mackinnon SE. Nerve transfers: indications, techniques, and outcomes. J Hand Surg Am 2010;35(2):332–41.

33. Nath RK, Mackinnon SE. Nerve transfers in the upper extremity. Hand Clin 2000;16(1):131–9, ix.

34. Seddon HJ, Medawar PB, Smith H. Rate of regeneration of peripheral nerves in man. J Physiol 1943; 102(2):191–215.

35. Novak CB, Mackinnon SE. Distal anterior interosseous nerve transfer to the deep motor branch of the ulnar nerve for reconstruction of high ulnar nerve injuries. J Reconstr Microsurg 2002;18(6):459–64.

36. Kobayashi J, Mackinnon SE, Watanabe O, et al. The effect of duration of muscle denervation on functional recovery in the rat model. Muscle Nerve 1997;20(7):858–66.

37. Brown JM, Yee A, Ivens RA, et al. Post-cervical decompression parsonage-turner syndrome represents a subset of c5 palsy: six cases and a review of the literature: case report. Neurosurgery 2010; 67(6):E1831–44.

38. Brown JM, Mackinnon SE. Nerve transfers in the forearm and hand. Hand Clin 2008;24(4):319–40, v.

39. Tos P, Artiaco S, Papalia I, et al. Chapter 14: end-to-side nerve regeneration: from the laboratory bench to clinical applications. Int Rev Neurobiol 2009;87: 281–94.

40. Krivolutskaia EG, Chumasov EI, Matina VN, et al. End-to-side type of plastic repair of the facial nerve branches. Stomatologiia (Mosk) 1989;68(6):35–8 [in Russian].

41. Lundborg G, Zhao Q, Kanje M, et al. Can sensory and motor collateral sprouting be induced from intact peripheral nerve by end-to-side anastomosis? J Hand Surg Br 1994;19(3):277–82.

42. May M, Sobol SM, Mester SJ. Hypoglossal-facial nerve interpositional-jump graft for facial reanimation without tongue atrophy. Otolaryngol Head Neck Surg 1991;104(6):818–25.

43. Viterbo F, Trindade JC, Hoshino K, et al. Lateroterminal neurorrhaphy without removal of the epineural sheath. Experimental study in rats. Rev Paul Med 1992;110(6):267–75.

44. Viterbo F, Trindade JC, Hoshino K, et al. End-to-side neurorrhaphy with removal of the epineurial sheath: an experimental study in rats. Plast Reconstr Surg 1994;94(7):1038–47.

45. Learmonth J. A technique for transplanting the ulnar nerve. Surg Gynecol Obstet 1942;75:792–3.

46. Tang PP, Bishai SK. Anterior submuscular transposition of the ulnar nerve. Tech Orthop 2006;21(4):318–24.

47. Finkelstein DI, Dooley PC, Luff AR. Recovery of muscle after different periods of denervation and treatments. Muscle Nerve 1993;16(7):769–77.

48. Ray WZ, Kasukurthi R, Yee A, et al. Functional recovery following an end to side neurorrhaphy of the accessory nerve to the suprascapular nerve: case report. Hand (N Y) 2009. [Epub ahead of print].

49. Brenner MJ, Dvali L, Hunter DA, et al. Motor neuron regeneration through end-to-side repairs is a function of donor nerve axotomy. Plast Reconstr Surg 2007;120(1):215–23.

50. Hayashi A, Pannucci C, Moradzadeh A, et al. Axotomy or compression is required for axonal sprouting following end-to-side neurorrhaphy. Exp Neurol 2008;211(2):539–50.

51. Haase SC, Chung KC. Anterior interosseous nerve transfer to the motor branch of the ulnar nerve for high ulnar nerve injuries. Ann Plast Surg 2002; 49(3):285–90.

52. Bain JR, Veltri KL, Chamberlain D, et al. Improved functional recovery of denervated skeletal muscle after temporary sensory nerve innervation. Neuroscience 2001;103(2):503–10.

53. Elsohemy A, Butler R, Bain JR, et al. Sensory protection of rat muscle spindles following peripheral nerve injury and reinnervation. Plast Reconstr Surg 2009; 124(6):1860–8.

54. Hynes NM, Bain JR, Thoma A, et al. Preservation of denervated muscle by sensory protection in rats. J Reconstr Microsurg 1997;13(5):337–43.

55. Papakonstantinou KC, Kamin E, Terzis JK. Muscle preservation by prolonged sensory protection. J Reconstr Microsurg 2002;18(3):173–82 [discussion: 183–4].

56. Wang H, Gu Y, Xu J, et al. Comparative study of different surgical procedures using sensory nerves or neurons for delaying atrophy of denervated skeletal muscle. J Hand Surg Am 2001;26(2):326–31.

57. Yoshitatsu S, Matsuda K, Yano K, et al. Muscle flap mass preservation by sensory reinnervation with end-to-side neurorrhaphy: an experimental study in rats. J Reconstr Microsurg 2008;24(7):479–87.

58. Michalski B, Bain JR, Fahnestock M. Long-term changes in neurotrophic factor expression in distal nerve stump following denervation and reinnervation with motor or sensory nerve. J Neurochem 2008; 105(4):1244–52.

59. Zhao C, Veltri K, Li S, et al. NGF, BDNF, NT-3, and GDNF mRNA expression in rat skeletal muscle following denervation and sensory protection. J Neurotrauma 2004;21(10):1468–78.

60. Bain JR, Hason Y, Veltri K, et al. Clinical application of sensory protection of denervated muscle. J Neurosurg 2008;109(5):955–61.

61. Oswald TM, Zhang F, Lei MP, et al. Muscle flap mass preservation with end-to-side neurorrhaphy: an experimental study. J Reconstr Microsurg 2004;20(6):483–8.

62. Tarasidis G, Watanabe O, Mackinnon SE, et al. End-to-side neurorrhaphy resulting in limited sensory axonal regeneration in a rat model. Ann Otol Rhinol Laryngol 1997;106(6):506–12.

63. Tarasidis G, Watanabe O, Mackinnon SE, et al. End-to-side neurorraphy: a long-term study of neural regeneration in a rat model. Otolaryngol Head Neck Surg 1998;119(4):337–41.

64. Kale SS, Glaus SW, Yee A, et al. Reverse End-to-side Nerve Transfer: from an animal model to clinical use. J Hand Surg 2011, in press.

65. Fujiwara T, Matsuda K, Kubo T, et al. Axonal supercharging technique using reverse end-to-side neurorrhaphy in peripheral nerve repair: an experimental study in the rat model. J Neurosurg 2007;107(4):821–9.

66. Brunelli GA, Vigasio A, Brunelli GR. Modified Steindler procedure for elbow flexion restoration. J Hand Surg Am 1995;20(5):743–6.

67. Vekris MD, Beris AE, Lykissas MG, et al. Restoration of elbow function in severe brachial plexus paralysis via muscle transfers. Injury 2008;39(Suppl 3):S15–22.

68. Moneim MS, Omer GE. Latissimus dorsi muscle transfer for restoration of elbow flexion after brachial plexus disruption. J Hand Surg Am 1986;11(1):135–9.

69. Zancolli E, Mitre H. Latissimus dorsi transfer to restore elbow flexion. An appraisal of eight cases. J Bone Joint Surg Am 1973;55(6):1265–75.

70. Ruhmann O, Schmolke S, Gossé F, et al. Transposition of local muscles to restore elbow flexion in brachial plexus palsy. Injury 2002;33(7):597–609.

71. Narakas AO. Muscle transpositions in the shoulder and upper arm for sequelae of brachial plexus palsy. Clin Neurol Neurosurg 1993;95(Suppl):S89–91.

72. Lin H, Hou C, Xu Z. Transfer of the superior portion of the pectoralis major flap for restoration of shoulder abduction. J Reconstr Microsurg 2009;25(4):255–60.

73. Carlsen BT, Bishop AT, Shin AY. Late reconstruction for brachial plexus injury. Neurosurg Clin N Am 2009;20(1):51–64, vi.

74. Bahm J, Noaman H, Becker M. The dorsal approach to the suprascapular nerve in neuromuscular reanimation for obstetric brachial plexus lesions. Plast Reconstr Surg 2005;115(1):240–4.

75. Colbert SH, Mackinnon S. Posterior approach for double nerve transfer for restoration of shoulder function in upper brachial plexus palsy. Hand (N Y) 2006;1(2):71–7.

76. Merrell GA, Barrie KA, Katz DL, et al. Results of nerve transfer techniques for restoration of shoulder and elbow function in the context of a meta-analysis of the English literature. J Hand Surg Am 2001;26(2):303–14.

77. Leechavengvongs S, Witoonchart K, Uerpairojkit C, et al. Nerve transfer to deltoid muscle using the nerve to the long head of the triceps, part II:

a report of 7 cases. J Hand Surg Am 2003;28(4): 633–8.

78. Novak CB, Mackinnon SE. Surgical treatment of a long thoracic nerve palsy. Ann Thorac Surg 2002;73(5):1643–5.

79. Tung TH, Novak CB, Mackinnon SE. Nerve transfers to the biceps and brachialis branches to improve elbow flexion strength after brachial plexus injuries. J Neurosurg 2003;98(2):313–8.

80. Mackinnon SE, Novak CB, Myckatyn TM, et al. Results of reinnervation of the biceps and brachialis muscles with a double fascicular transfer for elbow flexion. J Hand Surg Am 2005;30(5):978–85.

81. Bertelli JA. Lower trapezius muscle transfer for reconstruction of elbow extension in brachial plexus injuries. J Hand Surg Eur Vol 2009;34(4): 459–64.

82. Lieber RL, Fridén J, Hobbs T, et al. Analysis of posterior deltoid function one year after surgical restoration of elbow extension. J Hand Surg Am 2003;28(2):288–93.

83. Goubier JN, Teboul F. Transfer of the intercostal nerves to the nerve of the long head of the triceps to recover elbow extension in brachial plexus palsy. Tech Hand Up Extrem Surg 2007;11(2):139–41.

84. Narakas AO, Hentz VR. Neurotization in brachial plexus injuries. Indication and results. Clin Orthop Relat Res 1988;(237):43–56.

85. Moiyadi AV, Devi BI, Nair KP. Brachial plexus injuries: outcome following neurotization with intercostal nerve. J Neurosurg 2007;107(2):308–13.

86. Doi K, Sakai K, Kuwata N, et al. Reconstruction of finger and elbow function after complete avulsion of the brachial plexus. J Hand Surg Am 1991; 16(5):796–803.

87. Pet MA, Ray WZ, Yee A, et al. Nerve transfer to the triceps after brachial plexus injury: report of 4 cases. J Hand Surg Am 2011;36(3):398–405.

88. Mackinnon SE, Novak CB. Nerve transfers. New options for reconstruction following nerve injury. Hand Clin 1999;15(4):643–66, ix.

89. Samardzic MM, Grujicic DM, Rasulic LG, et al. The use of thoracodorsal nerve transfer in restoration of irreparable C5 and C6 spinal nerve lesions. Br J Plast Surg 2005;58(4):541–6.

90. Uerpairojkit C, Leechavengvongs S, Witoonchart K, et al. Nerve transfer to serratus anterior muscle using the thoracodorsal nerve for winged scapula in C5 and C6 brachial plexus root avulsions. J Hand Surg Am 2009;34(1):74–8.

91. Novak CB, Mackinnon SE, Tung TH. Patient outcome following a thoracodorsal to musculocutaneous nerve transfer for reconstruction of elbow flexion. Br J Plast Surg 2002;55(5):416–9.

92. Ray WZ, Mackinnon SE. Clinical outcomes following median to radial nerve transfers. J Hand Surg Am 2011;36(2):201–8.

93. Ustun ME, Oğün TC, Büyükmumcu M, et al. Selective restoration of motor function in the ulnar nerve by transfer of the anterior interosseous nerve. An anatomical feasibility study. J Bone Joint Surg Am 2001;83(4):549–52.

94. Ross D, Mackinnon SE, Chang YL. Intraneural anatomy of the median nerve provides "third web space" donor nerve graft. J Reconstr Microsurg 1992;8(3):225–32.

Current Status of Brachial Plexus Reconstruction: Restoration of Hand Function

Laurent Wehrli, MD[a], Chantal Bonnard, MD[a], Dimitri J. Anastakis, MD[b],*

KEYWORDS

- Brachial plexus • Hand • Reconstruction • Peripheral nerve
- Nerve transfer • Tendon transfer
- Free functioning muscle transfer

Brachial plexus injuries are devastating, and are associated with high levels of disability and decreased health status.[1] The hand is affected in the vast majority of injuries (**Fig. 1**).[2,3] Over the past decade, innovative applications of nerve transfers and free functioning muscle transfers (FFMT) have offered patients, particularly those with pan-plexus injuries, hope of regaining some hand function. Nevertheless, restoration of hand function in adult brachial plexus patients remains a formidable reconstructive challenge.

Several recent reviews describe the management and treatment of adult brachial plexus lesions.[4–8] The current status of nerve transfers, tendon transfers, and FFMT are reviewed in articles elsewhere in this issue. The purpose of this article is to focus on the reconstructive options available for the restoration of hand function (ie, prehension) in adult brachial plexus patients.

MOTOR AND SENSORY DEFICITS IN THE HAND FOLLOWING BRACHIAL PLEXUS INJURY

The root contribution to each upper extremity muscle is variable. In addition, a prefixed or post-fixed brachial plexus can further confound clinical

expression of a root lesion.[9,10] Following a stretch injury, each nerve fiber in the root, trunk, or peripheral nerve sustains a unique histologic lesion (ie, Sunderland 1–5)[11] such that one portion of a root may recover spontaneously and another portion may not. These factors contribute to significant variability in the expression of motor or sensory deficits following a root lesion(s). Each clinical case is unique and a detailed clinical examination is always required. Clinicians broadly group brachial plexus lesions into upper (C5C6) or lower (C8T1) plexus lesions with or without involvement of C7 (**Table 1**).

C5C6

In a C5C6 lesion the shoulder is paralyzed and elbow flexion is absent, which prevent the patient from positioning the hand in space. Forearm supination is weak but rarely requires reconstruction. Hand motor function and sensation are essentially normal.[2] Hypoesthesia of the thumb has been described in 17% of patients with a C5C6 lesion.[2]

C5C6C7

As in C5C6 lesions, the shoulder is paralyzed as are elbow flexion and extension. The hand

The authors have nothing to disclose.
a Service de Chirurgie Plastique et Reconstructive et Chirurgie de la main, Clinique de Longeraie, Université de Lausanne, 9 Avenue de la Gare, CH-1003 Lausanne, Switzerland
b Division of Plastic and Reconstructive Surgery, University of Toronto, 399 Bathurst Street, 2 EW Toronto, ON M5T 2S8, Canada
* Corresponding author.
E-mail address: dimitri.anastakis@uhn.on.ca

Clin Plastic Surg 38 (2011) 661–681
doi:10.1016/j.cps.2011.07.003

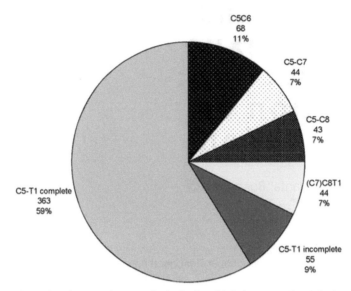

Fig. 1. Epidemiology of root involvement in supraclavicular brachial plexus traction injuries. Clinical presentation of palsy confirmed by surgical exploration of 617 cases of brachial plexus injury by Narakas and Bonnard[3] (467 cases) and Bertelli and colleagues[2] (150 cases). The root involvement includes either an avulsion or an extraforaminal rupture. "C5-T1 complete" is equivalent to a flail arm, whereas "C5-T1 incomplete" spares some finger flexion probably through T2 contribution. (*Data from* Narakas A, Bonnard C. Anatomopathological lesions. In: Alnot JY, Narakas A, editors. Traumatic brachial plexus injuries. Paris: Expansion Scientifique Française; 1996. p. 72–91; and Bertelli JA, Ghizoni MF, Loure Iro Chaves DP. Sensory disturbances and pain complaints after brachial plexus root injury: a prospective study involving 150 adult patients. Microsurgery 2011;31(2):93–7.

Table 1
Most frequent motor and sensory deficits in the hand following brachial plexus injuries

Roots	Muscles Affected	Functional Deficits	Hand-Specific Functional Deficits	Hand-Specific Sensory Deficits[2]
C5C6	Deltoid, supraspinatus, infraspinatus, biceps, brachialis, coracobrachialis, brachioradialis (± radial wrist extensors), clavicular pectoralis major	Shoulder external rotation, abduction and forward flexion, weak forearm supination, elbow flexion (± wrist extension)	Forearm supination (± wrist extension)	No, except thumb hypoesthesia in 17%
C5C7	As above, plus triceps, ECRL, ECRB, EDC, EPL, EPB, APL, supinator, PT (± FDS and FCR)	As above, plus elbow extension, prono-supination, wrist, finger, and thumb extension	Prono-supination, wrist, finger, and thumb extension	Thumb hypoesthesia, less marked in all other fingers
C5C8	As above, plus FCR, FDS, FDP, FPL (± FCU)	As above, plus complete wrist palsy	As above, plus thumb and index finger extrinsic flexion	Loss of protective sensation of thumb in 29%
(C7)C8T1	(± EDC, EPL) FDS, FDP, FPL, lumbricals and interossei, thenar and hypothenar muscles	(Finger extension) Finger and thumb flexion, median and ulnar intrinsic muscles	Finger and thumb flexion, median and ulnar intrinsic muscles	Loss of protective sensation in ring and little fingers
Pan-plexus	All above	Flail arm	Flail arm	Insensate hand

Abbreviations: APL, abductor pollicis longus; ECRB, extensor carpi radialis brevis; ECRL, extensor carpi radialis longus; EDC, extensor digitorum communis; EPB, extensor pollicis brevis; EPL, extensor pollicis longus; FCR, flexor carpi radialis; FDS, flexor digitorum superficialis; PT, pronator teres.

presents similar to radial nerve palsy with loss of wrist extension (extensor carpi radialis longus [ECRL] and extensor carpi radialis brevis [ECRB]) and loss of metacarpal phalangeal joint (MCPJ) extension except in cases where the extensor digitorum communis (EDC) is innervated by C8. The intrinsic muscles are normal. Prono-supination is weakened, due of loss of pronator teres (PT), supinator, and biceps function. The pronator quadratus is still preserved so the hand is maintained in a semipronated position. Finger flexion is intact through normal function of the flexor digitorum profundus (FDP). The flexor digitorum superficialis (FDS) may be partially paralyzed, and this may result in swan-neck deformities. The strength of the FDS must be tested if there are future plans to use the FDS as a transfer to restore wrist extension. There is hypoesthesia in all digits, predominantly in the thumb, but without any loss in protective sensation.[2] In cases of C5-C8 involvement, thumb anesthesia is present in 29%, with the intact T1 providing protective sensation in some fingers.[2]

C8T1 ± C7

In C8T1 lesions, both shoulder and elbow functions are intact. There is no intrinsic muscle function. Finger and thumb flexion are absent. The ring and small fingers are insensate.[2] If C7 is also involved, wrist extension may be weak, wrist flexion is weak, finger extension is absent, and the middle finger loses protective sensation.

Pan-Plexus (C5-T1)

In pan-plexus lesions the arm is flail and there is no protective sensation in the hand. Weak finger flexion may be present in a small subgroup for which there is T2 motor contribution to the lower trunk.[2,3,12,13]

PREVENTING HAND JOINT CONTRACTURES

The upper extremity is commonly overlooked during the early posttrauma period as emphasis is placed on life-threatening injuries. As such, patients may develop stiffness and contractures at all upper extremity joints (**Fig. 2**). Ideally the brachial plexus surgeon should be involved early in the patient's care and should ensure appropriate therapy to prevent joint contractures and strengthen functioning muscles in the affected limb. The hand should be splinted in a position of function, and passive range of motion started early following the injury.

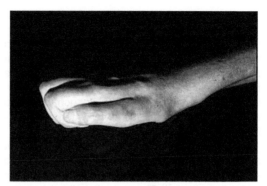

Fig. 2. A neglected hand following brachial plexus injury with typical adduction contracture of the thumb and metacarpal phalangeal joint and proximal interphalangeal joint contractures and stiffness.

RECONSTRUCTIVE STRATEGIES TO RESTORE HAND FUNCTION

Debate exists among surgeons regarding the priorities for upper extremity reconstruction. Each patient presents with a unique injury and pattern of paralysis. Each patient has different expectations and it is the authors' philosophy that all reconstructive options should be presented to the patient and that he or she should play an active role in formulating the final reconstructive plan. The authors' reconstructive strategy places priority on restoring elbow flexion, followed by shoulder stability and/or abduction, and then the restoration of hand function. A stable shoulder increases the function of the reinnervated elbow flexors and a functioning elbow increases shoulder use. Some surgeons perform arthrodesis of the glenohumeral joint, thereby allowing valuable donor nerves to be used for more distal functions.[14,15] Restoring protective hand sensation must be included in the reconstructive plan. Today, as part of their reconstructive armamentarium surgeons have the following options to restore hand function: (1) nerve repair; (2) nerve grafting; (3) nerve transfers from intraplexal or extraplexal sources; (4) tendon transfers (and tenodesis); (5) FFMT; (6) arthrodesis; and (7) a combination of these techniques.

SHORT NERVE GRAFTS FOR BRACHIAL PLEXUS RECONSTRUCTION (PLEXOPLEXAL GRAFTING)

Distal nerve transfers have become increasingly popular, especially after the publication of Oberlin's partial ulnar nerve transfer to the motor nerve of the biceps.[16] These transfers are easier to perform than a plexus dissection and repair, and the results are faster because of the short regeneration distance to the target muscle. A multinational survey of peripheral nerve surgeons performed in 2004 found that exploration of the brachial plexus is rarely performed.[17] One might speculate that exploration of the plexus with nerve grafting may not be the first choice even in cases of C5 and C6 rupture.[17] Nerve transfers are largely preferred, as is further highlighted in the recent review by Songcharoen and colleagues[18] of 1449 patients for whom they performed only 16 plexoplexal procedures.

Nevertheless, nerve grafts from a ruptured root allows one to bring a large number of motor and sensory axons into the target division, cord, or peripheral nerve.[19] The potential disadvantages of plexus grafting include: (1) the long regeneration distance; (2) co-contractions when antagonists are reinnervated with the same part of a root; (3) misdirected motor axons into sensory nerve fibers; and (4) dispersion of regenerating axons into many motor targets. Kline and colleagues[20,21] and Bertelli and Ghizoni[22] recommend exploration of the plexus, especially when there is no evidence of root avulsion on computed tomographic myelography and in gunshot or laceration injuries. The authors still believe the plexus should be explored to confirm that no upper root is amenable to nerve grafting.

C5C6 ± C7 Injuries

Recently, Bertelli and Ghizoni[23] demonstrated that the recovery of shoulder and elbow functions after distal nerve transfers are enhanced by associated repair of the plexus. In C5C6 ruptures, these investigators graft the anterior portion of C5C6 to the anterior portion of the upper trunk and the posterior portion of C5C6 to the posterior upper trunk. The spinal accessory nerve (SAN) is transferred to the suprascapular nerve (SSN), the long head of triceps branch to the anterior division of axillary nerve and teres minor branch, and the nerve to biceps is reinnervated with one fascicle of the ulnar nerve. Bertelli speculates that the reinnervation of the clavicular portion of the pectoralis major and the coracobrachialis through grafting from C5 to the anterior division of the upper trunk improves shoulder stability, which is necessary for good abduction. In terms of hand function, the C5C6 repair may improve the grip strength because of reinnervation of the ECRL. In C5C6 avulsion, only nerve transfers are possible.

C8T1 ± C7 Injury

With regard to lesions of the lower trunk, the authors' own experience allows one to say that it is almost always worthwhile repairing a laceration or a gunshot injury of the lower trunk with grafts no more than 5 cm length (recovery of useful finger flexion with minimal intrinsic recovery). In 2007, Haninec and colleagues[24] published a series of 95 patients treated with grafting of the plexus lesion (roots, cords, or trunks), intraplexal or extraplexal nerve transfers, and end-to-side neurorrhaphy. With regard to the hand these investigators did not graft the lower trunk, but in 5 cases grafted between the medial cord and the ulnar nerve. In 3 of 5 cases, there was recovery of flexor carpi ulnaris (FCU) and finger flexion but no intrinsic recovery. In 4 cases, Haninec and colleagues grafted the lateral and medial cord to the median nerve, which resulted in the recovery of the FDS in one case with no recovery of thenar muscle function. Finally, regarding the repair of a high-level radial nerve lesion (8 cases of posterior cord grafted to the radial nerve), triceps recovered in all cases, wrist extension in 3 cases, and fingers extension in 2 cases.

In isolated C8T1 avulsion or stretch injury, finger flexion, and intrinsic function (proximal interphalangeal joint [PIPJ] and distal interphalangeal joint [DIPJ] extension) are restored through tendon transfer surgery.[5,24] Grafting of the lower trunk in C8T1 rupture is not recommended.

LONG NERVE GRAFTS FOR BRACHIAL PLEXUS RECONSTRUCTION

In cases of complete palsy, long nerve grafts are required to bridge the long distance between the brachial plexus and upper arm.

Sural Nerve Grafts

When sural nerve grafts are used in plexus reconstruction, the length of the sural nerve graft does not have a significant effect on outcomes.[25,26] In complete palsies with C5C6 rupture, Bertelli and Ghizoni[25] recommend using long sural nerve grafts from C5 to the musculocutaneous nerve (MCN) and from C6 (or levator scapulae branch) to the radial nerve. According to Bertelli, there is little chance of useful hand function recovery with nerve grafting.

On the contrary, Chuang[5] recommends using long grafts from the available root(s) either to C8 or directly to the median nerve in an attempt to reanimate the hand. In complete avulsion, Chuang grafts the median nerve with the contralateral C7 (cC7). The results of grafting the median nerve or C8 root are not reported, but described by the author as M2 to M3 finger flexion.

Ulnar Nerve Grafts

Ulnar nerve grafts are used only in C8T1 avulsion or in an irreparable lesion of the medial cord.

These grafts are useful in large nerve gaps or in a scarred beds.[27] Endoscopic harvesting of the ulnar nerve has been described by Xu and colleagues.[28] The ulnar nerve must be vascularized to avoid central necrosis, and is used as either a pedicled graft or as a free microvascular transfer. The reported results of vascularized ulnar nerve grafts are variable. Bertelli and Ghizoni[22] report using a 30-cm long pedicled ulnar nerve graft from an intact root to the MCN in 8 cases. In this report, the investigators describe clinical failure in all 8 cases, and have since stopped using this technique. In 2009, Chuang[5] described the use of the C-loop of the ulnar nerve, but did not provide clinical results with this technique. Terzis and Kostopoulos[27] have published the largest series using vascularized ulnar nerve grafts, and report good results with either a pedicled or a free microvascular transfer. In ipsilateral intraplexal reconstruction, the nerve defect is short enough so that multiple segmented grafts may be done with the same vascularized ulnar nerve, for instance from C5 to the MCN and to the median nerve (Terzis' method).

NERVE TRANSFERS TO RESTORE HAND FUNCTION

Intraplexal nerve transfers (ie, from intact brachial plexus axons) have the advantage of bringing motor axons very close to the denervated muscle, and are usually performed without interpositional nerve grafts. The final functional benefits should always outweigh any donor loss. Nerve transfers from extraplexal sources serve as a complement to root repair in cases of root rupture.[13] Nerve transfers are the only means of providing motor axons in pan-plexus avulsions. Potential extraplexal donor nerves include the SAN, intercostal nerves (ICN), the phrenic nerve and the cC7 root.

Spinal Accessory Nerve

The SAN has been mostly used to restore elbow flexion and shoulder abduction by transfer to MCN[29,30] and SSN.[31,32] One must always remember that unlike elbow flexion, shoulder function is complex, and simple reinnervation of the SSN rarely results in good functional outcome. Improvement in shoulder function is directly related to the number of shoulder-specific nerve transfers performed.[23,32,33]

The posterior trapezius approach was initially described to avoid injury to the SAN when decompressing the SSN at the suprascapular notch.[34] A similar surgical approach has been described to harvest the maximum length of the descending branch of the SAN.[35–38] The medial root of the median nerve can then potentially be reached.[37] It is unknown whether the axonal loss of 38% (form 1380 down to 860 along the 10.5 extra centimeters)[37] counterbalances the disadvantage of using a nerve graft, as is done with the classic anterior approach. Overall, most surgeons commonly transfer the SAN to the SSN for shoulder abduction and do not use it as a donor for the restoration of hand function, except to innervate FFMT.[39,40]

Intercostal Nerves

Since Seddon's first case report[41] in 1963, the ICNs have been widely used to restore elbow flexion.[42–49] When elbow flexion and shoulder stabilization are addressed, the ICNs can be transferred to the median or ulnar nerve to provide protective hand sensation. In 31 patients with complete brachial plexus avulsion, Dolenc[50] transferred 3 ICNs to both the ulnar and radial nerves with interpositional nerve grafts. Dolenc reported no motor recovery in the hand, but protective sensation was noted in 52% of the cases. By transferring the fifth and sixth ICNs to the median nerve in 9 patients with root avulsions (mean age 18.6 years), Ogino and Naito[51] achieved wrist flexion M3 or greater in 67% and finger flexion M3 or greater in 44%. Of interest all 9 patients recovered light touch sensation without overresponse in the median nerve territory. In Nagano's series,[52] protective hand sensation was noted in 9 out of 10 patients (mean age 18 years) after transferring 2 ICNs to the median nerve. When comparing sensory outcome after ICN versus supraclavicular nerve transfer to the median nerve, Ihara and colleagues[53] concluded that the ICN transfers were associated with better sensory outcomes. Two-point discrimination has never been restored in this patient population. Additional hand sensory outcomes following nerve transfers are listed in **Table 2**. The complications following meticulous harvesting of ICN are minimal,[54,55] making the ICN a donor nerve of choice for the restoration of protective hand sensation. The lateral cord contribution to the median nerve can be neurotized in upper root injuries, and the medial cord contribution to the ulnar nerve neurotized in lower root injuries.

Phrenic Nerve

Lurje[56] described the phrenic nerve as a motor donor for neurotization in 1948. Gu and colleagues[57] have used the phrenic nerve since 1970, mainly to restore elbow flexion. For restoration of finger flexion, the phrenic nerve is

Table 2
Sensory outcomes in the hand following nerve transfers after root avulsions

Author	N	Procedure (n)	Patient Age (y)	Mean Follow-Up (mo)	Time to Initial Recovery (mo)	Some Tactile Sensation (≥S2)	Protective Sensation (≥S1)
Ihara et al,[53] 1996	15[a]	LCB to MN (3)	23.0	48	19	3/3	3/3
		SCN to MN (10)	24.5	32	22	2/10	8/10
		C5 to MN (2)	19.0	69	11	1/2	1/2
Doi et al,[40] 2000	21[b]	ICN to UN (9)	20.4	27	19	8/9	8/9
		ICN to MN (7)	21.4	47	24	6/7	7/7
		SCN to MN (5)	21.8	50	20	2/5	5/5
Hattori et al,[88] 2009	17[b]	ICN to MN (14)	24.7	49	19	10/14	14/14
		ICN to UN (3)	34.3	50	22	1/3	3/3

Abbreviations: ICN, intercostal nerves; LCB, lateral cutaneous branch of intercostal nerves; MN, median nerve; SCN, supra-clavicular nerves (cutaneous branches of cervical plexus); UN, ulnar nerve.
[a] All patients had C7C8T1 root avulsions; 5 patients had C5 and 12 patients had C6 root avulsion.
[b] All patients had complete root avulsions.

transferred with an interpositional graft to the lateral division of the medial cord.

Direct nerve coaptation is only possible if the phrenic nerve is harvested using a demanding thoracoendoscopic technique, which provides an additional 16 cm of phrenic nerve length.[58,59] Using this technique in 3 patients, Xu and colleagues[60] reported useful (M3 or more) recovery of thumb and finger flexion in all patients. Patients were young (24.3 years) and time to surgery was short (2.5 months).[60] Lin and colleagues[61] restored useful finger and thumb extension in 7 of 10 patients, with direct coaptation of an extrathoracic harvested phrenic nerve to the posterior division of the lower trunk.

In the arm, the posterior portion of the median nerve contributes to the anterior interosseous nerve (AIN). This portion is specifically targeted when planning to restore long finger and thumb flexors.[62] Transfer of the phrenic nerve to the posterior portion of the median nerve can be used in complete brachial plexus avulsions. The length of the required graft is shorter when the phrenic nerve is harvested using a video-assisted thoracic technique.[62] Zhao and colleagues[62] reported only one case of complete brachial plexus palsy with recovery of M4 strength in the FDP, flexor pollicis longus (FPL), and palmaris longus (PL) at 16 months following surgery.

The phrenic nerve is a major potential source of motor axons, but the current results when used as a nerve transfer to restore hand function are such that its use does not outweigh the theoretical risk of pulmonary complications. As such, the authors do not currently use the phrenic nerve as a transfer for the restoration of hand function.

Contralateral C7

The C7 root contains approximately 10 times more nerve fibers than the SAN. The harvesting of cC7 results in no described long-term motor or sensory deficit. Gu and colleagues[63] have been using the cC7 as an option for reinnervation of finger flexion since 1986.

Using a vascularized ulnar nerve or sural nerve grafts from cC7 to the median nerve is the most frequent procedure used to restore hand function. Graft length is often not specified in the literature, but the average distance via the subcutaneous anterior chest route to the ipsilateral axilla is approximately 36 cm.[64] A prespinal retrophrenic route intended to decrease that gap has been recently described.[65] Both scalenus anterior muscles are transected and the cC7 trunk then travels immediately posterior to the phrenic nerve and esophagus, and anterior to the vertebral body (**Fig. 3**). This procedure allows direct coaptation of cC7 to the ipsilateral C5 and C6 roots and short interpositional grafts when cC7 is transferred beyond the ipsilateral roots (3-cm grafts to upper trunk divisions and 8-cm grafts to the lateral and posterior cords).[65] Using a retroesophageal pre-phrenic route has allowed Zou and colleagues[66] to obtain tension-free nerve repair interposing the pedicled ulnar nerve to the radial and median nerves. Another recently described method to transfer cC7 directly to the lower trunk in slim patients consists of rerouting the ipsilateral low-er trunk and medial cord to the anterior chest from the axilla.[67] Some investigators advocate harvesting the entire cC7 root,[65,67–69] whereas others prefer using only the anterior division,[66]

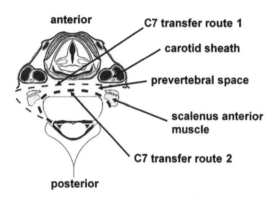

Fig. 3. Cross section of the neck illustrating the method of cC7 transfer through the transversely configured prespinal and retropharyngeal space after bilateral resection of scalenus anterior muscles as described by Xu and colleagues[65] (route 2) and the Mcguiness and Kay method of cC7 transfer (route 1). (*From* Xu L, Gu Y, Xu J, et al. Contralateral C7 transfer via the prespinal and retropharyngeal route to repair brachial plexus root avulsion: a preliminary report. Neurosurgery 2008;63(3):554; with permission.)

the posterior division,[64] or part of the divisions.[6,70] Of note, the size of the bridging ulnar nerve corresponds only to one division of C7.[63]

Overall, results of finger flexion graded M3 or greater have been reported in 20% to 50% of patients (**Table 3**). Comparing 64 patients with either entire cC7 harvesting using an anterior chest route in two stages or only the anterior division using a retroesophageal route in one stage, Zou and colleagues[66] were not able to identify a difference in motor results between these two groups. Three variables have been modified between the two groups: the route, the number of stages, and the donor part of cC7. The investigators concluded that harvesting only one division was adequate, allowing quicker recovery of the normal limb, and that two stages, as advocated by Gu[71] to enhance ulnar nerve graft vascularization, was not necessary. Published complications associated with cC7 harvesting are listed in **Table 4**.

Several brachial plexus surgeons no longer use cC7 as a donor nerve, because in their opinion the potential risks to the normal limb outweigh the functional hand improvement seen with this transfer.[4,6] The Mayo clinic group used the cC7 as a donor nerve in 21 patients and reported no result greater than M2 on composite grip, with none of the patients having useful hand function. The investigators concluded that harvesting the cC7 was not justified in reanimating the median nerve. Oberlin and colleagues[6] used the cC7 as a donor in 42 patients, using the MCN as a target in 22 cases. A 4-year follow-up of 34 patients

showed 11 (32%) patients with grade M3 or greater on reinnervated muscles. The investigators concluded the cC7 transfer to the MCN to be an unreliable procedure. The authors do not use the cC7 as a donor nerve to restore hand function.

Specific Nerve Transfers in Isolated Lower Brachial Plexus Injuries

As already discussed, the posterior part of the median nerve in the arm contributes to the AIN. These nerve fibers can be neurotized by the brachialis motor branch when C5-C6 are spared.[72,73] Zheng and colleagues[72] reported on this procedure in 6 patients who all recovered extrinsic finger flexion graded M3 or more. Potential risks include injury to the central portion of the median nerve in the arm with loss of sensation in thumb and damage to the epitrochlear branch, resulting in weakness of the PT and FCR. It is not yet clear whether this newly described distal nerve transfer offers a better outcome than classic tendon transfers.

In cases of C7 to T1 avulsion, finger and thumb extension have been restored by transferring the motor branch of the supinator to the posterior interosseous nerve. Dong and colleagues[74] described preliminary results with this transfer in 4 patients. None of the patients in this series had loss of supination and all had electrical signs of reinnervation by 6 months. Only one patient had a follow-up of 2 years, demonstrating motor strength graded M3 in the EDC, extensor carpi ulnaris (ECU), and extensor pollicis longus (EPL). Bertelli and Ghizoni[75] also reported on 4 patients using the same technique but harvesting the two branches of the supinator instead of one, and performing tendon transfers to restore finger flexion instead of transferring the brachialis motor branch to the AIN group in the arm. In this series all patients were able to extend their MCPJs with motor strength graded M3 at 12 months postoperatively. The radial deviation of the wrist in extension disappeared in all 4 patients, as the ECU was reinnervated.[75]

TENDON TRANSFERS

To be able to perform tendon transfers to restore hand function following brachial plexus injury, muscle units need to have been spared or sufficiently reinnervated. Most patients recover a few muscles that are available for transfer, although their strength is poor. Following primary nerve surgery it is important to wait at least 2 years for maximal recovery before contemplating tendon transfers. The reconstructive surgeon needs to be flexible and must be able to modify the

Table 3
Results of hand and wrist reanimation with use of cC7

Author	N	Follow-Up (y)	Amount of cC7 Harvested (n)	Bridging (n)	Route (n)	≥M3 (n)	≥S3 (n)
Songcharoen et al,[64] 2001	21	3.5	Posterior-superior half (21)	PUN (21) 1 stage to MN	Ant chest (21)	Median N: WF & FF (6/21)	(10/21)
Gu et al,[69] 2002	32	2	Entire (17) PD (12) AD (3)	PUN (20) FVUN (8) NG 4 2 stages (28) 1 stage (4)	Ant chest (32)	Median nerve: WF or FF (7/14) Radial N: WE or FE (4/6)	MCN (8/10) Radial N (5/6) Median N (12/14)
Chuang et al,[68] 1998	21	4.3	Entire (18) AD (2) PD (1)	PUN or FVUN		NA	NA
Terzis et al,[70] 2008	56	6.1	pPD & pAD (35) pPD (16) pAD (5)	NG (32/56) PUN or FVUN (24/56)	Ant chest (56)	25 pAD & 4pPD on median N: WF or FF >M3 (10/29) pPD on radial N: WF or FE >M3 (2/10)	Median N (12/29)
Xu et al,[65] 2008	8	1	Entire (8)	NG 6.3 cm × 6 (4) 8.6 cm × 6 (2) DA 2	Prespinal (8)	UT or LC & PC (shoulder and elbow reanimation)	C6 territory (8/8)
Feng et al,[67] 2010	4	2.5	Entire (4)	NG 4.5 cm (2) DA (2) 1 stage to ACRLT	ACRLT (4)	FCU (4/4) FDPrl (1/4)	(2/4)
Zou et al,[66] 2010	64	1.5	Entire (34) AD (30)	PUN (64) A: 2 stages B: 1 stage	A: Ant Chest (34) B: Retroesophageal (30)	Median N: GrB (12/26) Radial N: GrB (3/8)	NA
Hierner and Berger,[96] 2007	10	5	Partial (10)	PUN to MCN (6) PUN to MN (4)	Ant chest (10)	MCN: (6/6) Median nerve: (1/4)	NA

≥M3: at least active movement against gravity for wrist motion or weak resistance for finger grasping.
≥S3: at least superficial pain and partial sensation to touch (even with bad localization), without hyperesthesia.

Abbreviations: ACRLT, anterior chest rerouted lower trunk; AD, anterior division; Ant chest, anterior chest to axilla; DA, direct adaptation; FCU, flexor carpi ulnaris; FDPrl, flexor digitorum profundus of ring and little fingers; FE, finger extension; FF, finger flexion; FVUN, free vascularized ulnar nerve; LC, lateral cord; LT, lower trunk; MCN, musculocutaneous nerve; N, nerve; NA, not available; NG, nerve graft; pAD, part of anterior division; PC, posterior cord; PD, posterior division; pPD, part of posterior division; PT, pronator teres; PUN, pedicled ulnar nerve; UT, upper trunk; WF, wrist flexion.

Table 4
Complications of C7 harvesting in the healthy limb

Author	Numbness[a]	Time to Recover			Decreased Grip[b]	Time to Recover			Triceps Paresis	Time to Recover		
		<4 wk	≥4 wk	No Recovery		<8 wk	≥8 wk	No Recovery		<8 wk	≥8 wk	No Recovery
Gu et al,[63] 1992	42/49 26/26 entire C7 13/20 PD C7 3/3 AD C7	39	3	0	25/49 16/26 entire C7 8/20 PD C7 1/3 AD C7	25	—	0	8/49 6/26 entire C7 2/20 PD C7 0/3 AD C7	8	—	0
Terzis et al,[70] 2008	40/56	—	40	0	0/56	—	—	0	0/56	—	—	0
Songcharoen et al,[64] 2001	108/111	—	108	0	1 EDC/111	—	—	1 EDC M4 (3 y)	2/111	—	2	0
Chuang et al,[68] 1998	11/21	—	10	1 (16 mo)	2 EDC/21	—	2	0	4/21	—	4	0
Kus et al,[97] 1996	8/8	—	8	0	NA	NA	NA		6	NA	NA	NA
Liu et al,[98] 1997	2/2	—	2	0	2/2	—	2	0	2/2	—	2	0
Hierner and Berger,[96] 2007	10/10	—	10	0	0	NA	NA	0	0	NA	NA	0
Sammer et al,[99] 2009	21/21	—	21	0	8/21	—	—	1	3	NA	NA	—
Zou et al,[66] 2010	64/64	45	19	0	55/64	59	5	0	5/64	—	—	0

Abbreviations: AD, anterior division; EDC, extensor digitorum communis; FCR, flexor carpi radialis; NA, not available; PD, posterior division.
[a] Numbness of index pulp or median nerve innervated palm.
[b] Decreased grip or FCR/EDC paresis.

Table 5
FFMT procedures used to restore prehension

Authors	Description	First FFMT	Second FFMT	Sensory and Other Motor Reconstruction	Secondary Procedures
Doi et al,[40] 2000	Restore shoulder stability and function combined with flexion and extension of the elbow, hand sensibility, rudimentary hand grasp and release	Donor nerve: SAN Artery: TAT Origin: clavicle Pulley: under BR Insertion: radial wrist extensors and finger extensors Action: elbow flexion and finger extension	Donor nerve: motor ICN Artery: TDA Origin: second rib Pulley: routed subcutaneously along medial aspect of arm Insertion: finger flexor tendons Action: finger flexion	Sensory ICN transferred to the median nerve for sensation $ICN_{3,4}$ to motor branch of triceps	± arthrodesis thumb CMCJ ± glenohumeral joint arthrodesis ± flexor tenolysis
Bishop,[39] 2005	Restore shoulder stability and function combined with flexion and extension of the elbow, hand sensibility, rudimentary hand grasp and release	Donor nerve: SAN Artery: TAT Origin: clavicle Pulley: distal FCU used to create a pulley at level of proximal forearm Insertion: ECRB Action: elbow flexion and wrist extension	Donor nerve: $ICN_{3,4}$ Artery: thoracoacromial artery Origin: second rib Insertion: FDP + FPL Pulley: lacertus fibrosis Action: elbow flexion and finger flexion	Sensory ICN_{3-6} transferred to lateral cord contribution of the median nerve during second FFMT $ICN_{5,6}$ transferred to triceps motor branch	
Giuffre et al,[4] 2010	Single gracilis muscle transfer to restore elbow flexion and finger flexion	Donor nerve: ICN Artery: TDA Origin: clavicle Insertion: FDP + FPL Pulley: lacertus fibrosis Action: elbow flexion and finger flexion		Sensory ICN transferred to lateral cord contribution of the median nerve (1) 2 lower motor ICN transferred to Biceps in lower-case motor branch (2) XI transferred with interposed graft to triceps branches	Wrist arthrodesis

		Stage 1	Stage 2—FFMT	Stage 3
Gousheh and Arasteh,[91] 2010	Three-stage reconstruction to restore elbow and finger flexion	Sural nerve grafted from contralateral MPN to paralyzed arm	Donor nerve: MPN + sural nerve graft Artery: accessible axillary vessel Origin: coracoid process Insertion: biceps tendon Action: elbow flexion	Transfer of biceps tendon to FDP with TFL deep to forearm superficial fascia
Terzis and Kostopoulos,[90] 2009	Single FFMT transfers to restore finger flexion first then finger extension	Donor nerve: Banked cC7, ICN, SAN, ipsilateral upper plexus Artery: brachial artery Origin: 12–15 cm proximal to the elbow in the intermuscular septum Insertion: FPL + FDP or FPL + FDS Action: finger flexion	Donor nerve: Banked ICN, cC7, SAN, ipsilateral plexus Artery: brachial artery Origin: 12–15 cm proximal to elbow in the intermuscular septum Insertion: EPL + EDC Action: finger extension	Wrist arthrodesis performed before FFMT
Chuang,[89] 2008	Single FFMT to restore finger flexion	Donor nerve: ICN$_{3-5}$ Artery: TDA, lateral thoracic or circumflex humeral artery Origin: second rib Insertion: FPL + FDP Pulley: deep to PT and CFO Action: finger flexion		
Chuang,[89] 2008	Single FFMT to restore finger extension	Donor nerve: SAN Artery: brachial artery Origin: lateral clavicle Insertion: EDC Pulley: through BR and EDC Action: finger extension		

Abbreviations: BR, brachioradialis; cC7, contralateral C7; CFO, common flexor origin; EDC, extensor digitorum communis; EPL, extensor pollicis longus; FCU, flexor carpi ulnaris; FDP, flexor digitorum profundus; FDS, flexor digitorum sublimis; FFMT, free functioning muscle transfer; FPL, flexor pollicis longus; ICN, intercostal nerve; MPN, medial pectoral nerve; PT, pronator teres; SAN, spinal accessory nerve; TAT, thoracoacromial trunk; TDA, thoracodorsal artery; TFL, tensor fascia lata.

reconstructive plan according to available motor units. The classic tendon transfers described for combined median and ulnar nerve palsy and radial nerve palsy are typically performed.

Restoration of Wrist Extension

The aim of tendon transfers is to actively stabilize the wrist in extension to improve grip function.

Retroclavicular injury of the posterior cord

Patients with lesions isolated to the posterior cord have clinical findings similar to a high radial nerve palsy (including the triceps). In such cases, the usual high radial nerve tendon transfer for wrist extension using the PT to the ECRB is recommended.

C5C6 injury

In C5C6 root lesions, tendon transfers are not required. In almost every case, the wrist extensors are normal (ie, ECRB and ECU).

C5C6C7 injuries

In C5C6C7 root lesions, the PT is commonly paralyzed and is not available for tendon transfer. The first choice for tendon transfer is 1 or 2 FDS tendons ran through the interosseous membrane.[76] As the FDS may be completely innervated by C7, a preoperative electromyogram (EMG) may be necessary to confirm normal innervation. The use of the FDS requires a normal functioning FDP otherwise finger flexion will be adversely affected by the transfer. In patients with joint laxity, the harvesting of FDS may result in a swan-neck deformity that may require secondary correction. If there is concern regarding the strength of the FDS, an alternative is to use the FCU.[77] The FCR or the PL must be normal before using the FCU, otherwise active wrist flexion with the subsequent tenodesis effect is lost. Of course FCU is not a synergistic transfer but it functions well in cases where global reinnervation has occurred. Bertelli and Ghizoni[78] recommend transferring the reinnervated brachialis to the ECRB if the usual motors are not valid.

C7C8T1 injuries

In C7C8T1 root lesions, wrist extension is usually strong and is the only motor of the hand.

Restoration of Finger Extension

Retroclavicular injury of the posterior cord

In lesions of the posterior cord, the same tendon transfers as in a high radial palsy are commonly performed, and include transfer of the FCU to the EDC and EPL, and transfer of the PL (through the interosseous membrane) to the abductor pollicis

longus (APL) and extensor pollicis brevis (EPB). Some surgeons prefer using the FCR instead of the FCU.[79]

C5C6 injury

Finger extension is normal.

C5C6C7 injuries

Finger extension may be deficient when C7 is a major contributor to the EDC. Either the FCU or FCR can be used as tendon transfers to restore finger extension. If either the FCU or FCR is paralyzed, it is best not to use the remaining wrist flexor as it would compromise the tenodesis effect. In such cases, transfer of an FDS tendon to the EDC or tenodesis of the EDC to the radius is recommended. When using an ulnar nerve fascicle to neurotize the biceps, Bertelli and Ghizoni[23] recommend using a motor fascicle intended for the intrinsic muscles or the FDP, in order to later be able to use the FCU for tendon transfer; they did not observe any decrease in hand strength.

Restoration of Finger Flexion in Lower Plexus Injuries

In C8T1 root lesions, restoration of finger flexion is performed by transferring the ECRL to the FDP through the interosseous membrane. This transfer is reliable and allows the patient to use the hand as a strong hook. This transfer requires that the ECRB have normal function as confirmed with an EMG. If the ECRB is denervated or weak, wrist extension will be lost and the ECRL to FDP transfer will not function well. Other transfers described to restore finger flexion include using the FCR to the FDP[5] or using the brachialis for finger and thumb flexion.[78] In cases where finger extension is absent, the EDC can be tenodesed on the radius or sutured to the paralyzed FDS through the interosseous membrane.[80]

Pinch Reconstruction in Lower Brachial Plexus Palsies

The brachioradialis is the best transfer to reanimate thumb opposition. It is transferred to the FPL (with interphalangeal joint [IPJ] arthrodesis)[5] or to a paralyzed FDS, which is then rerouted to function as an opponensplasty.[77] For abduction of the thumb, the APL and EPB can be fixed to the radius if required. Pinch is activated through the tenodesis effect using active wrist flexion to open pinch and the active wrist extension to close it. Bertelli and colleagues[81] have described transfer of the supinator to the EPB to open the pinch. Active or passive Zancolli lasso procedure (tenodesis of the FDS around the A1 pulley) improves the clawing hand.

During the activities of daily living, the patient uses his or her normal hand to place an object he or she wants to hold in his or her reconstructed hand. The reconstructed grip can maintain the object in the hand. This type of reconstruction allows the patient the ability to perform bimanual activities. However, active and spontaneous prehension is present only if wrist, finger, and thumb extension are normal.

Restoration of Finger Flexion in Complete Palsy (C5-T1)

Transfer of a reinnervated biceps can be used for finger flexion. In this transfer, an interpositional tensor fascia lata graft bridges the detached biceps tendon to the FDP and FPL tendons passing deep to the PT and the FDS arcade.[82] No loss of elbow flexion has been reported.

ARTHRODESIS

In a few select cases, arthrodesis may be useful. For example, fusion of the thumb IPJ is indicated when the brachioradialis is transferred to the FPL, to improve pinch strength. Wrist arthrodesis may be considered when the wrist is unstable and flexes together with the fingers.[83] In this situation, finger flexion improves with a wrist fusion. Before performing a wrist fusion, the authors recommend that the patient be fitted with a wrist extension splint to mimic wrist and hand position following wrist fusion. However, the authors rarely recommend wrist fusion as a first option because it abolishes the tenodesis effect. Wrist fusion is currently performed when FFMTs are used to reanimate the finger flexion and extension.

FUNCTIONING FREE MUSCLE TRANSFER FOR RESTORATION OF HAND FUNCTION

Primary nerve surgery for the restoration of shoulder and elbow function provides the brachial plexus patient with good functional results. Unfortunately, there has been little change in the outcomes following nerve grafting or nerve transfer for the restoration of hand function in patients

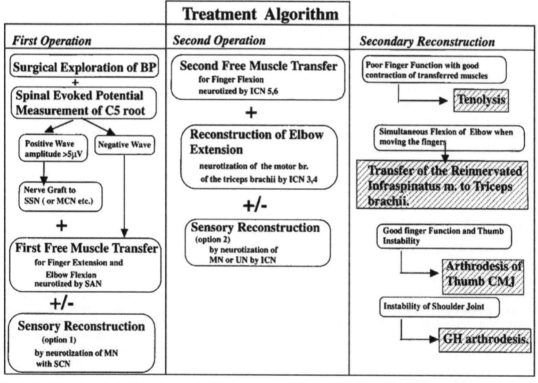

Fig. 4. Doi's treatment algorithm for the double free muscle technique. BP, brachial plexus; CMJ, carpometacarpal joint; GH, glenohumeral joint; ICN, intercostal nerve; MCN, musculocutaneous nerve; MN, median nerve; SAN, spinal accessory nerve; SCN, supraclavicular nerve; SSN, suprascapular nerve; UN, ulnar nerve. (*From* Doi K, Muramatsu K, Hattori Y, et al. Restoration of prehension with the double free muscle technique following complete avulsion of the brachial plexus. Indications and long-term results. J Bone Joint Surg Am 2000; 82(5):654; with permission.)

with pan-plexus lesions.[39] Over the past decade, there has been increasing experience with the restoration of hand function using FFMT motored by extraplexal donor nerves. This reconstructive option is typically reserved for long-standing or failed reconstruction cases.

The principles of FFMT in brachial plexus reconstruction are similar to those described for FFMT in general upper extremity reconstruction,[84–86] and include: (1) no simpler solution for the patient's problem; (2) good patient motivation and awareness; (3) available, undamaged motor nerve, artery, and vein at the site of muscle transplantation; (4) adequate skin coverage for the distal half of the muscle; and (5) supple joints and gliding tendons. Adding to the complexity of brachial plexus reconstruction is the absence of hand sensation and intrinsic muscle function.

Surgeons know that an insensate hand is prone to injury and is rarely incorporated into the activities of daily living. It is now known that sensory input may be an important modulator of motor plasticity and that without sensory input from the hand, relearning a motor skill may be difficult.[87] Given the importance of sensation, every effort should be made to restore protective sensation before or at the time of FFMT. Most FFMT reconstructive strategies include nerve transfers to restore protective hand sensation. Typically this involves transfer of the sensory portion of the ICN to the lateral cord contribution to the median nerve.[88] Restoration of intrinsic hand muscle function is not possible with either primary nerve surgery or FFMT. Most patients require secondary procedures to the hand following FFMT.

The gracilis muscle is most commonly used for restoration of hand function. Chuang[89] provides an excellent description of the extraplexal donor nerves commonly used with FFMT. Potential donor nerves commonly used to motor FFMT for restoration of hand function include the spinal accessory nerve (SAN), ICNs, phrenic nerve, and cC7. A major technical advantage of FFMT is the coaptation of the donor nerve in close proximity to the muscle, minimizing reinnervation time.

FFMT used to restore hand function can be broadly divided into two techniques: (1) double FFMT and (2) single FFMT. Multiple staged reconstructions involve interpositional nerve grafting to bring donor nerve from the normal contralateral arm to the paralyzed arm. The delay between the grafting and subsequent FFMT is usually 1 year. Some of the various FFMT strategies used to restore hand function are listed in **Table 5**.

Doi and colleagues[40] first described the double FFMT to restore multiple functions including rudimentary hand grip and release. Doi's treatment algorithm is shown in **Fig. 4**. The first FFMT, used to restore elbow flexion and finger extension, is transferred and reinnervated by the SAN (**Fig. 5**). The second FFMT, transferred to restore finger flexion, is reinnervated by the fifth and sixth ICN (**Fig. 6**). **Fig. 7** illustrates the transfer of ICNs to the triceps to restore elbow extension. Overall, Doi and colleagues reported that this procedure resulted in excellent to good elbow flexion in 96% of patients. Close to two-thirds of

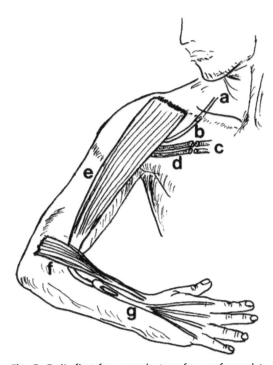

Fig. 5. Doi's first free muscle transfer, performed to restore finger extension and elbow flexion simultaneously. The transferred muscle is placed on the anterior surface of the upper arm. The nutrient vessels are anastomosed to the thoracoacromial artery and the cephalic vein, and the motor nerve is coapted to the spinal accessory nerve. The muscle is anchored to the acromion and the lateral aspect of the clavicle proximally, passed underneath the pulley of the brachioradialis and the wrist extensors, and sutured distally to the extensor digitorum communis tendon in the forearm. a, spinal accessory nerve; b, motor branch of muscle transplant; c, thoracoacromial artery and branches of cephalic vein; d, nutrient artery and veins of muscle transplant; e, muscle transplant; f, brachioradialis and wrist extensors serving as pulley; g, extensor digitorum communis tendon. (*From* Doi K, Muramatsu K, Hattori Y, et al. Restoration of prehension with the double free muscle technique following complete avulsion of the brachial plexus. Indications and long-term results. J Bone Joint Surg Am 2000;82(5):655; with permission.)

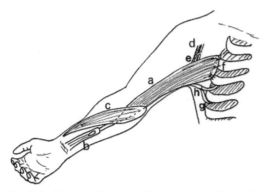

Fig. 6. Doi's second free muscle transfer, performed to restore finger flexion. The transferred muscle is placed on the medial surface of the upper arm. The nutrient vessels are anastomosed to the thoracodorsal artery and vein, and the motor nerve is coapted to the fifth and sixth intercostal nerves. The muscle is anchored to the second and third ribs proximally and to the flexor digitorum profundus tendons distally, passing beneath the pulley of the pronator teres and the wrist flexors. a, muscle transplant; b, flexor tendons of long finger; c, pronator teres and wrist flexors serving as pulley; d, thoracodorsal artery and vein; e, nutrient artery and veins of muscle transplant; f, second and third ribs; g, fifth and sixth intercostal nerves; h, motor branch of muscle transplant. (*From* Doi K, Muramatsu K, Hattori Y, et al. Restoration of prehension with the double free muscle technique following complete avulsion of the brachial plexus. Indications and long-term results. J Bone Joint Surg Am 2000;82(5):655; with permission.)

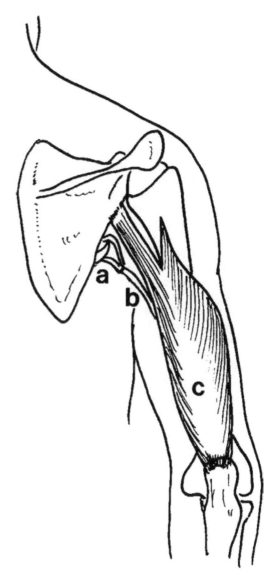

Fig. 7. Doi's transfer of the third and fourth intercostal nerves to the motor branch of the triceps brachii muscle, performed to restore elbow extension and stability. This procedure is done at the time of the second free muscle transfer. a, third and fourth intercostal nerves; b, motor branch of triceps brachii; c, triceps brachii. (*From* Doi K, Muramatsu K, Hattori Y, et al. Restoration of prehension with the double free muscle technique following complete avulsion of the brachial plexus. Indications and long-term results. J Bone Joint Surg Am 2000; 82(5):658; with permission.)

patients achieved more than 30° of total active motion of the fingers following the second FFMT. Doi's double FFMT can provide reliable and useful hand function in cases of complete brachial plexus avulsion.

Bishop[39] described modifications to the double FFMT originally described by Doi. In stage 1, Bishop secures the gracilis muscle to the ECRB as opposed to the finger extensors. In doing so, the transfer capitalizes on the tenodesis effect that promotes finger flexion. To prevent the bow-stringing at the elbow he detaches the distal portion of the FCU and creates a pulley at the level of the proximal forearm.

When reporting on his results on 8 of 9 patients having a minimum 1-year follow-up, Bishop was not able to replicate the hand prehension results described in many Asian studies, attributing their differing results to patient-related factors. He also describes scarring of the wrist and finger tendons as a major postoperative problem. Following double FFMT, Bishop described weaker elbow flexion compared with single FFMT for elbow flexion. Also, grip function was less reliable, with 5 of 8 patients having 30° total active motion in the digits with the second FFMT.

Giuffre and colleagues[4] described using a single FFMT to restore elbow flexion and finger flexion. When performed along with other nerve transfers and secondary procedures, this approach results in proximal joint stability and balance at the shoulder, elbow, and wrist, which is essential in restoring hand function.

Terzis and Kostopoulos[90] described the results of 71 single FFMTs for hand reanimation. In this series, the investigators make use of banked donor nerve tissue to motor the FFMT. The investigators describe a statistically significant difference between preoperative and postoperative muscle strength grading and range of motion. The distal SAN was found to be the strongest donor motor nerve for finger extension. The ICNs were useful for finger flexion, and the cC7 was useful for finger extension.

Gousheh and Arasteh[91] describe the results in 19 patients following a 3-staged surgical reconstruction to provide both elbow flexion and finger flexion. In this procedure, the investigators first used a sural nerve graft from contralateral medial pectoral nerve (MPN) to paralyzed arm. One year later, they performed FFMT for finger flexion. In this study, 6 out of 17 patients achieved M4 finger flexion with good grip and an ability to hold a 2-kg weight. The investigators describe overall functional results of the limb as being good in 6, satisfactory in 11, and failed in 2 patients.

The described double and single FFMTs can provide reliable and useful hand function in cases of complete brachial plexus avulsion. The reported results following FFMT vary from center to center. This variability may be due to patient factors as described by Bishop or due to inconsistencies in our grading systems as proposed by Chuang.

MOTOR RELEARNING AND CORTICAL PLASTICITY

Cortical plasticity occurs in the sensorimotor cortex in response to anything from learning to make a fist following tendon transfer to flexing the elbow with FFMT. Every brachial plexus patient who undergoes a nerve transfer, tendon transfer, or FFMT will need to relearn a motor skill. Studies of the human brain during motor relearning have shown that at the onset of learning a new motor skill, there is an expansion of motor cortical representation along with increased excitability and decreased intracortical inhibition (**Fig. 8**). This phenomenon may represent a "priming" of the cortex to learn a new motor skill. As the patient practices the motor skill, there is an increase in the amount of cortical representation. As the skill is mastered, the degrees of cortical representation

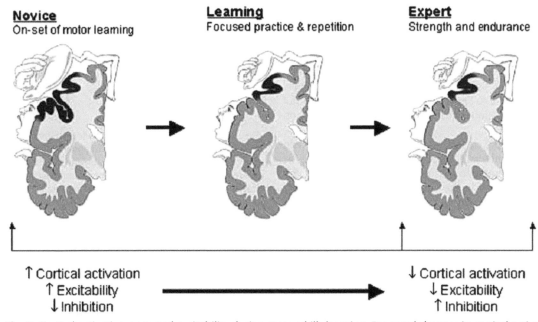

Fig. 8. Cortical activation maps and excitability during motor skills learning. Proposed changes in cortical activation, excitability, and inhibition as seen in functional magnetic resonance imaging and transcranial magnetic stimulation during motor skills learning. As the subject learns and becomes an expert, decreased cortical activation, decreased cortical excitability, and increased inhibition occur. (*Adapted from* Anastakis DJ, Chen R, Davis KD, et al. Cortical plasticity following upper extremity injury and reconstruction. Clin Plast Surg 2005;32:618; with permission.)

and excitability decrease and approach normal levels.[87,92]

Sensory input is an important modulator of cortical plasticity during motor learning. Also, sensory reeducation may not only be important in the recovery of protective sensation but may also play a role in optimizing gains in motor function following reconstruction of the upper extremity. The authors speculate that the absence of sensory input contributes to aberrant cortical plasticity during motor relearning, ultimately affecting functional outcomes.[93] Hence, efforts should be made to restore sensory function. Ensuring optimal sensory function before motor reconstruction may be an important strategy to consider in the reconstructive plans for patients with combined motor and sensory deficits. Reconstructive failures that occur despite intact neuromuscular connections in the periphery might be explainable by a lack of cortical sensorimotor network recruitment. That is, there may be a "central" mechanism of treatment failure.

Several strategies can be used to optimize motor relearning following reconstruction to restore prehension, and include: (1) preoperative training and practice of the movements required to activate the nerve transfer, tendon transfer, or FFMT; (2) reinforce with the patient the importance of early and long-term practice and repetition; (3) immediate sensory and motor reeducation following reconstruction[94,95]; (4) early activation of the motor movement with gravity removed; (5) focused practice and repetition with a therapist during early stages of motor learning; and (6) strengthening and endurance exercises for up to and possibly beyond 2 years following motor reinnervation.

In the future, surgeons may work with neuroscientists to establish a patient's ability to learn a new motor skill following reconstruction. We may see the augmentation of cortical plasticity through pharmacologic manipulation (ie, priming the brain's ability to learn a new motor skill). Further investigations into the cortical plasticity that appears during both motor and sensory recovery will affect the timing and types of rehabilitation strategies used. In the future, cortical plasticity and its manipulation may be an important contributor to functional outcome following reconstruction.

SUMMARY

Although restoration of hand function in brachial plexus patients remains a formidable challenge, the past decade has brought significant improvement in our ability to restore hand function in cases that were previously deemed as not reconstructable. A systematic approach to reconstruction of brachial plexus injuries places priority on restoring elbow flexion, followed by shoulder stability and/or abduction, then the restoration of hand function. The restoration of sensory function in the hand is of paramount importance in terms of motor relearning and if the hand is to be used for daily activities over the long term.

Today, we have as part of our reconstructive armamentarium the following options to restore hand function: (1) direct nerve repair; (2) nerve grafting; (3) nerve transfers from intraplexal or extraplexal sources; (4) tendon transfers (and tenodesis); (5) FFMT; (6) arthrodesis; and (7) a combination of these techniques. Distal nerve transfers provide innovative solutions to complex reconstructive problems. Potential extraplexal donor nerves used to restore hand function include the SAN, ICN, the phrenic nerve, and the cC7 root.

Transfer of the sensory portion of the ICN to the median or ulnar nerve is useful in restoration of sensory function in the hand. The phrenic nerve is a major potential source of motor axons, but the current results of functional benefit for restoration of hand function may not outweigh the potential risk of pulmonary complications. Debate around the routine use of the cC7 as a donor nerve in brachial plexus reconstruction persists, and there are several brachial plexus surgeons who no longer use cC7 as a donor nerve for the restoration of hand function. Though this debate exists, cC7 remains a viable option both as a nerve transfer and as an extraplexal donor nerve for FFMT.

Tendon transfers continue to enhance hand function in patients with brachial plexus lesions. For the patient with a pan-plexus injury, FFMT remains the most promising reconstructive option to restore hand function. Innovative applications of FFMT and the use of extraplexal donor nerves have provided patients with reliable and useful outcomes for hand function. Opportunity for future improvement exists, and the next decade will no doubt bring further innovation and functional improvement in restoration of hand function.

REFERENCES

1. Novak CB, Anastakis DJ, Beaton DE, et al. Patient-reported outcome after peripheral nerve injury. J Hand Surg Am 2009;34(2):281–7.
2. Bertelli JA, Ghizoni MF, Loure Iro Chaves DP. Sensory disturbances and pain complaints after brachial plexus root injury: a prospective study involving 150 adult patients. Microsurgery 2011;31(2):93–7.
3. Narakas A, Bonnard C. Anatomopathological lesions. In: Alnot JY, Narakas A, editors. Traumatic

brachial plexus injuries. Paris: Expansion Scientifique Française; 1996. p. 72–91.

4. Giuffre JL, Kakar S, Bishop AT, et al. Current concepts of the treatment of adult brachial plexus injuries. J Hand Surg Am 2010;35(4):678–88 [quiz: 688].

5. Chuang DC. Adult brachial plexus reconstruction with the level of injury: review and personal experience. Plast Reconstr Surg 2009;124(Suppl 6): e359–69.

6. Oberlin C, Durand S, Belheyar Z, et al. Nerve transfers in brachial plexus palsies. Chir Main 2009;28(1):1–9.

7. Doi K. Management of total paralysis of the brachial plexus by the double free-muscle transfer technique. J Hand Surg Eur Vol 2008;33(3):240–51.

8. Terzis JK, Kostopoulos VK. The surgical treatment of brachial plexus injuries in adults. Plast Reconstr Surg 2007;119(4):73e–92e.

9. Johnson EO, Vekris MD, Zoubos AB, et al. Neuroanatomy of the brachial plexus: the missing link in the continuity between the central and peripheral nervous systems. Microsurgery 2006;26(4):218–29.

10. Pellerin M, Kimball Z, Tubbs RS, et al. The prefixed and postfixed brachial plexus: a review with surgical implications. Surg Radiol Anat 2010;32(3): 251–60.

11. Sunderland S. A classification of peripheral nerve injuries producing loss of function. Brain 1951; 74(4):491–516.

12. Loukas M, El-Zammar D, Tubbs RS, et al. A review of the T2 segment of the brachial plexus. Singapore Med J 2010;51(6):464–7.

13. Narakas A. Neurotization in the treatment of brachial plexus injuries. In: Gelberman RH, editor, Operative nerve repair and reconstruction, vol. 2. Philadelphia: J. B. Lippincott company; 1991. p. 1329–58.

14. Rouholamin E, Wootton JR, Jamieson AM. Arthrodesis of the shoulder following brachial plexus injury. Injury 1991;22(4):271–4.

15. Chammas M, Goubier JN, Coulet B, et al. Glenohumeral arthrodesis in upper and total brachial plexus palsy. A comparison of functional results. J Bone Joint Surg Br 2004;86(5):692–5.

16. Oberlin C, Beal D, Leechavengvongs S, et al. Nerve transfer to biceps muscle using a part of ulnar nerve for C5-C6 avulsion of the brachial plexus: anatomical study and report of four cases. J Hand Surg Am 1994;19(2):232–7.

17. Belzberg AJ, Dorsi MJ, Storm PB, et al. Surgical repair of brachial plexus injury: a multinational survey of experienced peripheral nerve surgeons. J Neurosurg 2004;101(3):365–76.

18. Songcharoen P, Wongtrakul S, Spinner RJ. Brachial plexus injuries in the adult. nerve transfers: the Siriraj Hospital experience. Hand Clin 2005;21(1):83–9.

19. Narakas AO. Lesions found when operating traction injuries of the brachial plexus. Clin Neurol Neurosurg 1993;95(Suppl):S56–64.

20. Kline DG, Tiel RL. Direct plexus repair by grafts supplemented by nerve transfers. Hand Clin 2005;21(1): 55–69, vi.

21. Ranalli NJ, Kline DG, McGarvey ML, et al. Clinical problem-solving: brachial plexus closed injury and reconstruction. Neurosurgery 2008;62(6):1330–8 [discussion: 1338–9].

22. Bertelli JA, Ghizoni MF. Results of c5 root grafting to the musculocutaneous nerve using pedicled, vascularized ulnar nerve grafts. J Hand Surg Am 2009; 34(10):1821–6.

23. Bertelli JA, Ghizoni MF. Nerve root grafting and distal nerve transfers for C5-C6 brachial plexus injuries. J Hand Surg Am 2010;35(5):769–75.

24. Haninec P, Samal F, Tomas R, et al. Direct repair (nerve grafting), neurotization, and end-to-side neurorrhaphy in the treatment of brachial plexus injury. J Neurosurg 2007;106(3):391–9.

25. Bertelli JA, Ghizoni MF. Reconstruction of complete palsies of the adult brachial plexus by root grafting using long grafts and nerve transfers to target nerves. J Hand Surg Am 2010;35(10):1640–6.

26. Kandenwein JA, Kretschmer T, Engelhardt M, et al. Surgical interventions for traumatic lesions of the brachial plexus: a retrospective study of 134 cases. J Neurosurg 2005;103(4):614–21.

27. Terzis JK, Kostopoulos VK. Vascularized ulnar nerve graft: 151 reconstructions for posttraumatic brachial plexus palsy. Plast Reconstr Surg 2009;123(4): 1276–91.

28. Xu W, Lu J, Xu J, et al. Full-length ulnar nerve harvest by means of endoscopy for contralateral C7 nerve root transfer in the treatment of brachial plexus injuries. Plast Reconstr Surg 2006;118(3):689–93 [discussion: 694–5].

29. Allieu Y, Privat JM, Bonnel F. Paralysis in root avulsion of the brachial plexus. Neurotization by the spinal accessory nerve. Clin Plast Surg 1984;11(1):133–6.

30. Songcharoen P, Mahaisavariya B, Chotigavanich C. Spinal accessory neurotization for restoration of elbow flexion in avulsion injuries of the brachial plexus. J Hand Surg Am 1996;21(3):387–90.

31. Bonnard C, Narakas A. Neurotization using the spinal accessory nerve in the brachial plexus lesions. In: Alnot JY, Narakas A, editors. Traumatic brachial plexus injuries. Paris: Expansion Scientifique Française; 1996. p. 156–66.

32. Chuang DC, Lee GW, Hashem F, et al. Restoration of shoulder abduction by nerve transfer in avulsed brachial plexus injury: evaluation of 99 patients with various nerve transfers. Plast Reconstr Surg 1995;96(1):122–8.

33. Cardenas-Mejia A, O'Boyle CP, Chen KT, et al. Evaluation of single-, double-, and triple-nerve transfers for shoulder abduction in 90 patients with supraclavicular brachial plexus injury. Plast Reconstr Surg 2008;122(5):1470–8.

34. Jobe CM, Kropp WE, Wood VE. Spinal accessory nerve in a trapezius-splitting surgical approach. J Shoulder Elbow Surg 1996;5(3):206–8.

35. Colbert SH, Mackinnon S. Posterior approach for double nerve transfer for restoration of shoulder function in upper brachial plexus palsy. Hand (N Y) 2006;1(2):71–7.

36. Pruksakorn D, Sananpanich K, Khunamornpong S, et al. Posterior approach technique for accessory-suprascapular nerve transfer: a cadaveric study of the anatomical landmarks and number of myelinated axons. Clin Anat 2007;20(2):140–3.

37. Vathana T, Larsen M, de Ruiter GC, et al. An anatomic study of the spinal accessory nerve: extended harvest permits direct nerve transfer to distal plexus targets. Clin Anat 2007;20(8):899–904.

38. Guan SB, Hou CL, Chen DS, et al. Restoration of shoulder abduction by transfer of the spinal accessory nerve to suprascapular nerve through dorsal approach: a clinical study. Chin Med J (Engl) 2006;119(9):707–12.

39. Bishop AT. Functioning free-muscle transfer for brachial plexus injury. Hand Clin 2005;21(1):91–102.

40. Doi K, Muramatsu K, Hattori Y, et al. Restoration of prehension with the double free muscle technique following complete avulsion of the brachial plexus. Indications and long-term results. J Bone Joint Surg Am 2000;82(5):652–66.

41. Seddon HJ. Nerve grafting. J Bone Joint Surg Br 1963;45:447–61.

42. Bhandari P, Sadhotra L, Bhargava P, et al. Effectiveness of intercostal nerves in restoration of elbow flexion in devastating brachial plexus injuries. IJNT 2009;6(1):53–8.

43. Chuang DC, Yeh MC, Wei FC. Intercostal nerve transfer of the musculocutaneous nerve in avulsed brachial plexus injuries: evaluation of 66 patients. J Hand Surg Am 1992;17(5):822–8.

44. Coulet B, Boretto JG, Lazerges C, et al. A comparison of intercostal and partial ulnar nerve transfers in restoring elbow flexion following upper brachial plexus injury (C5-C6+/-C7). J Hand Surg Am 2010;35(8):1297–303.

45. Merrell GA, Barrie KA, Katz DL, et al. Results of nerve transfer techniques for restoration of shoulder and elbow function in the context of a meta-analysis of the English literature. J Hand Surg Am 2001;26(2):303–14.

46. Nagano A, Tsuyama N, Ochiai N, et al. Direct nerve crossing with the intercostal nerve to treat avulsion injuries of the brachial plexus. J Hand Surg Am 1989;14(6):980–5.

47. Minami M, Ishii S. Satisfactory elbow flexion in complete (preganglionic) brachial plexus injuries: produced by suture of third and fourth intercostal nerves to musculocutaneous nerve. J Hand Surg Am 1987;12(6):1114–8.

48. Narakas AO. Thoughts on neurotization or nerve transfers in irreparable nerve lesions. Clin Plast Surg 1984;11(1):153–9.

49. Millesi H. Surgical management of brachial plexus injuries. J Hand Surg Am 1977;2(5):367–78.

50. Dolenc VV. Intercostal neurotization of the peripheral nerves in avulsion plexus injuries. Clin Plast Surg 1984;11(1):143–7.

51. Ogino T, Naito T. Intercostal nerve crossing to restore elbow flexion and sensibility of the hand for a root avulsion type of brachial plexus injury. Microsurgery 1995;16(8):571–7.

52. Nagano A. Treatment of brachial plexus injury. J Orthop Sci 1998;3(1):71–80.

53. Ihara K, Doi K, Sakai K, et al. Restoration of sensibility in the hand after complete brachial plexus injury. J Hand Surg Am 1996;21(3):381–6.

54. Kovachevich R, Kircher MF, Wood CM, et al. Complications of intercostal nerve transfer for brachial plexus reconstruction. J Hand Surg Am 2010;35(12):1995–2000.

55. Giddins GE, Kakkar N, Alltree J, et al. The effect of unilateral intercostal nerve transfer upon lung function. J Hand Surg Br 1995;20(5):675–6.

56. Lurje A. Concerning surgical treatment of traumatic injury of the upper division of the brachial plexus (Erb's-type). Ann Surg 1948;127(2):317–26.

57. Gu YD, Wu MM, Zhen YL, et al. Phrenic nerve transfer for brachial plexus motor neurotization. Microsurgery 1989;10(4):287–9.

58. Lijie T, Zhenglang X, Xu W, et al. Mobilization of the phrenic nerve in the thoracic cavity by video-assisted thoracic surgery. Techniques and initial experience. Surg Endosc 2001;15(10):1156–8.

59. Xu WD, Gu YD, Xu JG, et al. Full-length phrenic nerve transfer by means of video-assisted thoracic surgery in treating brachial plexus avulsion injury. Plast Reconstr Surg 2002;110(1):104–9 [discussion: 110–1].

60. Xu WD, Lu JZ, Qiu YQ, et al. Hand prehension recovery after brachial plexus avulsion injury by performing a full-length phrenic nerve transfer via endoscopic thoracic surgery. J Neurosurg 2008;108(6):1215–9.

61. Lin H, Hou C, Chen A, et al. Transfer of the phrenic nerve to the posterior division of the lower trunk to recover thumb and finger extension in brachial plexus palsy. J Neurosurg 2011;114(1):212–6.

62. Zhao X, Lao J, Hung LK, et al. Selective neurotization of the median nerve in the arm to treat brachial plexus palsy. Surgical technique. J Bone Joint Surg Am 2005;87(Suppl 1(Pt 1)):122–35.

63. Gu YD, Zhang GM, Chen DS, et al. Seventh cervical nerve root transfer from the contralateral healthy side for treatment of brachial plexus root avulsion. J Hand Surg Br 1992;17(5):518–21.

64. Songcharoen P, Wongtrakul S, Mahaisavariya B, et al. Hemi-contralateral C7 transfer to median nerve in the treatment of root avulsion brachial plexus injury. J Hand Surg Am 2001;26(6):1058–64.

65. Xu L, Gu Y, Xu J, et al. Contralateral C7 transfer via the prespinal and retropharyngeal route to repair brachial plexus root avulsion: a preliminary report. Neurosurgery 2008;63(3):553–8 [discussion: 558–9].

66. Zou YW, Wang ZJ, Yu H. Treatment of brachial plexus injury with modified contralateral C7 transfer. Orthop Surg 2010;2(1):14–8.

67. Feng J, Wang T, Gu Y, et al. Contralateral C7 transfer to lower trunk via a subcutaneous tunnel across the anterior surface of chest and neck for total root avulsion of the brachial plexus: a preliminary report. Neurosurgery 2010;66(6 Suppl Operative):252–63 [discussion: 263].

68. Chuang DC, Cheng SL, Wei FC, et al. Clinical evaluation of C7 spinal nerve transection: 21 patients with at least 2 years' follow-up. Br J Plast Surg 1998;51(4):285–90.

69. Gu Y, Xu J, Chen L, et al. Long term outcome of contralateral C7 transfer: a report of 32 cases. Chin Med J (Engl) 2002;115(6):866–8.

70. Terzis JK, Kokkalis ZT, Kostopoulos E. Contralateral C7 transfer in adult plexopathies. Hand Clin 2008; 24(4):389–400, vi.

71. Gu YD. Contralateral C7 root transfer over the last 20 years in China. Chin Med J (Engl) 2007;120(13): 1123–6.

72. Zheng XY, Hou CL, Gu YD, et al. Repair of brachial plexus lower trunk injury by transferring brachialis muscle branch of musculocutaneous nerve: anatomic feasibility and clinical trials. Chin Med J (Engl) 2008;121(2):99–104.

73. Gu Y, Wang H, Zhang L, et al. Transfer of brachialis branch of musculocutaneous nerve for finger flexion: anatomic study and case report. Microsurgery 2004; 24(5):358–62.

74. Dong Z, Gu YD, Zhang CG, et al. Clinical use of supinator motor branch transfer to the posterior interosseous nerve in C7-T1 brachial plexus palsies. J Neurosurg 2010;113(1):113–7.

75. Bertelli JA, Ghizoni MF. Transfer of supinator motor branches to the posterior interosseous nerve in C7-T1 brachial plexus palsy. J Neurosurg 2010; 113(1):129–32.

76. Bincaz LE, Cherifi H, Alnot JY. Palliative tendon transfer for reanimation of the wrist and finger extension lag. Report of 14 transfers for radial nerve palsies and ten transfers for brachial plexus lesions. Chir Main 2002;21(1):13–22 [in French].

77. Bonnard C, Narakas A. Restoration of hand function after brachial plexus injury. Hand Clin 1995;11(4): 647–56.

78. Bertelli JA, Ghizoni MF. Brachialis muscle transfer to reconstruct finger flexion or wrist extension in

79. Ropars M, Dreano T, Siret P, et al. Long-term results of tendon transfers in radial and posterior interosseous nerve paralysis. J Hand Surg Br 2006;31(5): 502–6.

80. Goubier JN, Teboul F, Oberlin C. Extensor tenodesis for plexic hands with C7 to T1 or C8, T1 root avulsions: a new technique. Tech Hand Up Extrem Surg 2006;10(4):252–4.

81. Bertelli JA, Ghizoni MF, Tacca CP. Transfer of the supinator muscle to the extensor pollicis brevis for thumb extension reconstruction in C7-T1 brachial plexus palsy. J Hand Surg Eur Vol 2010; 35(1):29–31.

82. Oberlin C, Durand S, Fox M, et al. Transfer of the recovered biceps to the long flexors of the digits to restore grip function following complete traumatic brachial plexus palsy. Chir Main 2010; 29(3):167–71.

83. Terzis JK, Barmpitsioti A. Wrist fusion in posttraumatic brachial plexus palsy. Plast Reconstr Surg 2009;124(6):2027–39.

84. Chuang DC. Functioning free-muscle transplantation for the upper extremity. Hand Clin 1997;13(2): 279–89.

85. Doi K, Hattori Y, Tan SH, et al. Basic science behind functioning free muscle transplantation. Clin Plast Surg 2002;29(4):483–95, v–vi.

86. Manktelow RT, Zuker RM. The principles of functioning muscle transplantation: applications to the upper arm. Ann Plast Surg 1989;22(4):275–82.

87. Anastakis DJ, Chen R, Davis KD, et al. Cortical plasticity following upper extremity injury and reconstruction. Clin Plast Surg 2005;32(4):617–34, viii.

88. Hattori Y, Doi K, Sakamoto S, et al. Sensory recovery of the hand with intercostal nerve transfer following complete avulsion of the brachial plexus. Plast Reconstr Surg 2009;123(1):276–83.

89. Chuang DC. Nerve transfer with functioning free muscle transplantation. Hand Clin 2008;24(4): 377–88, vi.

90. Terzis JK, Kostopoulos VK. Free muscle transfer in posttraumatic plexopathies: part III. The hand. Plast Reconstr Surg 2009;124(4):1225–36.

91. Gousheh J, Arasteh E. Upper limb functional restoration in old and complete brachial plexus paralysis. J Hand Surg Eur Vol 2010;35(1):16–22.

92. Anastakis DJ, Malessy MJ, Chen R, et al. Cortical plasticity following nerve transfer in the upper extremity. Hand Clin 2008;24(4):425–44, vi–vii.

93. Manduch M, Bezuhly M, Anastakis DJ, et al. Serial fMRI of adaptive changes in primary sensorimotor cortex following thumb reconstruction. Neurology 2002;59(8):1278–81.

94. Lundborg G. Richard P. Bunge memorial lecture. Nerve injury and repair–a challenge to the plastic brain. J Peripher Nerv Syst 2003;8(4):209–26.

95. Rosen B, Lundborg G. Training with a mirror in rehabilitation of the hand. Scand J Plast Reconstr Surg Hand Surg 2005;39(2):104–8.

96. Hierner R, Berger AK. Did the partial contralateral C7-transfer fulfil our expectations? Results after 5 year experience. Acta Neurochir Suppl 2007;100:33–5.

97. Kus H, Pielka S, Rutowski R. Transfer of nerve fibres from C7 of the contralateral side to neurotisize segments of completely avalsed brachial plexus. J Hand Surg 1996;21B(1):20.

98. Liu J, Pho RW, Kour AK, et al. Neurologic deficit and recovery in the donor limb following cross-C7 transfer in brachial-plexus injury. J Reconstr Microsurg 1997;13(4):237–42 [discussion: 242–3].

99. Sammer DM, Kircher MF, Bishop AT, et al. Hemi-contralateral C7 transfer to the median nerve: outcomes and complications. Paper presented at: Combined ASSH and ASHT Annual Meeting. San Francisco, September 4, 2009.

Treatment of Nonunion and Malunion Following Hand Fractures

Warren C. Hammert, MD

KEYWORDS

- Nonunion • Malunion • Phalanx • Metacarpal
- Hand fracture complication

Fractures in the upper extremity are common, accounting for about 1.5% of emergency department visits, with hand fractures comprising 40% of all upper extremity fractures.[1] Complications can and do occur, making their diagnosis and treatment an important part of caring for patients with these injuries.

Malunions are common in the metacarpals and phalanges, although not all are clinically significant. The common fifth metacarpal neck, or boxer's fracture, usually heals with an apex dorsal deformity, but this is rarely problematic. By contrast, those with rotational or angular deformities often affect hand function, and treatment is necessary. Nonunions, on the other hand, are uncommon, but when they occur are often significant and inevitably require treatment. Nonunions are often associated with other conditions such as tendon and nerve injuries, and as a result sometimes salvage procedures, such as arthrodesis or amputation, are the best treatment.[2]

NONUNION

Delayed unions often occur in the hand, but will eventually heal and do not require intervention, whereas nonunions are more common with infection and open fractures, and these will inevitably require operative treatment. Occasionally they may result from metabolic abnormalities, such as low calcium or vitamin D, but once the metabolic abnormality is corrected, union will typically follow. Radiographic appearance alone is not a reliable indicator of nonunion, but with clinical instability or deformity, treatment should be considered because prolonged immobilization is poorly tolerated and permanent stiffness will occur.

Timing for the diagnosis of nonunion is variable, but generally requires consecutive radiographs without signs of progressive healing for a period of 4 to 6 months. The pathophysiology of the nonunion is hypertrophic or atrophic, with atrophic being much more common in the hand.[3] Hypertrophic nonunions display callous formation, but without bridging callous between fracture segments. With rigid fixation, union will typically occur. Atrophic nonunions do not exhibit callous and often reveal resorption at the site of the fracture. Resorption may be secondary to impaired blood supply, infection, metabolic conditions such as smoking or diabetes, or soft-tissue interposition between the fracture ends. Technical difficulties from a previous operative procedure, such as overdistraction of the fracture site, devascularization from exposure, or inadequate fixation can also lead to nonunion. Preoperative blood work, including a white blood cell count, erythrocyte sedimentation rate, and C-reactive protein, can be helpful and provide a means to follow recovery in the event of an infection. Intraoperative bone cultures should be obtained to determine specific organisms and to guide antibiotic choice. Surgical principles include eradication of any residual infection, debridement of nonviable bone, and stabilization of the fracture segments. Bone graft is often required to achieve union.[3]

I have no conflicts of interest and nothing of financial interest to disclose.
Department of Orthopaedic Surgery, University of Rochester Medical Center, 601 Elmwood Avenue, Box 665, Rochester, NY 14642, USA
E-mail address: Warren_Hammert@URMC.Rochester.edu

Clin Plastic Surg 38 (2011) 683–695
doi:10.1016/j.cps.2011.08.001

Arthrodesis is useful for articular nonunions associated with joint stiffness. This digit is likely to remain stiff following healing of the nonunion, and arthrodesis allows for internal fixation to cross the joint, allowing for a longer implant and more stability. Both the joint and nonunion site should be debrided, bone grafted, and stabilized (**Fig. 1**).[2]

Nonunions commonly occur in the tuft of the distal phalanx, but are rarely symptomatic. These fractures are typically the result of crush injuries and are associated with nail bed injuries. Despite nail bed repair some of these will fail to unite, which may result in an unstable tip of the finger and, depending on the digit, may be problematic for the patient. When a significant amount of bone is missing, amputation revision may be the best treatment, as bone grafting on the tip of the phalanx is prone to resorb.

When the nonunion is in the shaft of the distal phalanx, this can often be treated with compression across the nonunion site, either through an open approach or with percutaneous compression screw placement (**Fig. 2**).

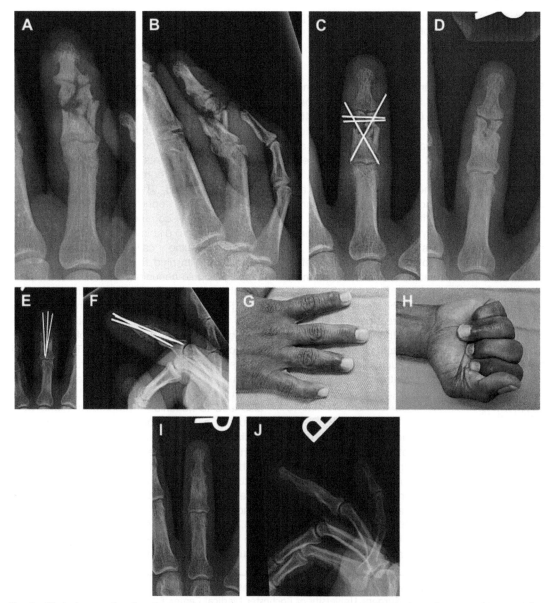

Fig. 1. Clinical example of patient with comminuted open fracture of middle phalanx. Preoperative posterior-anterior (*A*) and oblique (*B*) radiographs. Initial stabilization was with Kirschner (k)-wires (*C*). Persistent painful nonunion 8 months following injury (*D*) treated with correction of nonunion with bone graft and arthrodesis or arthritic distal interphalangeal (DIP) joint (*E, F*). Final clinical (*G, H*) and radiographic (*I, J*) appearance.

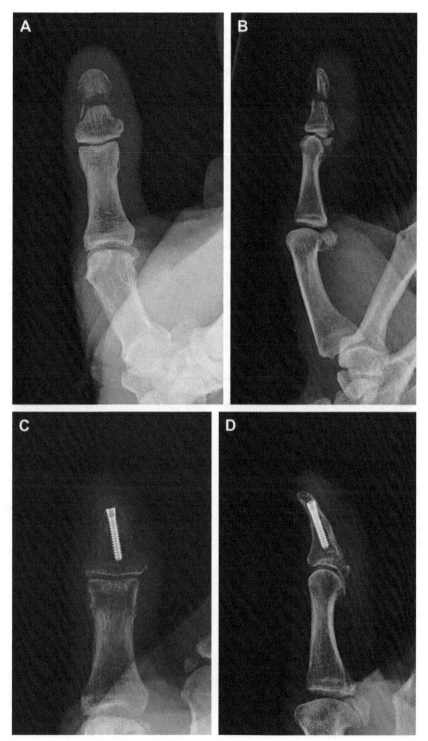

Fig. 2. Clinical example of distal phalanx nonunion in a thumb. The patient had pain and instability with pinch. Preoperative posterior-anterior (*A*) and lateral (*B*) radiographs. Postoperative radiographs (*C*, *D*) following open curettage of the nonunion site and placement of headless compression screw (no bone graft was used).

Metacarpal, Proximal, and Middle Phalanges

For shaft nonunions, rigid fixation is preferred when there is adequate soft-tissue coverage. The plate size is typically larger than would be used for an acute fracture in the same location. Unfortunately, especially in the phalanges, the soft tissue is often compromised, making plate fixation impossible (**Fig. 3**). The nonunion site is exposed and nonviable bone is debrided. The void is filled with bone graft and fixation is applied. Early motion is preferred to promote tendon gliding and to minimize adhesions, as these digits are typically stiff from the previous injury.

Amputation should be considered for cases with sensory loss, stiffness, persistent infection, or poor soft-tissue coverage. A stiff digit is often a liability to hand function and, even if the nonunion were to heal, the digit remains stiff and can impair hand function (**Fig. 4**). Recovery following amputation is often rapid, and leads to improvement in function of the hand.

Nonsurgical treatment of nonunions with bone stimulators has been described. An external bone stimulator is applied over the skin or cast, and ultrasonic or pulsed electromagnetic waves are used to induce healing. Current evidence for the effectiveness of external bone stimulation in the hand is limited to case reports, therefore further evidence is needed to determine the true efficacy of this treatment.

MALUNION

Malunions occur when a fracture heals in nonanatomic position; this can result in rotation, angulation, or shortening to varying degrees. Rotational deformities manifest with scissoring or crossing of the fingers in flexion (**Fig. 5**). This appearance is often not evident with the fingers in extension, but can result in weakness and difficulty with dexterity. These rotational deformities typically occur following oblique or spiral fractures. Lateral angular deformities result from either intraarticular malunion with displacement of one condyle or with comminution and collapse on one side. These deformities are often evident with the digits in extension and are exacerbated with flexion, resulting in scissoring of the digit. When the fracture is inadequately treated, these deformities may result in a malunion.

Metacarpal fractures and malunions typically have an apex dorsal angulation secondary to the pull of the intrinsic tendons. Proximal phalanx fractures and malunions typically have apex volar angulation, whereas fractures of the middle phalanx have variable angulation depending on their location in relation to the flexor digitorum superficialis (FDS) insertion, with those proximal to the FDS insertion typically apex dorsal and those distal being apex volar.

Shortening of the digit typically occurs following healing of a comminuted fracture or those with segmental bone loss. Angular deformity (dorsal-volar direction) can create relative shortening (without actual bone loss), affecting the extensor mechanism. Strauch and colleagues[4] demonstrated that 2 mm of metacarpal shortening results in 7° extensor lag, but this may not be as relevant because of the ability of the metacarpophalangeal (MCP) joint to hyperextend. Proximal phalanx malunions with apex volar angulation may result in pseudoclawing, with hyperextension of the MCP and extension lag at the proximal interphalangeal (PIP) joint. Vahey and colleagues[5] reported that 1 mm of shortening results in 12° of lag when the shortening is in the proximal phalanx, with increasing angulation resulting in increased lag.

Malunions Involving the Distal Interphalangeal Joint

Malunions of the distal phalanx articular surface are common as mallet fractures heal, many times as fibrous union, but these tend to remodel. Long-term osteoarthritis is possible radiographically, but there is no evidence to determine the incidence of clinical symptoms. When an extension lag is present at the distal interphalangeal (DIP) joint and volar plate laxity allows hyperextension at the PIP, a swan-neck deformity results that can adversely affect hand function. Treatment is directed at restoring the articular surface and thus minimizing the extension lag at the DIP joint, which will correct the secondary PIP joint hyperextension (**Fig. 6**).

Malunions Around the Proximal Interphalangeal Joint

When the fracture is in or near the joint and heals in a malunited position, deformity will result. Such deformity can include stiffness, pain, and rotational or angular deformities, affecting the function of the entire hand. Depending on the presence of arthritis, treatment may be with corrective osteotomy, arthrodesis, or arthroplasty, with autogenous tissue or a prosthetic implant. Arthrodesis and prosthetic arthroplasty are typically reserved for patients who have developed arthritis. Arthrodesis is preferred in the index finger because of the lateral stress from pinch, whereas arthroplasty is generally preferred in the other fingers to preserve motion and grip strength. Arthroplasty can be

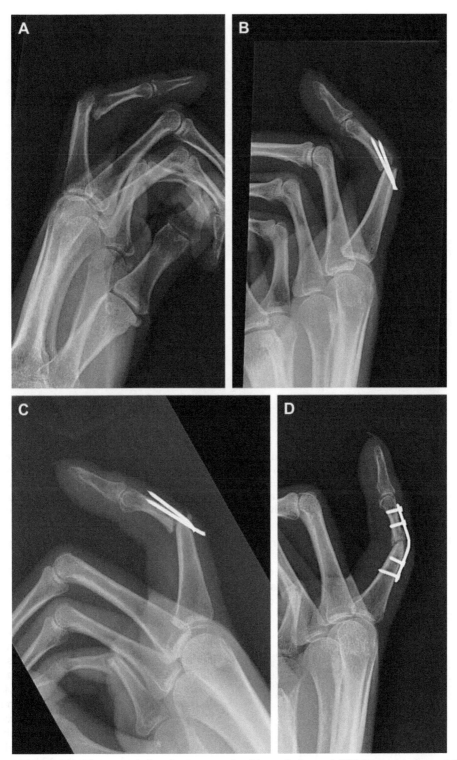

Fig. 3. Patient with scleroderma and chronic open proximal interphalangeal (PIP) joint dislocation (*A*) initially treated by attempted arthrodesis with k-wires (*B*) secondary to poor quality of soft tissue. Subsequent failure of k-wires and persistent nonunion (*C*) led to revision with bone graft and rigid fixation. (*D*) Early postoperative radiograph without evidence of union.

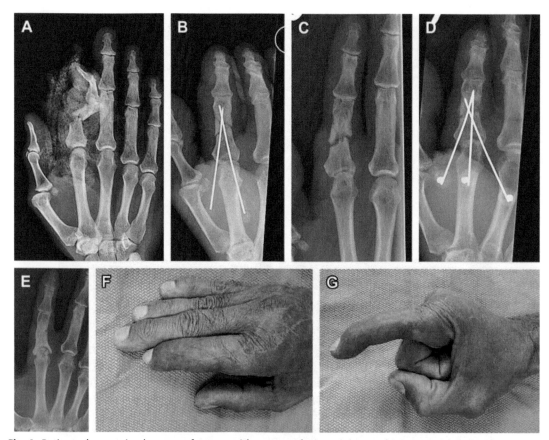

Fig. 4. Patient who sustained an open fracture with severe soft-tissue injury and injury to radial digital nerve and artery (*A*) initially treated with fracture debridement and stabilization with k-wires (*B*). Persistent symptomatic nonunion at was treated at 4 months (*C*) with bone grafting. The poor quality of the soft tissue prevented the use of rigid fixation, therefore k-wires were used for stabilization (*D*). Although the proximal phalanx healed, postoperative infection led to subsequent metacarpophalangeal (MCP) joint arthrosis (*E*) and a stiff painful digit (*F, G*). The patient was initially reluctant to have the finger amputated, but now has requested amputation.

expected to relieve pain, but postoperative motion is similar to preoperative motion.

Intra-articular malunions at the base of the middle phalanx are often the result of dorsal fracture dislocations, whereby the contour of the middle phalanx is lost and resultant dorsal

Fig. 5. Right middle finger with rotational malunion following nonoperative management of metacarpal fracture.

subluxation of the middle phalanx is present. When addressed early, before the onset of arthritis, this can be treated by resurfacing the base of the middle phalanx. The most common forms are volar plate arthroplasty hemi-hamate arthroplasty.

The indications are the same for both procedures and the decision is based on the surgeon's preference, but the current trend seems to be for the hemi-hamate arthroplasty, based on the greater number of articles in the recent literature. Both procedures are performed through the volar approach using a Brunner (zig-zag) incision. The digital neurovascular bundles are mobilized to prevent injury when the joint is exposed. The flexor sheath is opened between the A2 and A4 pulleys, and the flexor tendons are retracted to expose the volar aspect of the PIP joint. The volar plate is released distally and the collateral ligaments are released from the middle phalanx. The joint is exposed by retracting the neurovascular bundles

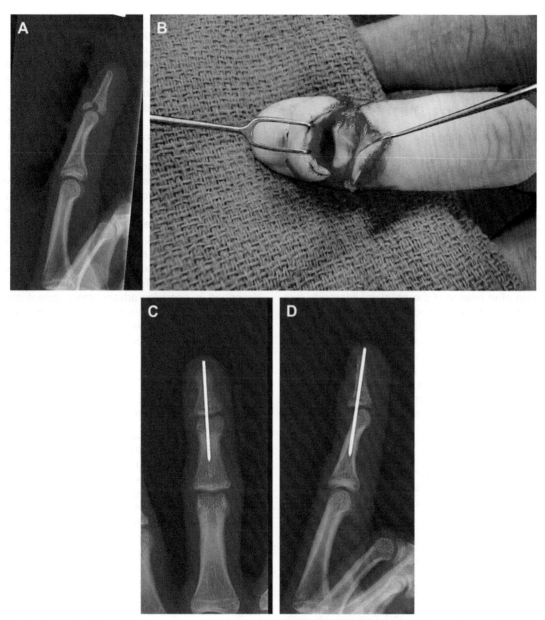

Fig. 6. Nonunion (fibrous) union of a mallet fracture 2 months following injury. (*A*) The patient had PIP joint hyperextension and early swan-neck deformity secondary to the mallet fracture. The nonunion was corrected through an open approach (*B*), and stabilized with k-wire through the fracture segment and across the DIP joint (*C, D*).

and flexor tendons, and hyperextending the digit ("shotgunning"), allowing the dorsal aspect of the proximal and middle phalanges to come together and thus allow visualization of the entire articular surface (**Fig. 7**).

For volar plate arthroplasty, it is important to excise the collateral ligaments.[6] A transverse mark is made in the middle phalanx, and the volar base is removed to create a trough where the volar plate can be advanced. The bone is cut, and the remaining bone is debrided to create a smooth surface into which the volar plate can be advanced. The joint is repositioned, and the volar plate is advanced and secured with transosseous sutures and tied over the dorsal aspect of the middle phalanx. The joint is pinned in slight flexion for 3 weeks and then motion is begun with an extension-blocking splint.[7,8]

The hemi-hamate arthroplasty is performed through the same exposure, shotgunning the joint

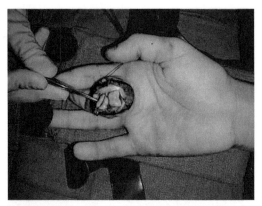

Fig. 7. Example of PIP joint exposure with the joint "shotgunned" open. Flexor tendons and digital neurovascular bundles are mobilized and retracted to protect them during exposure.

open after release of the collateral ligaments (not excised, as they are used during closure to provide additional lateral stability) and retraction of the flexor tendons. A transverse mark is made in the middle phalanx and bone is removed, creating a ledge on which to place the hamate graft. Dimensions of the graft are measured in dorsal-volar, radial-ulnar, and proximal-distal dimensions. Following preparation of the middle phalanx, the hand is pronated and the carpometacarpal joint of the fourth and fifth finger is confirmed with fluoroscopy. Following exposure of the dorsal hamate through a dorsal transverse incision, the dimensions of the defect are transferred to the hamate and the graft is harvested (**Fig. 8**).

It is preferable to harvest a graft slightly larger than anticipated, and trim it to fit the middle phalanx. A portion of the proximal dorsal hamate can be removed to allow proper contour as the graft is harvested. The graft is secured with small screws or headless compression screws, providing stable fixation and allowing for early motion. The thickness of the cartilage on the hamate is often thicker than the base of the middle phalanx, giving the radiographic appearance of malpositioned graft, but this can be ignored as the positioning is confirmed visually during placement of the graft and confirmed following fixation.[9] Care must be taken when placing the graft to recreate the curvature of the base of the middle phalanx. If the graft is placed too vertical, the middle phalanx will sublux in a dorsal direction—stability for this joint is based on the recreation of the contour of the base of the middle phalanx (**Fig. 9**). Postoperatively, motion is begun around the fifth day with a figure-of-8 splint to provide lateral stability and to block the final 20° of

extension. Biomechanical cadaver studies have demonstrated this graft to be suitable, with minimal donor site morbidity.[10]

Intra-articular malunions of the proximal phalanx are challenging to treat. It is easier to correct the malunion with larger articular segments and while the fracture site is visible. These malunions often present with angular deformity and digital stiffness. Concomitant procedures, such as capsulotomy and tenolysis, are often necessary and can be completed at the same time. For mature malunions, these may be addressed with an extra-articular osteotomy to improve alignment if the surgeon is willing to accept the intra-articular incongruity and subsequent arthrosis. With intra-articular osteotomies, the small fragments are challenging to stabilize and the blood supply can be compromised, leading to resorption. For unicondylar malunions, Teoh and colleagues[11] have described a condylar advancement osteotomy, which involves an intra-articular wedge resection and proximal extension into the shaft, allowing stabilization with interfragmentary screws in the diaphyseal bone. This approach creates a large fragment that is much easier to rigidly stabilize (**Fig. 10**).

Malunions Around the Metacarpophalangeal Joint

Malunions involving the MCP joint are less common than those at the PIP joint, but when they occur can be more difficult to treat. The principles for treatment are the same as for addressing malunions around the PIP joint. Early correction of a malunion is addressed with an intra-articular osteotomy. Mature malunions often have arthritic changes and, when symptomatic, can be addressed with arthroplasty or arthrodesis. Arthroplasty is preferred in the middle, ring, and small fingers. The index finger creates a special challenge because the lateral pinch forces can lead to implant failure, but arthrodesis of the MCP joint precludes placing the hand flat and reaching into tight places such as a pants pocket, so the decision must be individualized, taking into account the probable need for revision surgery when arthroplasty is chosen.

Shaft Malunions

The middle phalanx has a higher ratio of cortical to cancellous bone, and thus is slower to heal. Malunions in the shaft often result in a combination of deformities, including rotation, angulation, and shortening, but the deformity on one plane is usually the predominant functional problem that leads to consideration of operative treatment.

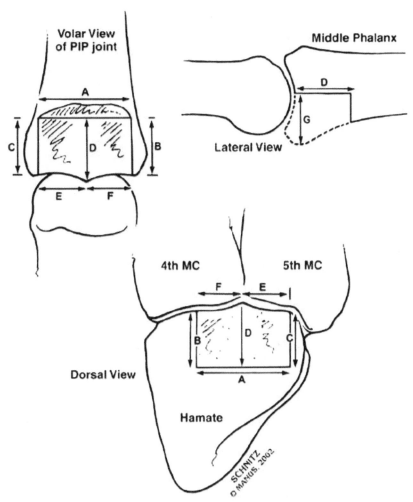

Fig. 8. Schematic of the prepared base of the middle phalanx (dimensions of the defect shown) and the corresponding donor site on the hamate (note the central ridge and dimensions on the required graft). (*From* Williams RM, Kiefhaber TR, Sommerkamp TG, et al. Treatment of unstable dorsal pip joint fracture dislocations with the hemi-hamate autograft. J Hand Surg Am 2003;28:859; with permission.)

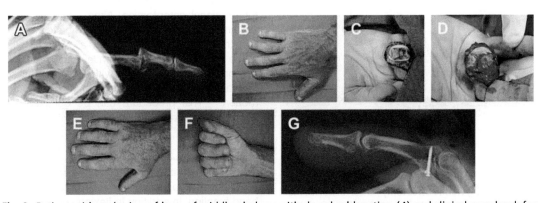

Fig. 9. Patient with malunion of base of middle phalanx with dorsal subluxation (*A*) and clinical angular deformity (*B*). Exposure of the joint before creating the graft recipient site (*C*) (note there is early arthrosis on the head of the proximal phalanx) and following fixation of the hemi-hamate graft (*D*). Postoperative clinical (*E*, *F*) and radiographic (*G*) appearance.

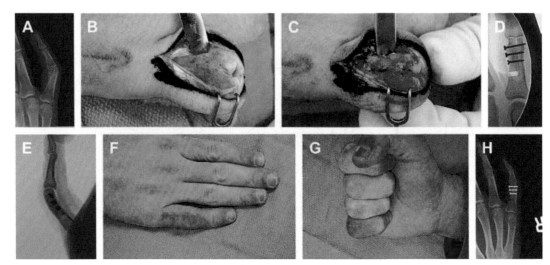

Fig. 10. Case of proximal phalanx unicondylar malunion resulting in angular deformity. (*A*) Preoperative radiograph demonstrating deformity. (*B*) Dorsal exposure of PIP joint and nonunion of radial condyle. (*C*) Appearance following condylar advancement osteotomy and stabilization with screws. Fluoroscopic images confirming adequate alignment and stabilization (*D, E*). Postoperative clinical (*F, G*) and radiographic (*H*) appearance.

Shortening needs to be corrected with an osteotomy through the fracture site to regain length, which requires rigid fixation and bone grafting. Angular deformities can be treated with an opening or closing wedge osteotomy. The closing wedge is technically easier, but can result in shortening of the digit (**Fig. 11**). The opening wedge is technically more demanding and will require bone grafting, and depending on fixation may require a structural graft, but is the only method that restores length (**Fig. 12**). Rotational deformities can be approached at the site of the malunion (**Fig. 13**) or in the proximal metacarpal region, with advocates for both.[12,13]

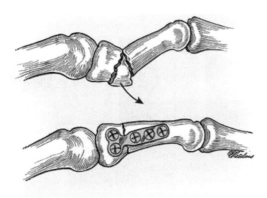

Fig. 11. Closing wedge osteotomy for correction of malunion of the proximal phalanx with volar angulation. (*From* Wolfe SW, Hotchkiss RN, Pederson WC, et al. Green's operative hand surgery. 6th ed. Philadelphia: Elsevier/Churchill Livingstone; 2011; with permission.)

Correction at the site of the deformity, whether in the phalanx or metacarpal, can allow for secondary procedures, such as tenolysis or capsulotomy, and prevent a zig-zag deformity, which occurs when correcting at a distant site. It can be technically more challenging when located near a joint. In the phalanges, treatment will require exposure through tendons, which must glide for adequate motion. Distant correction at the base of the metacarpal is technically easier, allows the osteotomy to be completed through metaphyseal bone, and avoids the extensor mechanism over the proximal phalanx, but has a limited amount of correction (<20°) secondary to the intermetacarpal ligament.[14]

Fixation is often achieved with plates and screws, with newer implants specifically designed for rotational osteotomies. Alternatively, Manktelow and Mahoney[15] have described a step osteotomy through the diaphysis, which allows correction at the site of the deformity with larger surface area for bony healing and fixation with wires or interfragmentary screws, allowing rigid fixation and early motion.[16] This procedure can be completed in the metacarpal or the phalanx (**Fig. 14**).

Thumb

The thumb has a different functional role from the other digits and is the most important digit for hand function. In addition to flexion and extension, the ability to pronate out of the plane of the palm allows for opposition. This greater degree of motion allows malunion to be better tolerated, and in the

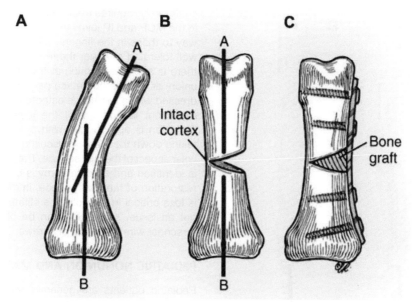

Fig. 12. Technique for lateral opening wedge phalangeal osteotomy. (*A*) Angular deformity in frontal plane. Lines A and B show alignment of proximal and distal portions of phalanx. (*B*) Corrective osteotomy leaving opposite cortex intact. (*C*) Corticocancellous graft inserted with lateral plate fixation. (Copyright Elizabeth Martin). (*From* Wolfe SW, Hotchkiss RN, Pederson WC, et al. Green's operative hand surgery. 6th ed. Philadelphia: Elsevier/Churchill Livingstone; 2011; with permission.)

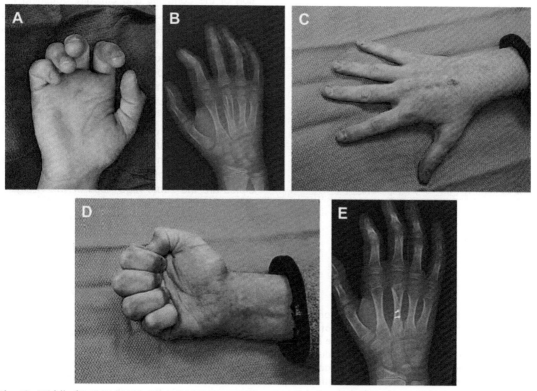

Fig. 13. Middle finger metacarpal malunion corrected at site of malunion following closed treatment of the fracture for 4 weeks. Preoperative clinical (*A*) and radiographic (*B*) appearance. Postoperative clinical (*C, D*) and radiographic appearance (*E*).

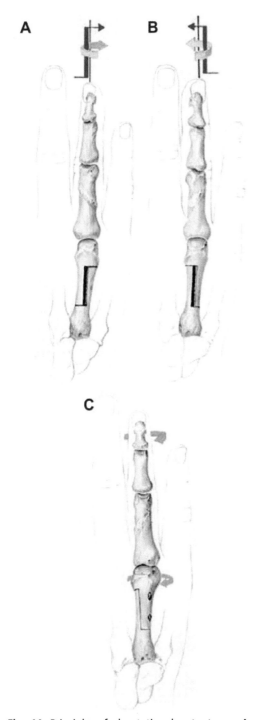

Fig. 14. Principle of derotational osteotomy. A z-shaped osteotomy is made with removal of a dorsal wedge of bone. (*A, B*) The direction of the distal cut dictates the rotation of the digit. (*C*) Reducing the gap rotates the distal part of the finger. (*From Jawa A, Zucchini M, Lauri G, et al. Modified step-cut osteotomy for metacarpal and phalangeal rotational deformity. J Hand Surg Am 2009;34:337; with permission.*)

shaft rarely requires treatment. Articular malunions in the MCP and IP joints are addressed in a similar way to those in the fingers, with arthrodesis being well tolerated at either the IP or MCP joints when there is adequate motion at the other joints. Malunion at the carpometacarpal joint can be addressed with a corrective osteotomy when there is significant incongruity of the joint surface. This condition is approached with a Wagner incision, taking down the thenar musculature to expose the volar aspect of the joint surface. The site of malunion is identified and an osteotomy is created to allow restoration of the joint surface. Immediate motion is less critical in this joint, as stiffness is typically not an issue, so fixation can be obtained using Kirschner wires (k-wires) or screws.

PEDIATRIC NONUNION AND MALUNION

Pediatric patients are generally thought to have significant capacity to remodel following fracture healing, and therefore can often tolerate malunion with minimal functional consequences. Fractures are often the result of the digit being caught or closed in locations such as a door or chair. Initial diagnosis may be compromised because of the younger age of the patient with incomplete ossification of the condyles and difficulty obtaining true lateral radiographs.[17] Delay in presentation and difficulty with clinical examination may also contribute to the development of malunion or nonunion.

Phalangeal neck fractures are a special subset, and have limited potential to remodel because of the distance from the physis, although case reports exist indicating complete remodeling and good function.[18,19] In addition, the loss of the retrocondylar fossa can create a block to flexion, compromising motion.

Nonunion of the thumb is more commonly involved than the other digits,[17] but treatment principles are the same regardless of which digit is affected. Nonunion typically requires open reduction and stabilization with the possible addition of bone graft. When treated early, Waters and colleagues[20] have described percutaneous reduction and stabilization. This technique involves inserting a k-wire into the malunion site through the dorsal callous and using it to mobilize and reduce the fracture, which is then stabilized by an additional wire.

In general, avascular necrosis involving these fractures is not common, although it can occur. Whereas nonunion is more common in the thumb, avascular necrosis associated with nonunion is more common in the small finger, presenting with stiffness.[21] Treatment and long-term outcomes for this condition have not been clearly delineated.

The decision to intervene must be carefully considered, as postoperative motion is unlikely to improve.

REFERENCES

1. Chung KC, Spilson SV. The frequency and epidemiology of hand and forearm fractures in the United States. J Hand Surg Am 2001;26(5):908–15.
2. Ring D. Malunion and nonunion of the metacarpals and phalanges. Instr Course Lect 2006;55:121–8.
3. Jupiter JB, Koniuch MP, Smith RJ. The management of delayed union and nonunion of the metacarpals and phalanges. J Hand Surg Am 1985; 10(4):457–66.
4. Strauch RJ, Rosenwasser MP, Lunt JG. Metacarpal shaft fractures: the effect of shortening on the extensor tendon mechanism. J Hand Surg Am 1998;23(3):519–23.
5. Vahey JW, Wegner DA, Hastings H 3rd. Effect of proximal phalangeal fracture deformity on extensor tendon function. J Hand Surg Am 1998;23(4): 673–81.
6. Eaton RG, Malerich MM. Volar plate arthroplasty of the proximal interphalangeal joint: a review of ten years' experience. J Hand Surg Am 1980;5(3): 260–8.
7. Burton RI, Campolattaro RM, Ronchetti PJ. Volar plate arthroplasty for osteoarthritis of the proximal interphalangeal joint: a preliminary report. J Hand Surg Am 2002;27(6):1065–72.
8. Blazar PE, Robbe R, Lawton JN. Treatment of dorsal fracture/dislocations of the proximal interphalangeal joint by volar plate arthroplasty. Tech Hand Up Extrem Surg 2001;5(3):148–52.
9. Williams RM, Kiefhaber TR, Sommerkamp TG, et al. Treatment of unstable dorsal proximal interphalangeal fracture/dislocations using a hemi-hamate autograft. J Hand Surg Am 2003;28(5):856–65.
10. Capo JT, Hastings H 2nd, Choung E, et al. Hemicondylar hamate replacement arthroplasty for proximal interphalangeal joint fracture dislocations: an assessment of graft suitability. J Hand Surg Am 2008;33(5):733–9.
11. Teoh LC, Yong FC, Chong KC. Condylar advancement osteotomy for correcting condylar malunion of the finger. J Hand Surg Br 2002;27(1):31–5.
12. Buchler U, Gupta A, Ruf S. Corrective osteotomy for post-traumatic malunion of the phalanges in the hand. J Hand Surg Br 1996;21(1):33–42.
13. Gollamudi S, Jones WA. Corrective osteotomy of malunited fractures of phalanges and metacarpals. J Hand Surg Br 2000;25(5):439–41.
14. Gross MS, Gelberman RH. Metacarpal rotational osteotomy. J Hand Surg Am 1985;10(1):105–8.
15. Manktelow RT, Mahoney JL. Step osteotomy: a precise rotation osteotomy to correct scissoring deformities of the fingers. Plast Reconstr Surg 1981;68(4):571–6.
16. Jawa A, Zucchini M, Lauri G, et al. Modified step-cut osteotomy for metacarpal and phalangeal rotational deformity. J Hand Surg Am 2009;34(2):335–40.
17. Al-Qattan MM, Cardoso E, Hassanain J, et al. Nonunion following subcapital (neck) fractures of the proximal phalanx of the thumb in children. J Hand Surg Br 1999;24(6):693–8.
18. Hennrikus WL, Cohen MR. Complete remodelling of displaced fractures of the neck of the phalanx. J Bone Joint Surg Br 2003;85(2):273–4.
19. Mintzer CM, Waters PM, Brown DJ. Remodelling of a displaced phalangeal neck fracture. J Hand Surg Br 1994;19(5):594–6.
20. Waters PM, Taylor BA, Kuo AY. Percutaneous reduction of incipient malunion of phalangeal neck fractures in children. J Hand Surg Am 2004;29(4): 707–11.
21. Al-Qattan MM. Nonunion and avascular necrosis following phalangeal neck fractures in children. J Hand Surg Am 2010;35(8):1269–74.

Thumb Reconstruction

Jeffrey B. Friedrich, MD[a,b,*], Nicholas B. Vedder, MD[a,b]

KEYWORDS

- Thumb - Reconstruction - Microsurgery - Hand
- Amputation

When thumb loss occurs because of trauma, replantation is the best method of reconstruction for most patients. When replantation is not possible, thumb reconstruction is necessary. The level of thumb amputation guides the type of reconstruction, and the level is based on physical examination and radiographic results. The reconstruction should be tailored to the patient's personal and professional needs. Because significant rehabilitation may be required, the patient must be a willing participant in the reconstruction and rehabilitation.

Functional compensation after distal third thumb loss is easily achieved; therefore, reconstruction at this level typically involves soft tissue only. Techniques such as the neurovascular advancement (Moberg) flap and the cross-finger flap reconstruction are reliable methods for reconstruction at this level. For losses in the middle third of the thumb, restoration of length is a priority. This priority can be addressed via absolute length restoration with metacarpal lengthening, osteoplastic reconstruction, or toe transfer; or via relative length restoration using phalangization of the thumb. Proximal third thumb losses are best treated with microsurgical reconstruction. However, in some cases, microsurgical reconstruction may not be possible. In these situations, transfer of another finger can provide an excellent thumb replacement. A normal finger (typically the index) can be pollicized to become a thumb. A damaged index finger can also be transferred (on-top plasty) to become a stable post for opposition, pinch, and grip.

Hand rehabilitation after reconstruction is absolutely necessary, especially after middle and proximal third reconstructions. Rehabilitation can last for months, and, for some procedures, such as neurovascular island flap reconstruction and digit transfer, sensory reeducation is an important part of the rehabilitation.

By far, the most common cause necessitating thumb reconstruction is trauma. Within the larger trauma classification, thumb injury can be the result of a variety of mechanisms, which include sharp cut, avulsion, and crush. There are some mechanisms that have characteristics of more than 1 injury type. This phenomenon is best illustrated by saw and lawn mower injuries, which have both cutting and crushing components, resulting in a larger zone of injury.

Other insults that can result in thumb loss requiring reconstruction include infections and neoplasms. Thumb reconstruction planning for tumor can be more deliberate than traumatic reconstruction and can often be performed at the time of tumor extirpation.[1]

Because there are many ways to reconstruct a deficient thumb, patients must be educated about the various options so that they may make an informed decision as to which type of reconstruction will serve them best in both the personal and professional settings. In addition to patient input regarding reconstructive methods, the patient must also commit to the reconstructive process and must be a good candidate medically, socially, and psychologically.

In many patients, thumb injuries occur in the workplace, and these patients are affected by the injury because their work requires significant hand use. In these patients, it is essential to work toward a thumb that has adequate length for both gripping and pinching, is stable during activities, has reasonable motion, and is sensate to give tactile input during these actions and to prevent recurrent ulceration or injury. However, adequate length, stability, motion, and sensibility are the

The authors have nothing to disclose.
[a] Division of Plastic Surgery, University of Washington, Seattle, WA, USA
[b] Department of Orthopedics, University of Washington, Seattle, WA, USA
* Corresponding author. 325 9th Avenue, Box 359796 (FedEx: Room 7EH70), Seattle, WA 98104.
E-mail address: jfriedri@uw.edu

end goals for any patient requiring thumb reconstruction, regardless of profession or vocation.[2]

The most important factor in patient selection is the amount and nature of tissue loss that must be reconstructed. The level of amputation is the easiest way to classify thumb deficiencies and is listed in thirds.[3] The distal third extends from the interphalangeal (IP) joint to the thumb tip. The middle third is the portion between IP joint and the metacarpal neck, and the proximal third is from the metacarpal neck to the carpometacarpal joint. Each amputation level presents unique challenges for the patient and the physician, and each level can be reconstructed with multiple modalities.

TREATMENT OPTIONS BASED ON INJURY ZONE
Distal Third Thumb

Thumb distal third amputations rarely require restoration of length because a thumb amputated through the IP joint remains functional.[3] Therefore, the chief goals of thumb tip reconstruction are soft tissue coverage of bone and length preservation. When there is no bone exposed at the tip of the thumb, closure can be achieved with either healing by secondary intention or skin grafting. Secondary healing of tip amputations up to 1.5 cm diameter with no exposed bone has been shown to result in good 2-point discrimination and is therefore a fairly easy method of achieving coverage.[4] Secondary healing by wound contraction has the advantage of bringing stable sensate skin together to close the defect, as opposed to skin grafts, which can remain insensate. Daily washing and dressing changes with nonadherent gauze are relatively easy for patients. Larger defects with a stable base, however, require skin grafting. Full-thickness grafts are usually preferred because they are more durable and stable, especially in the contact areas subject to pressure and shear. Small full-thickness skin grafts can be harvested from the hypothenar eminence or the volar wrist crease, whereas larger grafts are easily harvested from the groin crease.

When phalangeal bone is exposed at the thumb tip, vascularized coverage is required to preserve length, and there are several flaps that can accomplish this. The main criteria for flap selection are defect size and location of soft tissue loss, specifically if it is volar, dorsal, or at the tip. The Atasoy V-Y advancement flap provides good coverage of the tip of the distal phalanx when only a very small amount of bone is exposed.[5] The technique involves incising the volar pulp of the thumb in a V shape. Scissors are then used to carefully spread

the subcutaneous tissue. The subcutaneous attachments deep to the flap, which provide the neurovascular supply to the flap, are left intact. The flap is then advanced distally to close the defect, and the proximal aspect of the V incision is closed side to side, thereby creating the Y shape of the final scar. In practice, this flap is useful for only small defects because of the limited advancement that is possible.

The Moberg or neurovascular volar advancement flap is well suited to cover volar and tip defects of the thumb.[2] It is described as an advancement flap, but the amount of advancement achieved with the conventional rectangular Moberg flap is limited (**Fig. 1**). Instead, elevation of the flap combined with flexion of the IP joint of the thumb allows the flap to appear to advance distally. To elevate the flap, the midlateral lines are incised on either side of the thumb down to the base of the proximal phalanx. The flap is then elevated from the deeper tissues (flexor sheath) with sharp dissection. The flap includes both neurovascular bundles and all the subcutaneous tissue down to the flexor tendon sheath. The IP joint is flexed, and the flap is inset at the tip. If necessary, a Kirschner wire can be placed across the IP joint to stabilize it. This flap can cover a defect of 1 to 2 cm². A variation of the Moberg flap is the island flap that is incised transversely across the proximal base, and the only remaining attachments are the 2 neurovascular bundles. Unlike the conventional Moberg flap, this method allows a small amount of actual advancement, thereby covering more distal defects. The proximal gap at the base of the flap requires a small skin graft.

The cross-finger flap from the index finger is an excellent reconstructive technique for larger volar and tip defects of the thumb (up to 2–3 cm²).[6] The tissue transferred is reliable and durable.[7] The chief disadvantages of this technique are thumb coaptation to the index finger for 2 to 3 weeks and the need for a skin graft on the index donor site. A radially based rectangular flap is marked on the dorsum of the index proximal phalanx (**Fig. 2**). The flap is incised and elevated ulnarly to radially in the plane between the subcutaneous tissues and the extensor mechanism. It is very important to leave the paratenon on the extensor to allow skin grafting. When the radial aspect of the flap is reached, Cleland's ligament must be released along the length of the base of the flap to prevent kinking at the flap hinge. The flap is then inset to the thumb. A full-thickness skin graft is sutured to the dorsum of the index finger. At 2 or 3 weeks, the flap is divided, and the inset to the thumb is completed. After division,

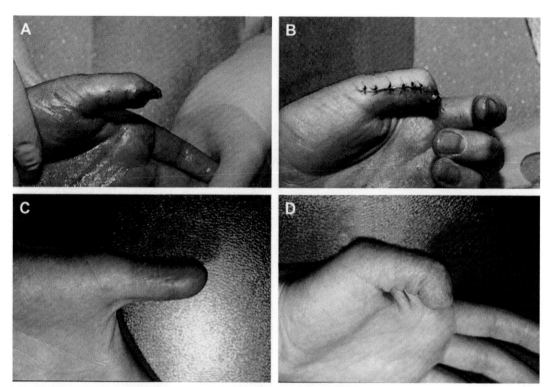

Fig. 1. (*A*) Thumb demonstrating tip amputation, (*B*) neurovascular advancement (Moberg) flap advanced to cover defect of tip, (*C, D*) healed thumb tip with good IP joint motion.

aggressive range of motion therapy for both the thumb and index finger should begin.

The Littler neurovascular island flap is a valuable tool in thumb reconstruction.[8] This flap is not typically used as a primary coverage flap, although it is possible to use it in that manner. The flap's most common use is for the restoration of sensation to the thumb pulp after reconstruction.[8,9] The flap is based on the ulnar neurovascular bundle of either the middle or ring finger. The ulnar side of the digit is chosen because its loss has minimal effect on grip and pinch activities. The dimensions of the flap needed are marked on the ulnar pulp of the chosen donor finger. Often, the flap requires harvesting of skin over the distal and middle phalanges of the donor finger. The flap is incised, and a midlateral or Bruner incision proceeding from the proximal aspect of the flap is made. The flap is elevated distally to proximally, and the entire ulnar neurovascular bundle is elevated in continuity with the flap. It is important to take the neurovascular bundle with a fairly thick sleeve of surrounding fatty tissue containing the vasa vasorum of the artery because that is the only source of venous outflow for the flap. Skeletonization of the artery results in venous congestion. The dissection must be done fairly proximally in the palm to allow adequate transposition to the thumb, and the

other branch of the common digital artery (the radial digital artery to the ring or small finger) must be divided. The common digital nerve can undergo intrafascicular splitting to allow adequate flap mobility. The flap is transposed to the thumb via subcutaneous tunnel, or a connecting incision from the donor site to the thumb can be made. The flap is then inset into the volar defect of the thumb. The donor site is grafted with full-thickness skin. In addition to postoperative restoration of motion, patients must work with a hand therapist on sensory re-education of the thumb.

The proximally based first dorsal metacarpal artery (FDMA) flap is very useful for thumb coverage, although it is better suited for dorsal thumb defects than palmar defects.[10,11] The flap's harvest causes virtually no donor site functional loss. The FDMA is found using a Doppler device, beginning proximally with the radial artery at the anatomic snuffbox. The radial artery then branches into the princeps pollicis artery radially and the FDMA ulnarly. The flap is centered over the FDMA. It is incised and dissected distally to proximally, leaving paratenon over the extensor mechanism for later skin grafting. To ensure inclusion of the FDMA with the flap, the thin fascia over the first dorsal interosseous muscle is included with the flap. Like the neurovascular island flap, the artery

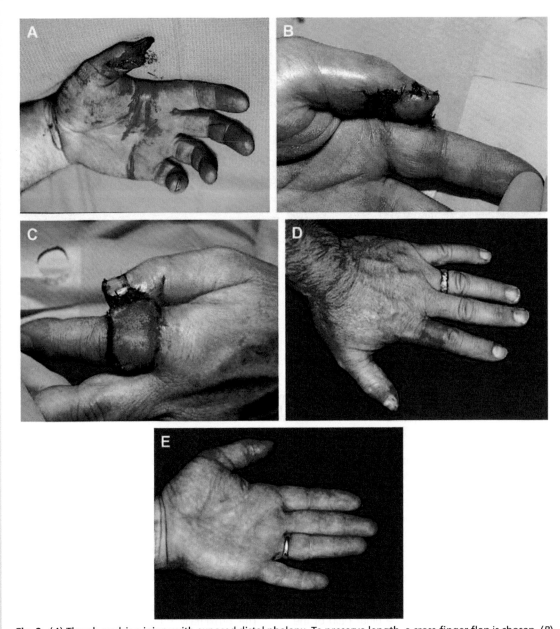

Fig. 2. (*A*) Thumb avulsion injury with exposed distal phalanx. To preserve length, a cross-finger flap is chosen. (*B*) Inset cross-finger flap. (*C*) Donor site of index finger covered with full-thickness skin graft. (*D, E*) Dorsal and volar views of reconstructed thumb and index finger donor site.

should not be skeletonized because this damages the venae comitantes. Once the flap is elevated, it can then be tunneled to the thumb in the subcutaneous plane or a connecting incision can be made. The donor defect is closed with a skin graft.

Middle Third Thumb

Loss in the middle third of the thumb is more functionally limiting than that of the distal third. Therefore, the priorities are both soft tissue coverage

and functional restoration. Commonly, the soft tissue coverage of amputations at this level will have been achieved acutely by revision amputation in which the skeletal components are shortened to allow primary closure.

Phalangization is a set of reconstruction techniques that increases the effective, rather than the absolute, length of the thumb. The chief component of phalangization is first webspace deepening.[3] Webspace deepening allows better thumb excursion, specifically both palmar and radial abduction, thereby improving the thumb's motion. First webspaces with mild or moderate tightness can be deepened with skin grafts or local tissue rearrangement (commonly Z-plasties). The main assessment of the webspace is whether the contracture is broad or a distinct linear band. If the contracture is broad, then scar contracture incision followed by skin grafting is used, whereas if the contracture is linear, local tissue rearrangement (usually Z-plasties) is the preferred treatment. Full-thickness skin grafts are usually used for the first web. A single Z-plasty can be used for a linear scar band, although 2 combined Z-plasties (4-flap Z-plasty or double-opposing Z-plasty) are uniquely suited to this anatomic area. When using either skin graft or Z-plasty for the first webspace, the adductor muscle is often tight due to scarring. A portion of the adductor muscle can be released to allow further thumb abduction before skin closure.

More significant first webspace contractures require transposition of a larger amount of vascularized tissue into the space. The dorsal hand flap can accomplish this task in a straightforward manner. This flap is proximally based on the dorsum of the hand and is vascularized by the metacarpal artery system. Unlike the FDMA flap, the dorsal hand flap is not an island flap and can include more than 1 metacarpal artery. The flap's distal extent is at the level of the metacarpal heads and is elevated in the plane between subcutaneous tissue and extensor tendon paratenon. The flap is then transposed radially into the first webspace after release of all constraining structures in the space. The donor site is skin grafted.

If the dorsal hand skin has been injured or if a larger amount of vascularized tissue is required to resurface both the first web and the thumb itself, then regional flaps are necessary. The radial forearm flap is an excellent choice for this. The utility of the radial forearm flap has been repeatedly demonstrated in a variety of hand reconstruction settings, including the thumb. The major drawback to use of a reverse-flow radial forearm flap is that its use may compromise future thumb reconstruction. Specifically, if a microvascular toe transfer is being considered for thumb reconstruction, the radial artery is the preferred recipient vessel, and the transposition of a pedicled radial forearm flap makes the later microvascular transfer difficult, if not impossible. It is, however, possible to use a radial artery perforator flap, leaving the radial artery intact.[12,13] Saint Cyr's group[14] has found with computed tomographic studies that a cluster of radial artery perforators exist just proximal to the wrist, making them quite suitable for thumb or first web reconstruction.

The radial forearm flap is extremity versatile and can be harvested as a fascia-alone flap, fasciocutaneous flap, or suprafascial skin flap. For thumb reconstruction, the use of the fascia-alone flap with skin grafts applied directly to the flap allows maintenance of the normal contour of the thumb, although it provides less padding than a fasciocutaneous flap.[15] An advantage of the fasciocutaneous flap is that the lateral antebrachial cutaneous nerve can be harvested with it and coapted to the ulnar digital nerve of the thumb, thus restoring some sensation. Because of their bulk, however, fasciocutaneous flaps usually require several debulking procedures. An Allen test is always performed to ensure that the digits will remain perfused by the ulnar artery. The pivot point of the flap pedicle is approximately at the radial styloid, although it can be more proximal than this. The flap should then be marked on the forearm such that the pivot point is midway between the distal end of the thumb or first web defect and the proximal end of the radial forearm flap. The flap is elevated on the radial and ulnar sides. On reaching the ulnar edge of the brachioradialis muscle on the radial side of the flap and the radial edge of the flexor carpi radialis tendon on the ulnar side of the flap, dissection then proceeds directly down to the radius. Dissection then proceeds under the deep aspect of the radial vascular bundle. Before dividing the proximal end of the radial artery, a microvascular clamp can be placed on the artery just proximal to the flap and the tourniquet released. After several seconds, if both the flap and all the digits are well perfused, the proximal radial artery can then be divided and the flap transposed to the thumb. Depending on the type of flap used, the donor site is primarily closed (fascia-alone flap) or skin grafted (fasciocutaneous or suprafascial). Because venous outflow from the reverse radial artery flap is retrograde through the venae comitantes against the venous valves, venous congestion can occur. It is imperative to include the venae comitantes and surrounding fatty tissue with the arterial pedicle when raising the flap. Performing an antegrade venous microvascular anastomosis with the cephalic vein of the flap to a vein in the hand can reduce venous congestion and flap swelling.

Metacarpal lengthening allows increase in the absolute length of the thumb ray (**Fig. 3**). This procedure is usually performed for more proximal losses in the middle third of the thumb and was pioneered by Matev.[16,17] Matev[18] reported that the only absolute contraindication to the procedure is less than 3 cm of remaining thumb metacarpal. It should be explained to the patient that this reconstruction technique requires a long period with

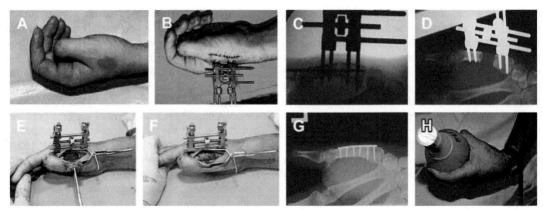

Fig. 3. (*A*) Thumb with healed amputation at IP joint level. (*B*) External distractor in place on thumb. (*C*) Radiograph of thumb at initiation of distraction. (*D*) Radiograph of completed distraction. (*E*) Bone graft placement into metacarpal defect created by distraction. (*F*) Bone graft in place. (*G*) Radiograph showing consolidation of bone graft. (*H*) Thumb demonstrating good grip function after distraction.

external fixation and multiple outpatient visits, and patient acceptance of the technique should be established before reconstruction. The pins for the distraction device are placed distally and proximally before osteotomy. Through a dorsal incision over the metacarpal, the distraction device is applied first, then the bone is cut at the diaphysis and the skin closed. Distraction is initiated at 1 millimeter per day until the desired length is achieved. Although in some patients, especially children, the bony gap of the metacarpal ossifies, most patients require bone grafting at a second surgery. This bone can be harvested from the iliac crest or, with small defects, from the distal radius. While the bone graft is consolidating, the original frame may be left in place or one may change the hardware to internal fixation. In Matev's[18] experience, several patients had first webspace creep because the distraction draws the first webskin distally. If this condition occurs, one of the first web -deepening techniques described previously may be used.

Osteoplastic thumb reconstruction allows restoration of good thumb length and, when combined with a neurovascular island flap, can result in fairly good thumb pulp sensation. Although not absolute prerequisites, the osteoplastic thumb reconstruction method works best when there is intact and functioning thenar musculature and a working thumb carpometacarpal joint. Conventional osteoplastic thumb reconstruction is performed in 3 stages:

1. Skeletal reconstruction with bone graft wrapped with a flap (typically a groin flap)
2. Groin flap division and serial thinning
3. Pulp reconstruction with a neurovascular island flap.

Some surgeons prefer to perform the groin flap procedure first and then do the bone grafting at a later surgery.

The groin flap is a versatile and reliable flap.[19] It is perfused by the superficial circumflex iliac artery, which runs parallel to and 2 cm below the inguinal ligament. The flap is centered over this line. It is incised and elevated laterally to medially just superficial to the muscle fascia. On reaching the lateral border of the sartorius, the sartorius muscle fascia is incised and elevated with the flap to prevent kinking of the pedicle. Typically, dissection to the medial border of the sartorius is sufficient length for a thumb groin flap. The proximal end of the flap is tubed. At this point, an iliac crest tricortical bone graft may be harvested from the lateral aspect of the groin flap incision. The bone graft is then fixed to the distal end of the thumb stump (either proximal phalanx base or distal metacarpal). Fixation can be provided in a variety of ways; however, plate and screw fixation allows early motion and results in less bone resorption. After bone graft fixation, the groin flap is wrapped around the graft and inset to the thumb. The groin flap is usually divided between 2 and 3 weeks after inset. Several stages of flap thinning are usually required. At approximately 3 to 6 months after skeletal and soft tissue reconstruction, sensibility is supplied by transfer of the neurovascular island flap. The chief disadvantages of the osteoplastic reconstruction technique for the thumb are possible bone graft resorption, the multiple stages required, and the bulky appearance of the reconstructed thumb.

If a groin flap is contraindicated, or if a patient refuses, osteoplastic reconstruction can be accomplished in a single stage with a radial forearm osteocutaneous flap (**Fig. 4**). The fasciocutaneous radial forearm flap is elevated as described previously. In addition, a nutrient vessel to the radius is preserved, and a small portion of tricortical bone on the radial side of the radius is harvested with a saw. The bone graft is fixed to the thumb stump and then wrapped with the radial forearm flap. Again, the flap can be innervated by suturing a thumb digital nerve to the lateral antebrachial cutaneous nerve, but this provides protective sensation at best. The radius is plated to prevent later fracture. Although the reconstruction itself is performed in 1 stage, at least 1 flap debulking procedure is likely required to achieve an acceptable contour of the thumb.

Thumb amputations do not always happen in isolation- there is often damage to other fingers, especially the index. In the ultimate example of "spare parts" surgery, the damaged/amputated index finger stump can be transferred onto the thumb stump. This transfer is an excellent reconstructive option for patients with a middle third amputation of the thumb, especially at the proximal end of that zone.[3,20] The index transfer procedure has been variably referred to as pollicization and on-top plasty. On-top plasty is likely more accurate as the term pollicization is used to denote transfer of a normally functioning index to the thumb position. On-top plasty does not necessarily need to be accomplished with the index stump- the middle or ring finger stump may also be used.

On-top plasty is usually done with a racquet-type incision at the base of the index (**Fig. 5**). Perhaps the most important part of the surgery is the dissection of the dorsal veins of the index finger. At least 1 vein must be preserved, but, when possible, it is recommended that the majority of the dorsal vein arcade be taken with

the digit. Volarly, both neurovascular bundles to the index are carefully dissected. Either before or after index dissection, the thumb is prepared for receipt of the transferred digit. This preparation consists of soft tissue elevation and metacarpal exposure for bone fixation. Internal fixation is preferred because it does not need to be removed, and early motion can be instituted. At this time, a microvascular clamp is placed on the ulnar digital artery to the index and the tourniquet released. If the index stump perfuses, then the ulnar digital artery is divided. Alternatively, the radial digital artery to the middle finger may be ligated and the common digital artery taken with the index. The ulnar digital nerve needs to be separated from the common digital nerve to the second webspace to allow transposition. Because this is a damaged index stump, the flexor and extensor mechanisms are not usually transferred (in contrast to pollicization) and can be divided. The second metacarpal is cut at the appropriate length for the thumb reconstruction. The remainder of the second metacarpal (down to proximal metaphyseal flare) is removed to allow a full first webspace. Fixation of the index metacarpal neck to the thumb metacarpal shaft or base is then performed.

TOE TRANSFERS
Great Toe Transfer

The great toe has historically been the most common donor for microsurgical toe to thumb transfer. The great toe's advantages as a donor are the excellent size match it provides and its potential for good pinch strength and stability. The great toe can be used in its entirety, or it can be partially used as either a wraparound flap or a trimmed flap. Techniques using the latter 2 flaps

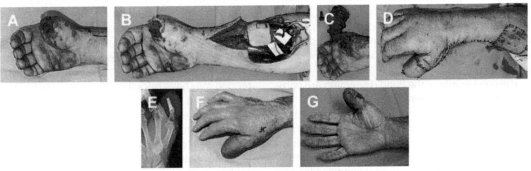

Fig. 4. (*A*) Thumb amputation through proximal phalanx with soft tissue loss near metacarpophalangeal joint. (*B*) Dissected radial forearm neuro-osteocutaneous flap (lateral antebrachial cutaneous nerve). (*C*) Interosseous wire fixation of radius segment onto end of proximal phalanx. (*D*) Inset radial forearm flap. (*E*) Radiograph of osteosynthesis of radius segment onto proximal phalanx. (*F*) Flap reconstruction before debulking. (*G*) Thumb appearance after debulking.

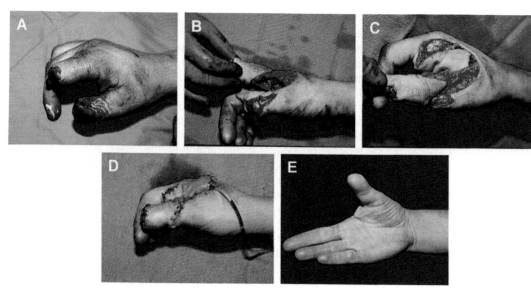

Fig. 5. (A) Amputation of thumb and tip of index finger. (B) Dissection and mobilization of damaged index finger for on-top plasty. (C) Index finger transposed to thumb tip. (D) Inset index transposition. (E) Healed result of on-top plasty.

are reserved for situations in which the use of the entire toe results in a bulky thumb reconstruction.

Maximizing the result of great toe to thumb transfer requires careful planning. As with any thumb reconstruction, the level of loss is important. This information is used to determine the need for inclusion of the metatarsophalangeal (MTP) joint in the donor toe. The maximum circumference of the contralateral thumb is also measured, usually just distal to the IP joint. This number is compared with the circumference of the great toe. If there is a significant discrepancy between these measurements, wraparound or trimmed toe techniques are used.

Dissection of both the hand and foot is done under tourniquet control and loupe magnification. Ideally, 2 surgical teams operate simultaneously to minimize operative time. In certain cases in which the anatomy of the recipient site is uncertain, dissection of the donor site may be delayed until it is determined that adequate recipient structures are present.

The chief points of the hand dissection are careful incision placement, identification of the anatomy of the recipient hand, and preparation of the skeletal, vascular, and neural structures of the recipient hand for toe transfer. Incision design varies from case to case depending on the nature of the original injury or congenital condition leading to thumb loss. Generally, incisions that create proximally based radial and ulnar flaps are preferred. In addition, the position of the radial artery should be identified by palpation or Doppler

examination and marked on the skin. Such an incision provides good access to both palmar and dorsal structures that must be exposed to complete the toe transfer. This positioning also provides for proper orientation of incisions to accept the dorsal and plantar flaps of the donor toe.

After elevation of the skin flaps, the digital nerves are identified and dissected free from surrounding soft tissues. The nerves must be dissected over an adequate length to allow for trimming of the nerve stumps back to healthy fascicles.[21] Sometimes this procedure may require dissection back to the level of the carpal tunnel. If no adequate nerve donor can be identified, nerve transfers from the radial sensory nerve or adjacent digital nerves may be necessary. Nerve ends are tagged with microsuture for later identification. Tendons are next addressed if a dynamic toe transfer is planned (static toe transfers, such as the wraparound procedure, do not require tendon repairs). If thumb loss is traumatic in nature, the flexor pollicis longus tendon may have retracted into the carpal tunnel or wrist and an extension of the thumb incision into the palm or a separate anterior wrist incision may be required to find this structure. The extensor pollicis longus tendon rarely retracts significantly and is usually easily identified, as is the extensor pollicis brevis. Next, the donor arterial supply must be addressed. The artery is located by extending the dorsal incision proximally toward the anatomic snuffbox, over the dorsal first webspace. Once identified, the artery is dissected free from surrounding soft tissues and is marked with a vessel loop. A recipient vein is then dissected. There is an abundance of veins on the dorsum of the hand that are suitable for toe transfer. When an adequate vein is identified, it is dissected in a similar manner to the artery and is marked with a vessel loop for later identification.

If the toe is to be transferred to the proximal phalanx of the recipient thumb, the metatarsal osteotomy is made in a transverse manner. If the recipient bone is the thumb metacarpal, the metatarsal osteotomy is made with a slight angle in a proximal-dorsal to distal-plantar direction. Alternatively, the thumb metacarpal osteotomy can be made with a slight volar inclination to overcome the natural tendency of the MTP joint of the transferred toe to assume an extended posture.[22] In cases in which the metacarpophalangeal (MCP) joint of the recipient thumb is preserved, dissection should preserve as much of the capsular soft tissues as possible for later attachment to the capsular soft tissues of the MTP joint of the donor toe.

Toe dissection is performed by a second operative team concurrent with the hand dissection. Preoperatively, the course of the dorsalis pedis artery and dorsal superficial veins of the foot are marked on the dorsal skin of the foot using a combination of palpation and Doppler device. Assessment of venous anatomy can be assisted by dependent positioning or the extremity and the use of a venous tourniquet, using a tourniquet pressure of approximately 80 to 100 mm Hg, with the venous anatomy marked out before skin preparation. Generally, foot incisions that create dorsal and plantar flaps, with a dorsal proximal extension for vessel dissection, are used. This incision provides for good access for dissection and creates flaps that are complementary to the radial and ulnar flaps of the hand.

After gravity exsanguination of the lower extremity and inflation of the tourniquet, incisions are made. Skin flaps are elevated laterally and medially on the dorsum of the foot to expose the underlying structures. Where possible, small sensory nerves are preserved. The superficial saphenous venous system is examined, and 1 or more veins of adequate size and length are identified as the donor vein. This vessel is dissected free from surrounding structures. The vein dissection should be carried proximally to an extent that allows for adequate donor vein length, which is determined by the venous anatomy at the recipient site in the hand. In general, 7 to 12 cm of donor vein is required.[23] The dissection is carried distally on to the dorsum of the great toe, where the vein gives off small branches dorsolaterally. In this region, a wide cuff of soft tissue should be included in the

dissection to preserve small venous branches crucial for adequate venous drainage of the flap. Small branches that course medially or laterally away from the toe are ligated and divided. In early descriptions of toe transfer, the arterial system was dissected proximally to distally. However, this method can make the distal dissection problematic, especially with a plantar-dominant arterial system. It is now generally accepted that the arterial dissection first begins in the first webspace, with the surgeon looking directly up the webspace.[24] After spreading through the subcutaneous tissues, the nexus of dorsal, plantar, medial (to the great toe), and lateral (to the second toe) arteries are found. This nexus has the appearance of a plus sign when looking up the foot. On reaching this nexus, the surgeon can then fairly easily determine whether the arterial system is dorsal dominant (most common) or plantar dominant and then adjust the skin incisions accordingly. If plantar dominant, the plantar incisions have to be made more proximally. The plantar artery to the great toe eventually rejoins with the dorsal system, but plantar dissection has to be done more proximally to get to that point. The artery to the second toe is ligated. Once the arterial and venous systems have been dissected, they can be tagged with vessel loops for later identification.

In cases in which reestablishment of dorsal sensory function of the transferred toe is desired, the deep peroneal nerve, which runs adjacent to the dorsalis pedis artery, is included in the flap. Dissection proceeds in a similar manner to the arterial dissection. Enough length must be harvested proximally for later repair to a branch of the radial sensory nerve in the hand.

The final structure that must be prepared on the dorsum of the foot is the extensor hallucis longus tendon. Once identified, this tendon is divided proximally, again preserving enough length for repair to the flexor pollicis longus tendon in the hand.

The digital nerves on the medial and lateral plantar toe must also be dissected. Once identified, the lateral plantar digital nerve to the great toe is dissected proximally to the common plantar digital nerve to the great and second toes. To gain more donor nerve length, intraneural dissection is used to separate the fascicles to the great toe from the second toe. Once an adequate length of nerve has been obtained (3–5 cm), the lateral plantar digital nerve to the great toe is divided. In a similar manner, the medial plantar digital nerve to the great toe is identified and dissected proximally over an adequate length. It is then also divided. Both nerves are tagged with microsuture for later identification.

At this point, the flexor hallucis longus tendon is identified over the plantar midaxis of the toe. Circumferential dissection of the tendon is undertaken in a distal to proximal direction. With careful retraction of the skin, the dissection can be continued proximally to provide the necessary length of donor tendon without having to significantly increase the length of the skin incision. In situations in which long lengths of tendon are required, the skin incision can be extended proximally on the plantar surface of the foot. Alternatively, the tendon can be exposed and divided through a separate incision posterior to the medial malleolus and then delivered into the distal plantar incision with traction. During this portion of the dissection, the flexor hallucis brevis muscle is also identified and divided near its insertion, distal to the sesamoid bones of the great toe.

With the neurovascular and tendinous dissections completed, attention is now turned to the skeleton of the toe. In situations in which the MTP joint of the donor toe is to be preserved, the metatarsal is exposed subperiosteally over its entire circumference proximal to this level. Unlike the second or third toes, using the great toe has the disadvantage of causing problems with ambulation because more metatarsal length is sacrificed. Because of this, only the minimum required amount of metatarsal should be taken with the donor toe. The osteotomy is performed with an oscillating saw. After completion of the osteotomy, the remaining attachments of the intrinsic muscles and intermetatarsal ligamentous structures attached to the donor toe distal to the osteotomy are divided. The insertion of the abductor hallucis muscle into the lateral aspect of the proximal phalanx can be preserved with an adequate length of tendon for later transfer into the abductor pollicis longus tendon of the donor hand. This can restore abduction of the reconstructed thumb.

When the toe dissection is complete, the tourniquet is deflated, allowing reperfusion of the toe. It should be noted that, because of arterial spasm resulting from dissection, the donor toe might remain pale for up to 20 or 30 minutes after release of the tourniquet. Spasm can be minimized by the application of topical drugs such as papaverine or concentrated lidocaine (20%). If the toe has not shown visible signs of reperfusion 20 to 30 minutes after release of the tourniquet and complete deflation of the tourniquet has been confirmed, the dissection should be carefully examined for evidence of damage to the donor vessels or presence of kinks or other obstacles to the flow of blood through these structures. Once reperfusion to the donor toe is established, it should be allowed to perfuse for approximately 20 minutes before completion of the harvest and transfer to the hand.

With the recipient site prepared and the toe dissected, transfer of the toe to the hand is next undertaken. At this point, with all structures in the hand and on the donor toe prepared, transfer should proceed fairly rapidly. The transfer is begun with reconstruction of the skeletal framework. If the toe has been harvested through the MTP joint and is to be transferred to the MCP joint of the thumb, repair of the capsular soft tissues must be carefully performed with absorbable sutures to maximize the function of the reconstructed joint. Care is taken to achieve proper axial alignment of the joint during this repair. The capsular repair is protected by skeletal stabilization with Kirschner wires, which are removed after the soft tissues of the joint have been given adequate time to heal. The MCP joint should be pinned in a position of slight flexion. More commonly, the toe is harvested at the level of the proximal portion of the metatarsal head, with planned transfer to the metacarpal in the hand. In such cases, osteosynthesis is performed. Rigid plate and screw fixation for osteosynthesis is preferred because of its strength and allowance of early active range of motion in the reconstructed thumb. If the transferred toe is harvested through the proximal phalanx and is to be transferred to the proximal phalanx of the thumb, a similar technique of osteosynthesis is used.

With the skeletal reconstruction complete, repair of soft tissues is then undertaken. A typical repair order is tendinous structures first, then nerves, followed by the artery, and finally the vein. The arterial and venous anastomoses are usually performed in an end-to-end manner because the size match of donor and recipient vessels is usually very good. Vascular clamps are then removed, and reperfusion of the transferred toe is established. If there is any question regarding the patency of any of the vascular anastomoses or excessive vessel length is noted in either the artery or vein after reestablishment of blood flow, revision should be performed immediately.

With perfusion established, skin closure must now be performed. Donor and recipient skin flaps are brought into approximation and trimmed as necessary. In children, absorbable suture, such as chromic gut, should be used to eliminate the need for later suture removal. In situations in which flaps cannot be closed without undue tension, a skin graft should be used for cover, provided that all vital structures, such as nerves, blood vessels, and tendons, are covered by healthy vascularized soft tissue. After placement of the usual sterile dressings, the extremity should be placed into a well-padded thumb spica splint with the tip of the toe flap visible for postoperative monitoring.

The final step in toe transfer is donor site repair. This procedure can be performed simultaneously with the toe transfer if a second operating team is available. Proper and careful donor site closure is critical in maintaining good ambulatory function. To provide for additional plantar soft tissue padding, the flexor hallucis brevis muscle can be advanced over the cut end of the metatarsal and fixed here. Skin flaps are then brought into approximation over a drain placed into the intermetatarsal space, and skin closure is then performed with simple interrupted monofilament sutures. Again, absorbable sutures should be used in young children. After placement of sterile dressings, a well-padded posterior splint is placed with the ankle positioned at 90°.

The chief disadvantage of great toe transfer is the donor site morbidity associated with this procedure. It is generally accepted that donor site morbidity is relatively minimal in properly planned and executed microsurgical toe to thumb transfer procedures.[24–27] However, many aspects of gait depend on adequate first metatarsal length. In situations in which the degree of thumb loss requires long skeletal length of the donor toe, harvesting of the first toe proximal to the metatarsal head to any significant degree affects gait. In addition, although harvesting of nonborder digits of the foot, such as the second or third toes, minimally affects the appearance of the foot (especially if a formal ray amputation webspace closure is completed after toe harvest), sacrifice of the great toe leaves a deformity that is readily apparent.

Wraparound Flap

Because the great toe is larger than the normal thumb, various modifications of great toe transfer for thumb reconstruction have been developed to create a better size match between the reconstructed thumb and the contralateral normal thumb. These modifications include the trimmed toe technique and the wraparound technique of great toe transfer.

The wraparound technique was first described by Morrison and colleagues[28] in 1980. In this procedure, the soft tissue and nail of the great toe only are transferred to the hand, without the metatarsal or proximal phalanx of the great toe. A bone graft, if required, provides skeletal support for the reconstructed thumb. The advantages of this flap include better size match with the opposite normal thumb and preservation of a portion of the great toe.[28,29] There are, however, several

disadvantages to this flap technique. Because this technique is an essentially static transfer when the use of a bone graft is required, it is useful only for thumb loss distal to the MCP joint. Another disadvantage of this flap is its lack of potential for growth because of the absence of an epiphysis. For this reason, this flap is not an appropriate choice for thumb reconstruction in children. Resorption of the bone graft is another potential problem but is relatively rare and minimized by the inclusion of the distal phalanx of the toe in the flap.

Indications for the procedure include reconstruction of the thumb with complete skin avulsion in which the skeleton and tendons remain intact and reconstruction of amputations distal to the MCP joint of the thumb. The former indication does not require the use of an iliac crest bone graft.

Because the ulnar vessels of the thumb tend to be dominant, the ipsilateral great toe is usually chosen for wraparound great toe transfer. The arterial supply to the flap tends to run in a medial direction as it courses distally on the foot, which corresponds to the course of the radial artery in the hand. Careful incision planning is required for successful wraparound toe transfer. The circumference of the contralateral normal thumb must be measured at its base and at the widest portion of the thumb pulp between the tip of the digit and the IP joint. The donor toe is measured in a similar manner, and the difference between corresponding measurements in the toe and thumb is determined.

Markings are made to design a flap that is based proximally and are made on the skin of the dorsal, lateral, and plantar skin of the great toe. At the completion of the dissection, a tongue of proximally based skin and subcutaneous tissue remains on the medial side of the great toe and is used for closure of the donor site. The width of this tongue roughly corresponds to the difference between the circumference of the great toe and the circumference of the thumb.

Dissection of neurovascular structures and tendons proceeds identically to the great toe transfer. The flap itself is essentially degloved from the skeleton of the great toe after incisions are made. Depending on the needs of the recipient site, the flap harvest may include the distal phalanx, flexor, and extensor tendons of the great toe. Inclusion of these structures is not necessary when reconstructing the thumb that has sustained avulsion of soft tissue only, with an intact skeleton and system of tendons.

Preparation of the recipient site for wraparound great toe transfer is similar to that for transfer of the whole great toe. In cases in which reconstruction of skeletal support is necessary, a tricortical iliac crest bone graft is used. The graft should be harvested to match the combined circumference of the normal thumb skeleton and adjacent tendons and trimmed to the appropriate length based on the size of the defect. Osteosynthesis to the stump of the recipient proximal phalanx and base of the donor distal phalanx is performed using Kirschner wires or interosseous wiring. The soft tissues of the flap are then wrapped around the skeletal framework. Repair of tendons and nerves and vascular anastomoses are then performed. The medial skin edges of the dorsal and plantar surfaces of the flap are then sutured together to complete the reconstruction. During closure, the nail width can be narrowed to match that of the opposite normal thumb, and the medial eponychial fold is also recreated.

Several techniques have been described for closure of the donor site after wraparound great toe transfer, and this remains the most vexing problem associated with this variety of toe transfer. The whole of the remaining skeletal framework can be preserved and the soft tissues reconstructed using a combination of the medial tongue of skin and soft tissue left behind by toe harvest and a cross toe flap from the plantar surface of the second toe.[28] Alternatively, the remaining skeleton can be shortened to allow donor site closure using only the medial great toe skin flap.

Trimmed Toe

The trimmed great toe flap was first described in the late 1980s.[30,31] This technique combines the advantages of the wraparound great toe flap, namely, better size match of the contralateral thumb while avoiding the disadvantage of lack of mobility and growth potential. Unlike the wraparound flap, the trimmed toe flap is harvested with both the proximal and distal phalanges. The circumferences of both the soft tissues and the bone are reduced to match the circumference of the contralateral normal thumb. With this technique, joints and physes are preserved. The indications for this technique include those for the whole great toe and wraparound techniques for which better size match of the contralateral normal thumb is desired.

Markings for the trimmed great toe technique are similar to those for the wraparound technique. The medial proximally based skin flap is elevated from the underlying periosteum, taking care to preserve the medial neurovascular structures of the toe. A proximally based flap consisting of periosteum and the medial collateral ligament of the IP

joint of the toe is then elevated from the underlying bony structures. The circumference of the phalanges is then reduced by making a longitudinal osteotomy in the sagittal plane, removing 3 to 4 mm of the medial portion of both bones. The toe is then harvested and inset in a manner similar to that of the great toe technique. Closure of the donor requires reconstruction of the IP joint medial collateral ligament that was taken down for osteotomy. Skin closure and management of the nail and eponychial fold are similar to those of the wraparound great toe flap. The donor site closure is identical to that for the wraparound flap.

Second Toe Transfer

Transfer of the second toe to the hand was first described in China in 1973.[32] This technique has multiple advantages that make it an excellent option for microsurgical thumb reconstruction. The second toe's minimal donor site impact, good appearance, and superb function after transfer into the thumb position make it an excellent option for toe to thumb transfer.

The use of the second toe minimizes donor site problems associated with toe transfer, which can be both functionally and socially significant. After transfer of the second toe, the overall contour of the foot is nearly normal and hardly noticeable.

Another advantage of second toe transfer is the available skeletal length of the donor toe (**Fig. 6**). Great toe donor length is limited by the functional loss that accompanies loss of the first metatarsal length. As longer lengths of metatarsal are taken and included with the great toe, balance and ambulation are adversely affected. Because the second metatarsal is not in a marginal position on the foot, its entire length and the MTP joint can be taken for transfer. This possibility makes the second toe an excellent choice for reconstruction of thumb amputations that are at the level of the proximal to middle portion of the thumb metacarpal.

Vascular dissection (artery and vein) of the second toe is essentially the same as that of the great toe, the only difference being that in the first webspace, the medial branch to the great toe is the artery that is ligated. Harvesting the second toe with a wide cuff of soft tissue to preserve vascular perforators is even more important than with great toe harvest. Preservation of both arterial and venous perforators is of paramount importance in maintaining second toe viability.

Second toe transfer is not without its disadvantages, chiefly the small size of the donor toe. This small size makes for a thumb that is narrower and weaker, and therefore potentially less functional,

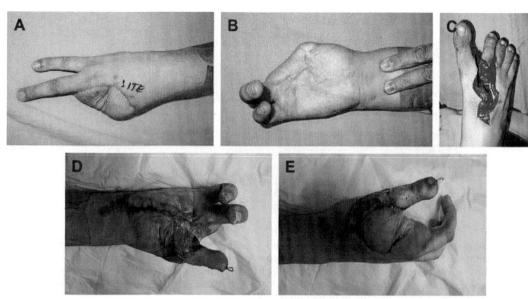

Fig. 6. (*A, B*) Dorsal and volar views of hand after amputation of thumb, index, and middle fingers and coverage with groin flap. (*C*) Dissected second toe. (*D, E*) Early postoperative results of second toe transfer. Note Kirschner wire preventing hyperextension of transferred toe.

than one reconstructed with a great toe. Another disadvantage of second toe transfer is the lack of soft tissue availability for coverage of interosseous muscles and bone when a long length of metatarsal is used. This lack can be dealt with by soft tissue augmentation of the recipient site before toe transfer, usually with a groin flap.

Certain details regarding insetting of the flap and donor site closure merit discussion. The arc of motion of the metatarsal joint of the second toe is mostly through dorsiflexion, and a hyperextension deformity of this joint after transfer to the thumb is possible. This deformity may lead to poor thumb function by limiting pinch strength. To minimize this risk, the osteotomies of the donor metatarsal and recipient metacarpal should be made with a slight palmar inclination to bring the thumb into a position of mild flexion at the MTP joint. In addition, the MTP and IP joints should be percutaneously pinned in a position of function for 6 weeks after transfer to minimize the risk of developing a hyperextension deformity and an extensor lag. Closure of the donor site in the foot also requires attention to detail. During harvest of the second toe, the intermetatarsal ligaments of the medial side of the third metatarsal and lateral side of the first metatarsal should be preserved. During closure of the donor site, these ligaments are sutured to each other. Ligament repair is reinforced with Kirschner wire fixation through the metatarsal necks of the great and third toes. These wires are removed 6 weeks postoperatively. By approximating the great and third toes, stability

of the foot is increased, and donor site appearance is minimized.

Toe Pulp Transfer

The versatile neurovascular anatomy of the great and second toes allows for the use of only portions of these structures to reconstruct complex partial thumb defects. Portions of the great and/or second toes can be used to reconstruct the palmer surface of the thumb, partial loss of the pulp of the thumb, or the dorsum of the digit, including the nailbed.[33–36] Great toe pulp transfer can be performed to restore a sensate pulp to the reconstructed thumb (**Fig. 7**). This pulp provides an alternative to the Littler neurovascular island flap and allows for sensibility restoration without sensory retraining. The disadvantage when compared with the neurovascular island flap is that the pulp obviously requires microsurgery, and the transfer can be a more involved surgery.[35]

Proximal Third

Loss of the thumb at the level of the proximal third is a challenge for reconstruction because this is essentially complete thumb loss. Although the divisions between middle third and proximal third loss are somewhat arbitrary, one chief difference is that loss at the proximal third can include loss of some or the entire cuff of thenar musculature. This muscle loss precludes use of previously mentioned techniques such as osteoplastic

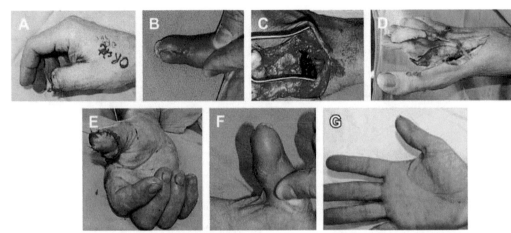

Fig. 7. (*A*) Amputation of thumb through IP joint caused by avulsion while cattle roping. (*B*) Volar view of thumb after replantation. The thumb was replanted with arterial inflow into the dorsal venous system with no venous outflow. This resulted in necrosis of the volar pulp while the rest of the thumb survived. (*C*) Dissection of recipient vessels for toe pulp transfer in the anatomic snuffbox. (*D*) Dissected toe pulp from great toe. (*E*) Inset of toe pulp flap to volar thumb. (*F, G*) Healed toe pulp flap on thumb.

reconstruction, distraction osteogenesis, and perhaps on-top plasty. Because of the paucity of local reconstruction options, microvascular techniques play a primary role in thumb reconstruction at this level. These techniques primarily are performed with various types of toe transfer and are mentioned in the previous sections.

There are some instances of proximal third loss in which on-top plasty may be appropriate. As stated, if some or all of the thenar musculature is missing, mobility of the transferred index is limited and may need to be augmented by an opponensplasty at a later time. In the adult, this opposition transfer can be accomplished with either the ring finger flexor digitorum superficialis tendon or the extensor indicis proprius tendon. The technique of on-top plasty is performed in the same manner as discussed in the section on middle third loss.

Index finger pollicization is another viable technique for proximal third thumb reconstruction. The procedure's utility in children with thumb hypoplasia or aplasia is undisputed. The procedure's use in adults is also fairly reliable, although it may be more difficult for adults to adapt to the new finger position. In Brunelli and colleagues'[37] description of pollicization in adults, the investigators highlight one of the chief differences in pollicization between children and adults: in children, the thenar musculature and the adductor pollicis are entirely missing, whereas in adults there may be at least a remnant. This occurrence slightly changes what is done with the index palmar interosseous (becomes the adductor pollicis) and the dorsal interosseous (becomes the thenar muscles). In children, these muscles are transferred with the index, but, in adults, the muscles themselves can be eliminated and their tendons sutured to the thenar and adductor remnants.

A variety of skin incision patterns can be used. Once the skin is incised, the dorsal veins are carefully dissected. Vein preservation is critically important and is often the most tedious portion of the pollicization surgery. Next, the neurovascular bundles to the index are dissected. The palmar and dorsal interosseous tendons are divided from the muscles. The flexor and extensor tendons are dissected after opening the first and second annular pulleys. The thumb is then prepared by dissection of the soft tissue and exposure of the metacarpal remnant. The thenar and adductor pollicis muscles or their remnants are also prepared. There are 2 possibilities for the ulnar digital artery of the index finger: it can be divided if the radial digital artery adequately perfuses the finger or the radial digital artery to the middle finger can be divided and the common digital artery to the second webspace can be taken with the index finger. The second metacarpal is then cut at the neck. The remainder of the second metacarpal down to the metaphyseal flare is removed to open the new first webspace. The index is transferred and rotated. The pulp of the new thumb should be facing the ring finger when bony fixation is completed. The tendon of the first dorsal interosseous muscle is sutured to the thenar muscle remnant (opponens pollicis if possible), and the tendon of the palmar interosseous muscle is sutured to the adductor pollicis muscle or its remnant. Some investigators recommend no shortening of the extrinsic extensor and flexor tendons, whereas others advocate tendon plication.[3,37] The MCP joint is pinned for 6 weeks in slight flexion to counteract the tendency of the index MCP joint to hyperextend. As with on-top plasty, the thenar musculature may be later found to be inadequate for functional opposition, and, in these cases, opposition transfer (ring finger flexor digitorum superficialis or extensor indicis proprius tendon) can be performed at a later time.

Prosthetics

Prostheses for thumb loss are a viable option for patients who do not wish to undergo reconstruction. Generally, prostheses are aesthetic in nature, meaning they have minimal or no function. Pillet's group[38] has the largest experience with upper extremity prosthetics, and their aesthetic results are quite impressive. There are scattered reports of osseointegrated digital and thumb prosthetics, which render them slightly more functional and durable.[39] In general, there must be at least a remnant of thumb proximal phalanx for an aesthetic prosthetic to remain on the thumb.[3] Otherwise, a hand-based extension may be required for prosthesis stabilization.

OUTCOMES, PROGNOSIS, COMPLICATIONS

Unfortunately, there is a scarcity of well-controlled outcomes studies related to the various types of thumb reconstruction. There are, however, several large retrospective series for each of the earlier-mentioned reconstruction methods that, in general, demonstrate good results.[2,5–7,10,18,20]

There are 5 goals when reconstructing a thumb. These are restoration of (1) functional length, (2) stability, (3) mobility (especially opposition), (4) sensibility, and (5) aesthetic appearance. The treating physician should help the patient choose the technique that allows restoration of (hopefully) all 5 of these aspects to the thumb. If all 5 are restored, then the prognosis for a functional thumb and a satisfied patient is good. If all 5 cannot be restored, then, at least, restoration of a stable thumb with adequate length allows some grip and pinch activities.

REFERENCES

1. Mehrara BJ, Abood AA, Disa JJ, et al. Thumb reconstruction following resection for malignant tumors. Plast Reconstr Surg 2008;121(4):1279–87.

2. Heitmann C, Levin LS. Alternatives to thumb replantation. Plast Reconstr Surg 2002;110(6):1492–503 [quiz: 1504–5].

3. Muzaffar AR, Chao JJ, Friedrich JB, et al. Posttraumatic thumb reconstruction. Plast Reconstr Surg 2005;116(5):103e–22e.

4. Bickel KD, Dosanjh A. Fingertip reconstruction. J Hand Surg Am 2008;33(8):1417–9.

5. Atasoy E, Ioakimidis E, Kasdan ML, et al. Reconstruction of the amputated finger tip with a triangular volar flap. A new surgical procedure. J Bone Joint Surg Am 1970;52(5):921–6.

6. Hynes DE. Neurovascular pedicle and advancement flaps for palmar thumb defects. Hand Clin 1997;13(2):207–16.

7. Woon CY, Lee JY, Teoh LC. Resurfacing hemipulp losses of the thumb: the cross finger flap revisited: indications, technical refinements, outcomes, and long-term neurosensory recovery. Ann Plast Surg 2008;61(4):385–91.

8. O'Brien B. Neurovascular island pedicle flaps for terminal amputations and digital scars. Br J Plast Surg 1968;21(3):258–61.

9. Thompson JS. Reconstruction of the insensate thumb by neurovascular island transfer. Hand Clin 1992;8(1):99–105.

10. Muyldermans T, Hierner R. First dorsal metacarpal artery flap for thumb reconstruction: a retrospective clinical study. Strategies Trauma Limb Reconstr 2009;4(1):27–33.

11. Gregory H, Heitmann C, Germann G. The evolution and refinements of the distally based dorsal metacarpal artery (DMCA) flaps. J Plast Reconstr Aesthet Surg 2007;60(7):731–9.

12. Page R, Chang J. Reconstruction of hand soft-tissue defects: alternatives to the radial forearm fasciocutaneous flap. J Hand Surg Am 2006;31(5):847–56.

13. Hansen AJ, Duncan SF, Smith AA, et al. Reverse radial forearm fascial flap with radial artery preservation. Hand (N Y) 2007;2(3):159–63.

14. Saint-Cyr M, Mujadzic M, Wong C, et al. The radial artery pedicle perforator flap: vascular analysis and clinical implications. Plast Reconstr Surg 2010; 125(5):1469–78.

15. Friedrich JB, Katolik LI, Vedder NB. Soft tissue reconstruction of the hand. J Hand Surg Am 2009; 34(6):1148–55.

16. Matev IB. Thumb reconstruction in children through metacarpal lengthening. Plast Reconstr Surg 1979; 64(5):665–9.

17. Matev IB. Thumb reconstruction through metacarpal bone lengthening. J Hand Surg Am 1980; 5(5):482–7.

18. Matev I. Thumb metacarpal lengthening. Tech Hand Up Extrem Surg 2003;7(4):157–63.

19. Friedrich J, Vedder N. Groin flap coverage of the hand and wrist. In: Cooney W, Moran S, editors. Soft tissue: master techniques in orthopaedic surgery series. Baltimore (MD): Lippincott, Williams & Wilkins; 2008. p. 233–44.

20. Bravo CJ, Horton T, Moran SL, et al. Traumatized index finger pollicization for thumb reconstruction. J Hand Surg Am 2008;33(2):257–62.

21. Maser B, Vedder N. Nerve repair and nerve grafting. In: Achauer B, Eriksson E, Guyuron B, et al, editors, Plastic surgery: indications, operations, and outcomes, vol. 4. St Louis (MO): Mosby, Inc.; 2000. p. 2103–14.

22. Shin AY, Bishop AT, Berger RA. Microvascular reconstruction of the traumatized thumb. Hand Clin 1999, 15(2):347–71.

23. Serafin D. The great toe flap. In: Serafin D, editor. Atlas of microsurgical composite tissue transplantation. Philadelphia: W.B. Saunders; 1996. p. 591–606.

24. Wei FC, el-Gammal TA. Toe-to-hand transfer. Current concepts, techniques, and research. Clin Plast Surg 1996;23(1):103–16.

25. Frykman GK, O'Brien BM, Morrison WA, et al. Functional evaluation of the hand and foot after one-stage toe-to-hand transfer. J Hand Surg Am 1986;11(1):9–17.

26. Poppen NK, Norris TR, Buncke HJ Jr. Evaluation of sensibility and function with microsurgical free tissue transfer of the great toe to the hand for thumb reconstruction. J Hand Surg Am 1983;8(5 Pt 1):516–31.

27. Lipton HA, May JW Jr, Simon SR. Preoperative and postoperative gait analyses of patients undergoing great toe-to-thumb transfer. J Hand Surg Am 1987; 12(1):66–9.

28. Morrison WA, O'Brien BM, MacLeod AM. Thumb reconstruction with a free neurovascular wraparound flap from the big toe. J Hand Surg Am 1980;5(6):575–83.

29. Serafin D. The great toe wrap-around flap. In: Serafin D, editor. Atlas of microsurgical composite tissue transplantation. Philadelphia: W.B. Saunders; 1996. p. 123–36.

30. Wei FC, Chen HC, Chuang CC, et al. Reconstruction of the thumb with a trimmed-toe transfer technique. Plast Reconstr Surg 1988;82(3):506–15.

31. Upton J, Mutimer K. A modification of the great-toe transfer for thumb reconstruction. Plast Reconstr Surg 1988;82(3):535–8.

32. Replantation surgery in China. Report of the American Replantation Mission to China. Plast Reconstr Surg 1973;52(5):476–89.

33. Serafin D. The partial toe flap. In: Serafin D, editor. Atlas of microsurgical composite tissue transplantation. Philadelphia: W.B. Saunders; 1996. p. 137–52.

34. Buncke HJ, Rose EH. Free toe-to-fingertip neurovascular flaps. Plast Reconstr Surg 1979;63(5):607–12.

35. Foucher G, Merle M, Maneaud M, et al. Microsurgical free partial toe transfer in hand reconstruction: a report of 12 cases. Plast Reconstr Surg 1980; 65(5):616–27.

36. Hamilton RB, Morrison WA. Microvascular segmental thumb reconstruction: a case report. Br J Plast Surg 1980;33(1):64–7.

37. Brunelli GA, Brunelli GR. Reconstruction of traumatic absence of the thumb in the adult by pollicization. Hand Clin 1992;8(1):41–55.

38. Pillet J, Didierjean-Pillet A. Aesthetic hand prosthesis: gadget or therapy? Presentation of a new classification. J Hand Surg Br 2001;26(6):523–8.

39. Manurangsee P, Isariyawut C, Chatuthong V, et al. Osseointegrated finger prosthesis: an alternative method for finger reconstruction. J Hand Surg Am 2000;25(1):86–92.

Reconstruction of the Rheumatoid Hand

Shimpei Ono, MD, PhD, Pouya Entezami, BS,
Kevin C. Chung, MD, MS*

KEYWORDS

• Rheumatoid hand • Treatment • Reconstruction

Rheumatoid arthritis (RA) affects the synovial tissue of the hand, resulting in the archetypal "rheumatoid hand" deformity. More than 70% of patients with RA complain of a loss in hand and wrist function, often restricting daily activities.[1] This condition has a substantial societal effect in terms of growing treatment cost[2,3] and productivity loss.[4–8] Although surgical treatment can improve the quality of life for patients with rheumatoid hand,[9] the indication for surgical intervention and the decision making among various treatment options are complex issues, for three main reasons.

First, RA is a polyarticular disease, and deformities in proximal joints will affect the position of the joints distally.[10] Therefore the order of priority among necessary treatment steps must be considered and any proximal deformities first must be corrected. A patient presenting with destruction of the metacarpophalangeal joint (MCPJ) and proximal interphalangeal joint (PIPJ) may gain sufficient enough motion at the MCPJ after surgery that the need for surgery to correct the PIPJ is alleviated.[11,12]

Second, the operative indication differs in each patient, which means an individual treatment plan must be formulated for each patient based on the status of the hand and the patient's particular needs. For example, the presence of a hand deformity is not an absolute indication for surgery, because many patients maintain good function despite significant physical manifestation. Alternatively, patients may want the deformity corrected only to improve the appearance. A previous study by Alderman and colleagues[13] using the Michigan Hand Outcomes Questionnaire showed that aesthetic consideration is a critical determinant of patient satisfaction in rheumatoid hand surgery.

Finally, rheumatologist and hand surgeons have different opinions regarding the indications, effectiveness, and outcomes of rheumatoid hand surgery.[14,15] Most patients with RA are seen by rheumatologists who generally view rheumatoid hand surgery as a less effective remedy. Therefore, many patients with RA who are unresponsive to medication are still not referred for hand surgery consultation.

These complexities make a standardized strategy to treat the rheumatoid hand difficult to develop. Previous studies have shown a large variation in the surgical rates across the United States for common surgical procedures for the rheumatoid hand.[16] The literature on treatment options and outcomes must be updated on a regular basis. The authors believe that this effort will help hand surgeons select proper treatment options tailored to each patient's desired outcome. This article provides a comprehensive review of surgical treatment options for rheumatoid hand reconstruction.

Supported in part by a grant from the National Institute of Arthritis and Musculoskeletal and Skin Diseases (R01 AR047328) and a Midcareer Investigator Award in Patient-Oriented Research (K24 AR053120) (to Dr Kevin C. Chung).
Disclosure: None of the authors has a financial interest to declare in relation to the content of this article.
Section of Plastic Surgery, Department of Surgery, The University of Michigan Health System, Ann Arbor, MI, USA
* Corresponding author. Section of Plastic Surgery, University of Michigan Health System, 2130 Taubman Center, SPC 5340, 1500 East Medical Center Drive, Ann Arbor, MI 48109-5340.
E-mail address: kecchung@umich.edu

MANAGEMENT OF THE RHEUMATOID HAND
Wrist

Pathology

Dorsal subluxation of the ulnar head (or more precisely, volar subluxation of the radius because the ulna is a fixed unit of the forearm); supination, palmar and ulnar translation, and collapse of the carpus; and radial deviation of the carpometacarpal joint represent the deformities at the wrist (**Fig. 1**). Synovitis often develops on the ulnar side of the wrist first. The synovial pannus progressively stretches the extensor carpi ulnaris (ECU) sheath and the capsuloligamentous apparatus of the distal radioulnar joint (DRUJ) and the radiocarpal, midcarpal, and carpometacarpal joints. Rupture of the ECU sheath results in palmar subluxation of the ECU. Furthermore, synovial proliferation within the DRUJ stretches the capsuloligamentous apparatus and eventually causes rupture of the triangular fibrocartilage complex (TFCC). With loss of the TFCC tether and the ECU restraint, the ulnar head dislocates dorsally, resulting in the classic caput ulnae. The palmarly subluxed ECU loses the ability to extend, and ulnarly deviates the hand. Along with the ECU, it becomes a wrist flexor and encourages palmar translation and supination of the carpus. The intact radial wrist extensors (extensor carpi radialis longus and extensor carpi radialis brevis) now act unopposed, causing the metacarpals to deviate radially. Degradation of the cartilage and interosseous cyst formation in the radius, scaphoid, and lunate, combined with radioscaphoid and midcarpal synovitis, leads to rupture of the scapholunate ligament, collapse of the scaphoid (scaphoid becoming horizontal with distal pole protruding into the carpal tunnel), bony destruction, and eventually carpal collapse. This loss in carpal height results in a relative lengthening of the flexor and extensor tendons and allows migration of the carpus toward the palmar and ulnar aspect of the radius (ulnar translation) (**Fig. 2**). This movement is hastened by the natural inclination of the articular surface of the radius.

Roughly 75% of patients with RA show wrist symptoms, making it the most commonly affected joint in RA.[17,18] During the early stages, patients develop wrist pain, tenderness, and bulging of the dorsal wrist. These symptoms may sometimes be alleviated through conservative treatment methods (eg, splinting). However, in advanced RA, several of the deformities described earlier may occur and restrict hand function through affecting the range of motion, grip strength, and overall function of the hand. The most commonly accepted indications of RA wrist surgery are when symptoms persist despite conservative treatment for at least 6 to 9 months, or when carpal deformity progresses.[19] Surgical treatment is undertaken primarily to alleviate wrist pain or correct wrist deformities that affect the fingers. Surgery resulting in a stable and functional wrist is tantamount for the success of future hand reconstruction endeavors. Surgical options include

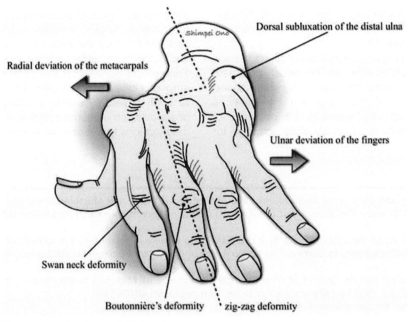

Dorsal subluxation of the distal ulna

Radial deviation of the metacarpals

Ulnar deviation of the fingers

Swan neck deformity

Boutonnière's deformity　zig-zag deformity

Fig. 1. Typical features of the rheumatoid hand.

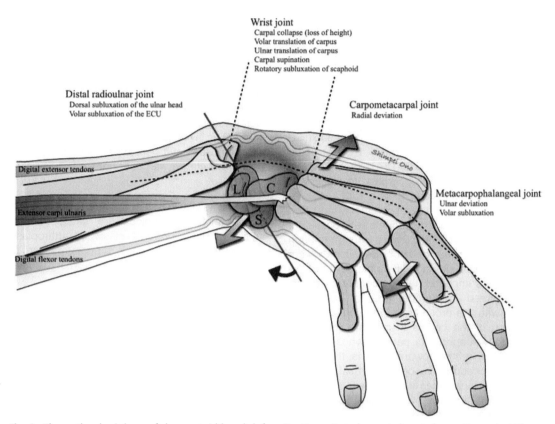

Fig. 2. The pathophysiology of rheumatoid hand deformity. C, capitate bone; L, lunate bone; S, scaphoid bone.

synovectomy, excision of the distal ulna (Darrach procedure), fusion of the DRUJ (Sauve-Kapandji procedure), wrist arthrodesis, and arthroplasty.

Synovectomy

Wrist synovectomy (**Fig. 3**) is usually recommended to treat refractory active synovitis or painful monoarthritis. However, the indications for it have never been clearly established. Lipscomb[20] recommended several months of conservative

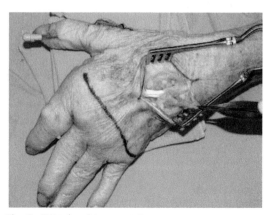

Fig. 3. Dorsal wrist synovectomy.

therapy before performing a synovectomy, but Hindley and Stanley[21] advocated early application of the procedure to prevent diseases progression. Ishikawa and colleagues[22] found that synovectomy procedures can provide significant pain relief even in advanced cases of the disease. Controversy also exists regarding the effectiveness of wrist synovectomy. The benefits of wrist synovectomy are difficult to evaluate properly because the procedure is usually performed in conjunction with other surgical procedures. No studies currently show conclusively that a synovectomy can change the natural course of RA. Several authors have reported that during the early stages of RA, the procedure provides pain relief and maintains grip strength with a lower probability of tendon rupture but may cause varying degrees of long-term loss of wrist motion.[23–28] Some investigators claim that the pain relief is ultimately transitory, with recurrence depending on the level of RA activity.[24] Wrist synovectomy cannot stop the progression of intra-articular cartilage destruction completely.[26,28–30]

Treatment of the DRUJ

Involvement of the DRUJ is a common cause of disability in the rheumatoid wrist, which may include wrist pain, restriction of pronation and supination, and compromised extensor tendons from a dorsally prominent ulnar head. Two procedures are commonly used to treat problems with the DRUJ.

Darrach procedure (distal ulna resection)

In 1912, Darrach[31,32] first described resecting the distal ulna in a patient with anterior ulnar subluxation. This resection is followed by significant reduction of pain caused by DRUJ problems and ulnar impingement on the carpus. Its efficacy in preventing extensor carpi tendon rupture is unclear. This procedure is most commonly indicated in low-demand or elderly patients with persistent ulnar-sided wrist pain and limited forearm rotation caused by a DRUJ problem.[33] Because forearm motion, grip strength, and lifting capability of the hand may be impaired, this procedure is usually not performed in high-demand patients. One concern with this procedure is the potential ulnar translation of the carpus in patients with weak ligamentous support. For patients whose lunates are already migrating toward the ulna, the Sauve-Kapandji procedure may be preferential, because the intact ulnar head can support the ulnar carpus. The other alternative would be to perform a concomitant radiolunate fusion alongside the Darrach procedure, provided that the midcarpal joint is intact. Combining the Darrach procedure with other surgical interventions is sometimes necessary to obtain optimal stabilization of the carpus.[34] These treatment options may be possible for patients whose symptoms are limited to the radioulnar joint and whose radiocarpal joint is stable and functional.

Sauve-Kapandji procedure

This procedure fuses the ulna head to the sigmoid notch of the radius and creates a pseudarthrosis by a proximal ulnar osteotomy to allow for rotation of the forearm (**Fig. 4**A).[35–37] This procedure is more appropriate for younger or high-demand patients or those who have ulnar translocation of their carpus.[38] A new joint is created farther down the ulna, stabilizing and preventing abnormal movement of the carpus at the DRUJ, while simultaneously unloading the ulna. This technique allows the ulna to be shortened, thereby transmitting more force across the radius rather than the damaged TFCC. Unfortunately, whether this method can prevent further dislocation of the carpus is still unclear, because robust studies on the long-term outcomes of the Sauve-Kapandji procedure are lacking.[9] A potential problem is the unpredictable fusion of the DRUJ when the bone stock in RA is insufficient. Fujita and

colleagues[39,40] reported on the Modified Sauve-Kapandji procedure (see **Fig. 4**B, C), which is designed to solve this problem. The modified procedure involves resecting the distal ulna and making a drill hole in the ulnar cortex of the distal part of the radius. The resected distal ulna is rotated 90°, inserted into the hole made in the distal radius, and secured with cancellous bone screw. The investigators concluded that the technique provides sufficient osseous support of the carpus in patients with poor bone quality.

Arthrodesis

For patients with symptoms arising from the radiocarpal joint, the choices are straightforward, involving either an arthrodesis or arthroplasty procedure. The arthrodesis procedures can be classified into either partial or total wrist fusion.

Partial wrist fusion

Partial wrist fusion is useful in patients with RA whose disease has destroyed the radiocarpal joints but has left the midcarpal joints unaffected. Limited arthrodesis of the involved joints combined with a synovectomy of the less-involved joints may relieve pain and preserve wrist motion. Radiolunate fusion, a representative of this kind of operation, was first described by Chamay and colleagues[41] and is performed in addition to a synovectomy and ulnar head resection when ulnar translation of the carpus is seen on radiographs. A radiolunate fusion will stabilize the wrist and allow motion through the midcarpal joint. Reported results include a decrease in pain and prevention of further ulnar carpal translocation, thus allowing for a satisfactory level of joint mobility. Borisch and colleagues[42] have shown long-term maintenance of the integrity of the midcarpal joint after radiolunate fusion.

Total wrist fusion

For patients with advanced arthritic changes in both the radiocarpal and midcarpal joints, total wrist fusion (TWF) is a well-established, safe, and reliable surgical option. TWF stabilizes the wrist and decreases pain, ultimately improving the patient's quality of life. This procedure is sometimes selected as a salvage procedure after a previous wrist surgery has failed. TWF can be achieved successfully either using pins or plates. Several articles compare the efficacy of various arthrodesis techniques, but no significant difference in outcomes between techniques was observed.[43–46]

Arthroplasty

Total wrist arthroplasty (TWA) is another motion-preserving alternative for patients with severe

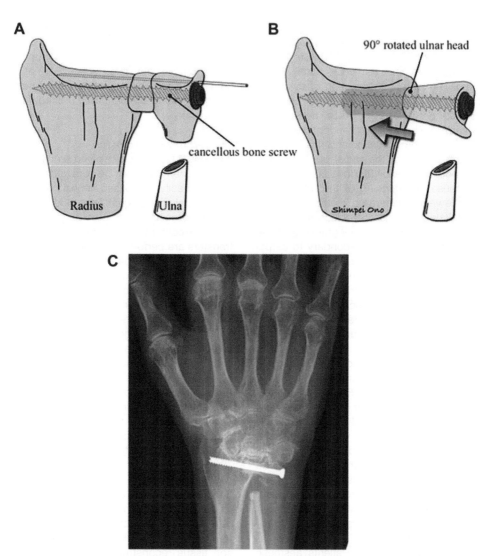

Fig. 4. Sauve-Kapandji procedure and a modified version. (*A*) Sauve-Kapandji procedure. (*B*) Modified Sauve-Kapandji procedure. The 90° rotated resected portion of the ulna is inserted into the distal part of the radius and fixed using a cancellous bone screw. (*C*) Radiograph of modified Sauve-Kapandji procedure.

deformities. Unsolved problems exist related to joint replacement prostheses, including loosening of the prosthesis, implant fracture, periprosthetic bone problems, and degenerative wear of the implants. Therefore, choosing between performing a TWF or a TWA is sometimes difficult. A systematic review comparing TWF and TWA showed that outcomes of TWF procedures were potentially more appealing than those of TWA,[47] but did not support the widespread application of TWA. Another decision analysis based on hand surgeon preferences assigned similar efficacies to TWF and TWA, showing that TWAs were only slightly preferred over TWFs.[48] Moreover, an economic analysis showed that a TWA incurred only a slightly higher cost over the traditional

TWF and that the incremental cost and quality-adjusted life-years for both treatment options were much lower than the acceptable range in the national criteria for adoption of a treatment strategy.[49] Other studies attempting to determine superiority between the procedures have also remained inconclusive.[50]

MCPJ

Pathology

Palmar subluxation, ulnar deviation, and flexion represent the deformities seen at the MCPJ. The synovial pannus in the MCPJ stretches the joint capsule, leading to rupture of the extensor tendon insertion over the base of the proximal phalanx, and resulting in palmar subluxation of the proximal phalanx on the metacarpal head. Progressive synovitis leads to elongation and rupture of the collateral ligaments and the volar plate, which exacerbates the palmar subluxation of the proximal phalanx. The ulnar deviation deformity (see **Fig. 1**) results partly from the radial deviation of the metacarpals. The extensor tendons subluxate into the intermetacarpal sulcus, and this is aggravated by attenuation of the radial portion of the extensor hood. The flexor tendons also translate ulnarly because of stretching of the MCPJ capsule, and the vector generated by the pull of the flexor is oblique and ulnar in relation to the axis of the A1 pulley. The relative lengthening of the flexor and extensor tendons secondary to carpal collapse leads to unopposed action of the intrinsics, resulting in a flexion deformity at the MCPJ. Over time, this results in intrinsic contracture. Fine pinch function also becomes disordered from ulnar drift because the index and long fingers can no longer oppose the thumb in a tip-to-tip pinch.

In the early stages of rheumatoid MCPJ disease, synovectomy sometimes combined with a crossed intrinsic transfer is sufficient. For a patient with chronic MCPJ subluxation or joint destruction, soft tissue reconstruction will not be effective and an arthroplasty procedure will be necessary. In patients who have collapsed wrists and radial deviation of the metacarpals, the wrist should be addressed first; otherwise radial deviation of the metacarpals will cause early postoperative ulnar subluxation of the fingers after MCPJ arthroplasty. Finger MCPJ should not be fused unless arthroplasty is not possible, because fusion causes considerable functional impairment. Patients' aesthetic consideration must be kept in mind, because the appearance of MCPJ is a prominent feature of the hand and shown to be important for men and women.[13]

Synovectomy

Before considering a synovectomy, the patient must have an adequate amount of conservative therapy, including systemic medication, splinting, and local intra-articular corticosteroid injections. Synovectomies are indicated for patients with resistance to medical treatment, persistent MCPJ synovitis, minimal joint deformity, and minimal radiographic manifestations of RA. Intermittent painful synovitis is an additional indication for a synovectomy. Although the available data do not indicate an interruption or a decrease in disease progression, a significant reduction of pain is generally achieved. Sekiya and colleagues[51,52] recently reported two case series regarding the usefulness of synovectomy procedures performed through arthroscopy of MCPJ and PIPJ in patients with RA. A recurrence of symptoms after the procedure is possible (30%–50% of patients undergo spontaneous remission), making the effectiveness of synovectomy procedures difficult to evaluate.

Crossed intrinsic transfer

If the MCPJ is not too involved and the fingers are drifted ulnarly but can be reduced to the natural posture easily, a crossed intrinsic transfer procedure is preferred (**Fig. 5**). Past studies have shown that the procedure can provide an effective long-term correction for ulnar drift.[53] Crossed intrinsic transfers are performed in conjunction with MCPJ synovectomy and soft tissue reconstruction (centering of extrinsic extensor tendons and repair or reefing of radial collateral ligaments and joint capsules). The ulnar lateral bands of the index, long, and ring fingers are transferred to the long, ring, and small finger extensor tendons or the radial lateral band in an effort to add more radial pull to the fingers. Rather than releasing the ulnar intrinsic tendons, the tendons may be used to reinforce the radial supporting structures of the adjacent fingers. The radial sagittal band of the affected finger is tightened to centralize its extensor tendon, because no ulnar intrinsic tendon is available for transfer.

MCPJ arthroplasty

Severe deformities at the MCPJ may manifest as joint destruction, chronic subluxation, and severe ulnar deviation. The ligamentous contractures around the joints cannot be corrected by soft tissue reconstruction alone. In most cases, silicone implants are the most reliable arthroplasty technique to replace destroyed joints. A recent prospective study showed significant improvement for patients with RA with poor baseline function treated with the silicone metacarpophalangeal arthroplasty (SMPA) compared with the nonsurgical group.[54] Significant pain unresponsive to conservative treatments and impaired function were strongly associated with patients who chose surgical treatment.[55] MCPJ arthroplasty must be limited to patients with severe functional impairments because some patients with major deformities can maintain a reasonable level of function, which may not improve significantly after joint reconstruction. MCPJ arthroplasty also has the advantage of shortening the bone at the MCPJ, decreasing the tension on the tendons and ligaments contributing to the ulnar deformity. Although various procedures are available for joint replacements, SMPA is the most widely used and

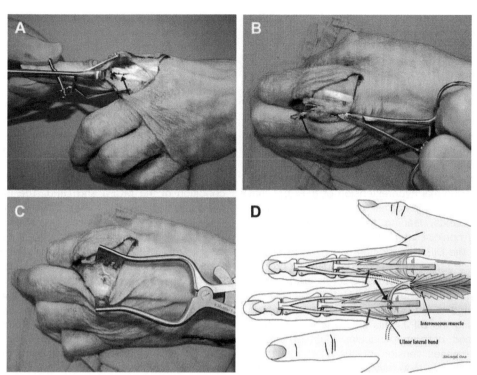

Fig. 5. Crossed intrinsic transfer. (*A*) Tightness of ulnar intrinsics necessitates release of ulnar lateral bands (*blue arrow*). The ulnar lateral band of index finger is identified in this picture. (*B*) The released ulnar lateral band of index finger (*blue arrow*) is transferred to the adjacent extensor mechanism (extensor tendon) of long finger for added stability. (*C*) Immediate postoperative view. (*D*) Illustration of this technique; red lines show the cutting sites. The ulnar lateral band of the index finger is transferred to the long finger (*black arrow*).

studied for the MCPJ.[56–58] Silicone implants are easy to place, can be revised without much difficulty, and are reasonable in cost.[59] These implants differ in fixation, articulation, and motion from other joint replacement prostheses.[60] The silicone prosthesis acts as a spacer between the metacarpal and proximal phalanx. The pistoning or gliding of the implant within the medullary canal is thought to add to the range of motion achieved by the arthroplasty and to disperse the forces along the implant–bone interface.[60,61] If an SMPA is performed, one of the most important considerations is the restoration of function. The literature indicates that one can anticipate an arc of motion within the 50° range, with improvement of extensor lag.[61] Improvement of ulnar deviation also occurs, although some ulnar drift tends to recur over time.[60–63] Recent studies have shown that outcomes for the ulnar digits seem to be worse than those for the radial digits after SMPA. Although the radial fingers can be aligned readily, achieving a satisfactory reduction for the ring and particularly the small finger may be difficult. To achieve sufficient correction of the deformities in the ulnar fingers, adequate bone resection and careful realignment of the extensor mechanism are essential, and the

abductor digiti minimi tendon is sometimes divided to release the small finger.[64] Another important outcome after MCPJ arthroplasty is the improvement in the appearance of the hand. The use of silicone implants have been shown to effectively correct ulnar drift deformities and improve the appearance of the rheumatoid hand. Short-term functional and aesthetic outcomes of the SMPA procedures are impressive,[65,66] but long-term studies have shown a high rate of breakage from imperfections of silicone used as an arthroplasty material.[67,68] Silicone implant fracture rates average at 2% of cases (range, 0%–38%).[69] Fortunately in most cases, implant fractures do not require revision of the prosthetic component; many authors report that most patients with fractured implants retain an acceptable level of function and do not require further surgery.[70]

PIPJ

The two main deformities at the PIPJ are the swan-neck deformity and the boutonniere deformity.

Swan-neck deformity
Swan-neck deformity is characterized by hyperextension of the PIPJ with reciprocal flexion of the

MCPJ and distal interphalangeal joint (DIPJ) (**Fig. 6**). A swan-neck deformity can occur from a disorder at the wrist, MCPJ, PIPJ, or DIPJ. The pathogenesis of wrist and MCPJ deformity was described earlier. At the PIPJ, the synovial pannus distends the joint and stretches the dorsal surface of the volar plate. This synovitis leads to stretching, weakening, and eventually destruction of the volar plate and collateral ligaments, and the insertion of the flexor digitorum superficialis (FDS), resulting in loss of palmar restraint at the PIPJ. This effect allows the normal extensor forces to cause abnormal hyperextension of the PIPJ that in turn relaxes the normal tension on the conjoint lateral bands, leading to dorsal migration. A relaxed conjoint lateral band loses the ability to extend the DIPJ. In addition, the hyperextension of the PIPJ stretches the flexor digitorum profundus (FDP) through increasing its flexor action of the DIPJ and causes the loss of the mechanical advantage of the oblique retinacular ligament in extending the DIPJ. This loss of conjoint lateral band and oblique retinacular ligament tension and increased tension of the FDP results in a DIPJ flexion deformity. Over time, adhesions develop between the central slip and the dorsally translated conjoint lateral bands, converting the flexible deformity to a fixed deformity. DIPJ synovitis can cause weakening and rupture of the terminal extensor tendon insertion, leading to the development of a mallet deformity. The proximal migration of the terminal extensor insertion will cause the lateral bands to become lax. All the power of the common extrinsic extensor will now be directed toward the central slip that inserts into the middle phalanx. Over time, the volar supporting structures of the PIPJ are weakened and the PIPJ is forced into hyperextension, resulting in a swan-neck deformity.

The treatment of a swan-neck deformity depends on the passive range of motion at the PIPJ and condition of the MCPJ and DIPJ. The MCPJ is evaluated to determine the condition of the articular surfaces and the presence of intrinsic muscle shortening. Treatment of the MCPJ (intrinsic release or MCPJ implant arthroplasty) should take precedence in patients with an abnormal MCPJ. The DIPJ is evaluated to determine the condition of the articular surfaces and whether the insertion of the terminal tendon into the base of the dorsum of the distal phalanx is preserved. Treatment of an abnormal DIPJ is DIPJ fusion. The surgical treatment of a flexible hyperextension deformity at the PIPJ has the goal of creating a palmar restraint that will allow flexion and extension but preventing hyperextension. A tenodesis is most often used for this purpose. This tenodesis can be performed using either the FDS

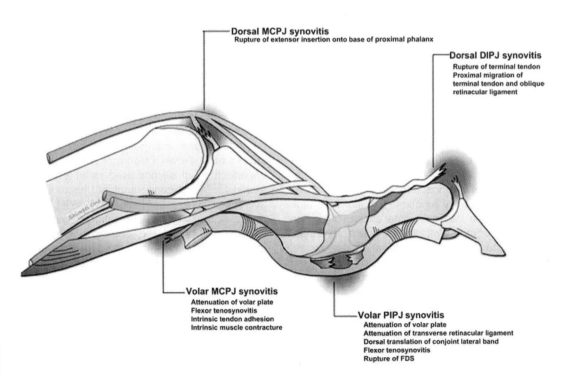

Dorsal MCPJ synovitis
Rupture of extensor insertion onto base of proximal phalanx

Dorsal DIPJ synovitis
Rupture of terminal tendon
Proximal migration of terminal tendon and oblique retinacular ligament

Volar MCPJ synovitis
Attenuation of volar plate
Flexor tenosynovitis
Intrinsic tendon adhesion
Intrinsic muscle contracture

Volar PIPJ synovitis
Attenuation of volar plate
Attenuation of transverse retinacular ligament
Dorsal translation of conjoint lateral band
Flexor tenosynovitis
Rupture of FDS

Fig. 6. Swan neck deformity. Swan neck deformity is characterized by hyperextension of the PIPJ with reciprocal flexion of the MCPJ and DIPJ.

(superficialis tenodesis)[71–73] or the conjoint lateral band.[74–76] The most important aspect of tenodesis is to fix the tendon to bone instead of soft tissue (eg, collateral ligament, pulley, flexor sheath), because a soft tissue attachment invariably attenuates over time. The authors prefer the superficialis tenodesis because it is simple, provides a sturdier check-rein against PIPJ hyperextension, and can be performed in the palm, thus avoiding dissection in zone two.[72] Superficialis tenodesis does not address the mallet deformity in patients with an intact terminal tendon insertion. Conjoint lateral band tenodesis corrects the PIPJ hyperextension and DIPJ flexion simultaneously. However, the quality of the conjoint lateral band can vary among patients, and dissecting it in a rheumatoid digit can be challenging. In patients with a limited range of PIPJ motion the goal is to restore flexibility, which is achieved by releasing the adhesions and soft tissue contractures through manipulation under anesthesia. A surgical release of the joint is considered only in select cases if manipulation is not successful. A surgical release will require compliance with a rigorous postoperative therapy regimen because surgery itself can lead to increased adhesions and scarring, and therefore patient selection is important. The presence of digital flexor tenosynovitis should also be determined, because this may restrict flexor tendon excursion. A patient with RA with flexor tenosynovitis will have good passive range of motion but limited active range of motion, whereas a patient with joint damage will have limitation in both passive and active motion.[77] In patients who have no passive motion at the PIPJ because of articular damage to the proximal interphalangeal joint surface or an unstable dislocated joint, the treatment choices are limited to joint fusion or implant arthroplasty. Although implant arthroplasty seems to be an attractive solution, the authors believe that joint fusion is the more reliable option in patients with RA. The ligamentous support of the PIPJ in RA is usually diseased and does not provide enough stability for implants. Implant arthroplasty of the PIPJ in RA is limited to the ring and small fingers (index and long fingers need good lateral stability, and flexion is less important) in patients with good adjacent joints (no MCPJ disease), good dorsal skin, intact flexor tendons, and good soft tissue support.[78]

Boutonniere deformity

Boutonniere deformity is characterized by a flexion deformity of the PIPJ with reciprocal extension of the MCPJ and DIPJ (**Fig. 7**).[79] Unlike swan-neck deformity, boutonniere deformity has only one factor contributing to its development (ie, synovitis of the PIPJ).[80,81] The synovial pannus distends the capsuloligamentous apparatus and the central band. It stretches the conjoint lateral bands laterally, breaking through between the central band and the conjoint lateral bands. This process combined with stretching of the central band leads to a volar displacement of the conjoint lateral bands over the convexity of the phalangeal condyles. The conjoint lateral bands are now volar to the axis of rotation of the PIPJ and become a flexor of the PIPJ instead of its normal role as

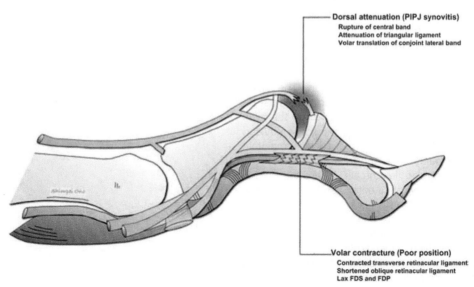

Dorsal attenuation (PIPJ synovitis)
Rupture of central band
Attenuation of triangular ligament
Volar translation of conjoint lateral band

Volar contracture (Poor position)
Contracted transverse retinacular ligament
Shortened oblique retinacular ligament
Lax FDS and FDP

Fig. 7. Boutonniere's deformity. Boutonniere's deformity is characterized by a flexion deformity of the PIPJ with reciprocal extension of the MCPJ and DIPJ.

an extensor. The stretched central band is no longer able to maintain full extension of the PIPJ, and the volarly subluxed conjoint lateral bands maintain persistent PIPJ flexion. Eventually, the head of the proximal phalanx prolapses through the attenuated central slip like a button through a button hole. The rupture of the central slip means that the interosseous and lumbrical muscles no longer have an insertion into the base of the middle phalanx, and their force is now transmitted via the lateral bands to the distal phalanx with resultant hyperextension of the DIPJ. The proximal migration of the extensor apparatus as a result of the boutonniere deformity allows the pull of the extensor tendon to be concentrated on its insertion into the base of the proximal phalanx, resulting in hyperextension of the MCPJ. Eventually, persistent PIPJ flexion leads to shortening and contracture of the volar plate, collateral ligaments, transverse retinacular ligament, and oblique retinacular ligaments. The shortening of the oblique retinacular ligaments maintains the hyperextension deformity at the DIPJ and limits active flexion of the DIPJ. MCPJ hyperextension is thereby exaggerated through compensating for the increasing PIPJ flexion deformity. Passive correction of the boutonniere deformity is possible in the early stage, but later becomes fixed because of fibrosis and contracture of the capsular structures.[59,82]

The soft tissue reconstruction of rheumatoid boutonniere deformity is unpredictable and often disappointing. A boutonniere deformity is not as functionally disabling as swan-neck deformity, and rarely compromises PIPJ flexion and grip strength. One should not trade extension at the PIPJ for a stiff finger and a weak hand. Like swan-neck deformity, the treatment of boutonniere deformity depends on the passive range of motion at PIPJ. Patients with a normal PIPJ and an early boutonniere deformity are best treated by splinting the PIPJ in extension. The splint should not extend to the DIPJ and care must be taken to avoid pressure necrosis of the skin around the PIPJ. The patients should be advised to continue to flex the DIPJ, which will maintain the lateral bands in a good position. In patients who are unable to flex the DIPJ while the PIPJ is maintained in complete extension by a tight oblique retinacular ligament, an extensor tenotomy will be required. Transecting the terminal tendon will permit the extensor tendon system to migrate proximally, which places additional tension on the PIPJ through the central tendon to the middle phalanx to partially overcome the flexion posture of the PIPJ. If patients have a limited range of PIPJ motion, they will need surgery to restore extensor force to the PIPJ using local tissues. Before considering any surgical treatment, the patient should undergo a trial of splinting to try to stretch out the collateral ligaments, volar plate, joint capsule, and volar skin. It is also important to establish that the flexor tendons are intact and functioning and that the joint surfaces are smooth on the radiograph. Surgery has the goal of excising and repairing the attenuated portion of the central band, while repositioning and maintaining the conjoint lateral bands dorsally. If patients have no passive motion at the PIPJ or have articular damage, surgical options are limited to joint fusion or implant arthroplasty. The indications for implant arthroplasty in boutonniere deformity are even more limited than for swan-neck deformity, because a significant resection of the proximal phalanx is required to seat the implants in the flexed boutonniere deformity, and this leads to instability because the collateral ligaments must be sacrificed. Additionally, an extensor reconstruction is needed, which adds to the period before mobilization can be started. The authors' preferred treatment for severe boutonniere deformity is fusion of the PIPJ.

Thumb Deformity

Thumb deformities are common manifestations of RA and represent a significant source of disability. The thumb is estimated to be responsible for 50% of the hand function. The thumb deformity can present as a boutonniere's posture, in which the MCPJ is flexed and the interphalangeal joint is hyperextended (**Fig. 8**), or the less-common swan-neck deformity, in which the MCPJ is extended and the interphalangeal joint is flexed.[83]

The goal of treatment is the restoration and maintenance of stable and painless motion.

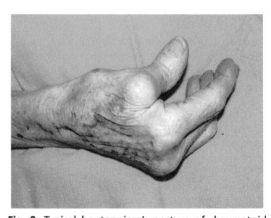

Fig. 8. Typical boutonniere's posture of rheumatoid thumb in which the MCPJ is flexed and the interphalangeal joint is hyperextended.

Treatment is based on the type and stage of the specific deformity. Early disease is amenable to nonsurgical measures or soft tissue procedures, such as synovectomy, rerouting of the extensor pollicis longus tendon, or capsulodesis. More severe joint involvement is best treated with arthroplasty or arthrodesis. Arthroplasty is the preferred procedure in low-demand patients or those requiring fine dexterity skills; arthrodesis may benefit more active patients.[84] Basically, fusion of two joints in tandem is considered the last stage because this will markedly limit the movement of the thumb. Interphalangeal joint fusion at 0° to 20° is tolerated extremely well and maintains function. MCPJ arthroplasty is recommended if the carpometacarpal and interphalangeal joints are to be fused so that the motion of the thumb can be preserved for prehensile tasks. In certain situations fusion of the thumb MCPJ should be considered the primary operation. Instability of the thumb at this level is distressing because the subluxation of the thumb MCPJ can greatly affect grip strength. During exposure for the fusion operation, the extensor mechanisms can be lengthened or shortened depending on the posture of the reconstructed thumb.

Tenosynovitis and Tendon Rupture

Tendons can be involved in RA wherever they are covered by tenosynovium or when they come in close contact with joints or bones affected by RA. Flexor tendons are covered by tenosynovium under the carpal tunnel and in the digital flexor sheath, whereas extensor tendons are covered by tenosynovium only under the extensor retinaculum. Synovitis involves the extensor tendons more frequently than the flexor tendons of the hand. As synovitis progresses, the tendon is infiltrated by the invasive synovium and structural changes occur in the tendinous tissue, which may include ischemic necrosis, eventually leading to loss of function and rupture without additional mechanical irritation. Synovitis of the extensor tendons commonly develops in the ulnar three extensor compartments, affecting the extensor digitorum communis, the extensor digiti quinti, and the ECU. The most common rupture is that of the extensors of the small finger, caused by attrition by the ulnar head. Other common tendon ruptures are to the extensor digitorum communis tendons to the ring and long fingers, followed by the extensor pollicis longus, and rarely the ECU.

Synovitis of the flexor tendons can present as isolated carpal tenosynovitis (20%), palmodigital tenosynovitis (50%), and diffuse tenosynovitis (30%). The index, long, and small fingers are most frequently involved. Rheumatoid nodules are three times more frequent in the flexor tendons than the extensor tendons and are usually confined to the profundus tendon.[85] The most common flexor tendon to be ruptured is the flexor pollicis longus, caused by bone spicules from the scaphoid, which may also rupture the FDP of the index finger. The distal ulna affects the FDP of the small finger. A flexor tendon rupture in the digital flexor sheath is almost always secondary to infiltrative synovitis, and usually involves the FDS at the PIPJ.[86]

Treatment of ruptured extensor tendons

The definitive treatment of tendon rupture is to address the offending causes through removing the head of the ulna and excising the hypertrophic synovial tissue over the extensor mechanism. Treatment options of extensor tendon rupture related to RA are as follows (**Fig. 9**):

- For patients with isolated small finger extensor tendon rupture, the distal end of the small finger extensor tendon can be transferred end-to-side to the intact extensor tendon of the ring finger.
- For patients with both ring and small finger extensor tendon ruptures, the extensor indicis proprius tendon can be transferred over to power both the ring and small finger extensor tendons. If the ring and small finger extensor tendons were sutured to the long finger extensor tendon, the oblique path of the transferred tendons could result in abduction of the small finger, causing functional problems.
- For patients with long, ring, and small finger extensor tendon ruptures, the extensor indicis proprius tendon can be transferred to power the ring and small finger, whereas the long finger can be sutured end-to-side to the index extensor tendon. Because all four fingers will be powered by the extensor tendons to the index finger, the strength of extension will be greatly diminished. An alternative strategy is to transfer the FDS tendon from either the long or the ring finger to power the ring and small fingers, whereas the extensor indicis proprius tendon is used to power the long finger.
- For patients with all four finger extensor tendon ruptures, using the FDS tendons of the long and ring fingers should be considered, with one tendon mobilizing the ring and small finger and the other powering the index and long fingers, respectively. The FDS of the long finger can be passed

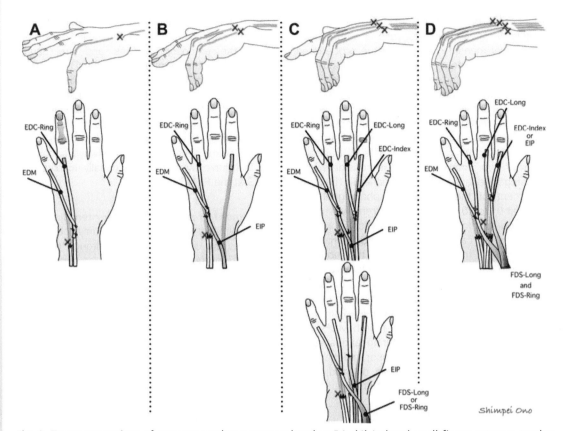

Fig. 9. Treatment options of extensor tendon rupture related to RA. (*A*) Isolated small finger extensor tendon rupture. Extensor digiti minimi (EDM) is transferred to extensor digitorum communis (EDC) of ring finger (EDC-Ring). (*B*) Both ring and small finger extensor tendon ruptures. Extensor indicis proprius (EIP) is transferred to EDC-Ring and EDM. (*C*) Long, ring, and small finger extensor tendon ruptures. (1) EIP transferred to the EDC-Ring and EDM, and EDC of long finger (EDC-Long) to EDC of index finger (EDC-Index). (2) Flexor digitorum superficialis (FDS) of long/ring transferred to EDC-Ring and EDM, and EIP to EDC-Long. (*D*) All four finger extensor tendon ruptures. FDS-Long transferred to EDC-Index/EIP, and FDS-Ring to EDC-Ring and EDM.

subcutaneously radially to power in the index and long fingers, whereas the FDS of the ring finger can be transferred from the ulnar direction to power the ring and small fingers. Although the FDS for finger extension is not a synergistic transfer, this tendon has more than 70 mm of excursion and is useful for tendon transfers in this situation.

Treatment of ruptured flexor tendons

Management of a flexor tendon rupture within the digit is difficult, and a flexor tenosynovectomy performed early can prevent this. Rupture of the FDS is frequently overlooked because the patient can still fully flex the finger, and therefore many surgeons do not routinely examine the integrity of the FDS tendons. Palpating the volar aspect of the finger and finding an empty sheath, usually at the level of the proximal phalanx, will establish the level of rupture. Treatment options of flexor tendon rupture related to RA are as follows:

- For rupture of the FDS, the FDS should be excised and tenosynovectomy of the FDP should be performed.
- For rupture of the FDP, it may be possible to advance and repair the rupture if it has occurred distal to the FDS insertion, because the proximal end is usually caught at the FDS chiasm. However if repair is not possible or the rupture has occurred proximally, it is better to excise the FDP and do an arthrodesis or tenodesis of the distal interphalangeal joint. Irrespective of what technique is chosen to repair the ruptured FDP, the most important consideration is that a complete flexor tenosynovectomy of the FDS is performed to protect it from rupture.

- Rupture of both the FDS and FDP presents a difficult situation, and the chances of obtaining active flexion at the PIPJ are severely limited. Two options are available: (1) perform a flexor tenosynovectomy, insert a silicone rod, and perform a tendon graft procedure at a later date, or (2) fuse the interphalangeal joints and suture one of the long flexors to the base of the proximal phalanx (flexor sheath or bone) to increase the strength of flexion at the MCPJ.

SUMMARY

Surgical treatment is clearly essential for improving the quality of life for patients with a rheumatoid hand; however, the indication for surgical intervention and the decision making among various treatment options are still complex issues. A major reason for this is that RA affects each individual differently. Therefore, it is important to consider the priority among necessary treatment steps and the patient's specific lifestyle needs, and to outline expectations for improvement. Although some patients with hand deformities may not necessarily need reconstructive surgery, others may seek functional or aesthetic improvement through surgery. The other reason for the complex decision process is the lack of well-established outcomes studies regarding the effectiveness of rheumatoid hand surgery, making clear-cut guidelines difficult to establish, and sometimes delaying referrals for hand surgery consultations from rheumatologists. Future outcomes research is vital to assessing the effectiveness of various surgical procedures and determining whether these techniques are effective in improving the quality of life for patients. An experienced rheumatoid hand surgeon will strive to understand the patient's needs and expectations for improvement, and the available surgical options that will allow the best outcome.

REFERENCES

1. de la Mata Llord J, Palacios Carvajal J. Rheumatoid arthritis: are outcomes better with medical or surgical management? Orthopedics 1998;21:1085–6.
2. Kavanaugh A. Economic consequences of established rheumatoid arthritis and its treatment. Best Pract Res Clin Rheumatol 2007;21:929–42.
3. Dunlop DD, Manheim LM, Yelin EH, et al. The costs of arthritis. Arthritis Rheum 2003;49:101–13.
4. Lajas C, Abasolo L, Bellajdel B, et al. Costs and predictors of costs in rheumatoid arthritis: a prevalence-based study. Arthritis Rheum 2003;49:64–70.
5. Griffith J, Carr A. What is the impact of early rheumatoid arthritis on the individual? Best Pract Res Clin Rheumatol 2001;15:77–90.
6. Waltz M. The disease process and utilization of health services in rheumatoid arthritis: the relative contributions of various markers of disease severity in explaining consumption patterns. Arthritis Care Res 2000;13:74–88.
7. das Chagas Medeiros MM, Ferraz MB, Quaresma MR. The effect of rheumatoid arthritis on the quality of life of primary caregivers. J Rheumatol 2000;27:76–83.
8. Neville C, Fortin PR, Fitzcharles MA, et al. The needs of patients with arthritis: the patient's perspective. Arthritis Care Res 1999;12:85–95.
9. Ghattas L, Mascella F, Pomponio G. Hand surgery in rheumatoid arthritis: state of the art and suggestions for research. Rheumatology (Oxford) 2005;44:834–45.
10. Neumann D. Kinesiology of the musculoskeletal system: foundations for physical rehabilitation. 1st edition. St Louis (MO): Elsevier Science; 2002.
11. Nalebuff EA, Millender LH. Surgical treatment of the boutonniere deformity in rheumatoid arthritis. Orthop Clin North Am 1975;6:753–63.
12. Nalebuff EA. Metacarpophalangeal surgery in rheumatoid arthritis. Surg Clin North Am 1969;49:823–32.
13. Alderman AK, Arora AS, Kuhn L, et al. An analysis of women's and men's surgical priorities and willingness to have rheumatoid hand surgery. J Hand Surg Am 2006;31:1447–53.
14. Alderman AK, Chung KC, Kim HM, et al. Effectiveness of rheumatoid hand surgery: contrasting perceptions of hand surgeons and rheumatologists. J Hand Surg Am 2003;28:3–11 [discussion: 12–3].
15. Alderman AK, Ubel PA, Kim HM, et al. Surgical management of the rheumatoid hand: consensus and controversy among rheumatologists and hand surgeons. J Rheumatol 2003;30:1464–72.
16. Alderman AK, Chung KC, Demonner S, et al. The rheumatoid hand: a predictable disease with unpredictable surgical practice patterns. Arthritis Rheum 2002;47:537–42.
17. Ilan DI, Rettig ME. Rheumatoid arthritis of the wrist. Bull Hosp Jt Dis 2003;61:179–85.
18. Flatt A. The care of the arthritic hand. 5th edition. Saint Louis (MO): Quality Medical Publishing; 1995.
19. Kim SJ, Jung KA. Arthroscopic synovectomy in rheumatoid arthritis of wrist. Clin Med Res 2007;5:244–50.
20. Lipscomb PR. Synovectomy of the wrist for rheumatoid arthritis. JAMA 1965;194:655–9.
21. Hindley CJ, Stanley JK. The rheumatoid wrist: patterns of disease progression. A review of 50 wrists. J Hand Surg Br 1991;16:275–9.
22. Ishikawa H, Hanyu T, Tajima T. Rheumatoid wrists treated with synovectomy of the extensor tendons

and the wrist joint combined with a Darrach procedure. J Hand Surg Am 1992;17:1109–17.

23. Trieb K. Treatment of the wrist in rheumatoid arthritis. J Hand Surg Am 2008;33:113–23.

24. Rosen A, Weiland AJ. Rheumatoid arthritis of the wrist and hand. Rheum Dis Clin North Am 1998;24: 101–28.

25. Adolfsson L, Frisen M. Arthroscopic synovectomy of the rheumatoid wrist. A 3.8 year follow-up. J Hand Surg Br 1997;22:711–3.

26. Brumfield R Jr, Kuschner SH, Gellman H, et al. Results of dorsal wrist synovectomies in the rheumatoid hand. J Hand Surg Am 1990;15:733–5.

27. Allieu Y, Lussiez B, Asencio G. Long-term results of surgical synovectomies of the rheumatoid wrist. Apropos of 60 cases. Rev Chir Orthop Reparatrice Appar Mot 1989;75:172–8 [in French].

28. Thirupathi RG, Ferlic DC, Clayton ML. Dorsal wrist synovectomy in rheumatoid arthritis–a long-term study. J Hand Surg Am 1983;8:848–56.

29. Millender LH, Nalebuff EA. Preventive surgery—tenosynovectomy and synovectomy. Orthop Clin North Am 1975;6:765–92.

30. Nakamura H, Nagashima M, Ishigami S, et al. The anti-rheumatic effect of multiple synovectomy in patients with refractory rheumatoid arthritis. Int Orthop 2000;24:242–5.

31. Darrach W. Anterior dislocation of the head of the ulna. Ann Surg 1912;56:802–3.

32. Lau FH, Chung KC. William Darrach, MD: his life and his contribution to hand surgery. J Hand Surg Am 2006;31:1056–60.

33. Garcia-Elias M. Failed ulnar head resection: prevention and treatment. J Hand Surg Br 2002;27:470–80.

34. Ishikawa H, Hanyu T, Saito H, et al. Limited arthrodesis for the rheumatoid wrist. J Hand Surg Am 1992; 17:1103–9.

35. Sauvé L, Kapandji M. Nouvelle technique de traitement chirurgical des luxations récidivantes isolées de l'extrémité inférieure du cubitus. J Chir 1936;47: 589–94 [in French].

36. Chantelot C, Fontaine C, Flipo RM, et al. Synovectomy combined with the Sauve-Kapandji procedure for the rheumatoid wrist. J Hand Surg Br 1999;24:405–9.

37. Vincent KA, Szabo RM, Agee JM. The Sauve-Kapandji procedure for reconstruction of the rheumatoid distal radioulnar joint. J Hand Surg Am 1993;18:978–83.

38. Millroy P, Coleman S, Ivers R. The Sauve-Kapandji operation. Technique and results. J Hand Surg Br 1992;17:411–4.

39. Fujita S, Masada K, Takeuchi E, et al. Modified Sauve-Kapandji procedure for disorders of the distal radioulnar joint in patients with rheumatoid arthritis. J Bone Joint Surg Am 2005;87:134–9.

40. Fujita S, Masada K, Takeuchi E, et al. Modified Sauve-Kapandji procedure for disorders of the distal

41. Chamay A, Della Santa D, Vilaseca A. Radiolunate arthrodesis. Factor of stability for the rheumatoid wrist. Ann Chir Main 1983;2:5–17.

42. Borisch N, Haussmann P. Radiolunate arthrodesis in the rheumatoid wrist: a retrospective clinical and radiological longterm follow-up. J Hand Surg Br 2002;27:61–72.

43. Toma CD, Machacek P, Bitzan P, et al. Fusion of the wrist in rheumatoid arthritis: a clinical and functional evaluation of two surgical techniques. J Bone Joint Surg Br 2007;89:1620–6.

44. Rehak DC, Kasper P, Baratz ME, et al. A comparison of plate and pin fixation for arthrodesis of the rheumatoid wrist. Orthopedics 2000;23:43–8.

45. Christodoulou L, Patwardhan MS, Burke FD. Open and closed arthrodesis of the rheumatoid wrist using a modified (Stanley) Steinmann pin. J Hand Surg Br 1999;24:662–6.

46. Howard AC, Stanley D, Getty CJ. Wrist arthrodesis in rheumatoid arthritis. A comparison of two methods of fusion. J Hand Surg Br 1993;18:377–80.

47. Cavaliere CM, Chung KC. A systematic review of total wrist arthroplasty compared with total wrist arthrodesis for rheumatoid arthritis. Plast Reconstr Surg 2008;122:813–25.

48. Cavaliere CM, Chung KC. Total wrist arthroplasty and total wrist arthrodesis in rheumatoid arthritis: a decision analysis from the hand surgeons' perspective. J Hand Surg Am 2008;33:1744–55, 55 e1–2.

49. Cavaliere CM, Chung KC. A cost-utility analysis of nonsurgical management, total wrist arthroplasty, and total wrist arthrodesis in rheumatoid arthritis. J Hand Surg Am 2010;35:379.e2–91.e2.

50. Murphy DM, Khoury JG, Imbriglia JE, et al. Comparison of arthroplasty and arthrodesis for the rheumatoid wrist. J Hand Surg Am 2003;28:570–6.

51. Sekiya I, Kobayashi M, Okamoto H, et al. Arthroscopic synovectomy of the metacarpophalangeal and proximal interphalangeal joints. Tech Hand Up Extrem Surg 2008;12:221–5.

52. Sekiya I, Kobayashi M, Taneda Y, et al. Arthroscopy of the proximal interphalangeal and metacarpophalangeal joints in rheumatoid hands. Arthroscopy 2002;18:292–7.

53. Oster LH, Blair WF, Steyers CM, et al. Crossed intrinsic transfer. J Hand Surg Am 1989;14:963–71.

54. Chung KC, Burns PB, Wilgis EF, et al. A multicenter clinical trial in rheumatoid arthritis comparing silicone metacarpophalangeal joint arthroplasty with medical treatment. J Hand Surg Am 2009;34:815–23.

55. Chung KC, Kotsis SV, Kim HM, et al. Reasons why rheumatoid arthritis patients seek surgical treatment for hand deformities. J Hand Surg Am 2006;31: 289–94.

radioulnar joint in patients with rheumatoid arthritis. Surgical technique. J Bone Joint Surg Am 2006; 88(Suppl 1 Pt 1):24–8.

56. Linscheid RL. Implant arthroplasty of the hand: retrospective and prospective considerations. J Hand Surg Am 2000;25:796–816.

57. Sollerman CJ, Geijer M. Polyurethane versus silicone for endoprosthetic replacement of the metacarpophalangeal joints in rheumatoid arthritis. Scand J Plast Reconstr Surg Hand Surg 1996;30:145–50.

58. el-Gammal TA, Blair WF. Motion after metacarpophalangeal joint reconstruction in rheumatoid disease. J Hand Surg Am 1993;18:504–11.

59. Feldon P, Terrono AL, Nalebuff EA, et al. Rheumatoid arthritis and other connective tissue diseases. In: Green DP, Hotchkiss RN, Pederson WC, et al, editors. Green's operative hand surgery. Philadelphia: Elsevier/Churchill Livingstone; 2005. p. 2049–136.

60. Swanson AB. Flexible implant arthroplasty for arthritic finger joints: rationale, technique, and results of treatment. J Bone Joint Surg Am 1972;54:435–55.

61. Stirrat CR. Metacarpophalangeal joints in rheumatoid arthritis of the hand. Hand Clin 1996;12:515–29.

62. Bieber EJ, Weiland AJ, Volenec-Dowling S. Silicone-rubber implant arthroplasty of the metacarpophalangeal joints for rheumatoid arthritis. J Bone Joint Surg Am 1986;68:206–9.

63. Beckenbaugh RD, Dobyns JH, Linscheid RL, et al. Review and analysis of silicone-rubber metacarpophalangeal implants. J Bone Joint Surg Am 1976;58:483–7.

64. Chung KC, Kotsis SV, Wilgis EF, et al. Outcomes of silicone arthroplasty for rheumatoid metacarpophalangeal joints stratified by fingers. J Hand Surg Am 2009;34:1647–52.

65. Chung KC, Kowalski CP, Myra Kim H, et al. Patient outcomes following Swanson silastic metacarpophalangeal joint arthroplasty in the rheumatoid hand: a systematic overview. J Rheumatol 2000;27:1395–402.

66. Chung KC, Kotsis SV, Kim HM. A prospective outcomes study of Swanson metacarpophalangeal joint arthroplasty for the rheumatoid hand. J Hand Surg Am 2004;29:646–53.

67. Burgess SD, Kono M, Stern PJ. Results of revision metacarpophalangeal joint surgery in rheumatoid patients following previous silicone arthroplasty. J Hand Surg Am 2007;32:1506–12.

68. Bass RL, Stern PJ, Nairus JG. High implant fracture incidence with Sutter silicone metacarpophalangeal joint arthroplasty. J Hand Surg Am 1996;21:813–8.

69. Foliart DE. Swanson silicone finger joint implants: a review of the literature regarding long-term complications. J Hand Surg Am 1995;20:445–9.

70. Mannerfelt L, Andersson K. Silastic arthroplasty of the metacarpophalangeal joints in rheumatoid arthritis. J Bone Joint Surg Am 1975;57:484–9.

71. Swanson A. Surgery of the hand in cerebral palsy and swan neck deformity. J Bone Joint Surg Am 1960;42:951–64.

72. Nalebuff EA. The rheumatoid swan-neck deformity. Hand Clin 1989;5:203–14.

73. Milford L. Sublimis tenodesis technique by Curtis. 6th edition. St Louis (MO): Mosby; 1980.

74. Thompson JS, Littler JW, Upton J. The spiral oblique retinacular ligament (SORL). J Hand Surg Am 1978; 3:482–7.

75. Littler JW. The finger extensor mechanism. Surg Clin North Am 1967;47:415–32.

76. Zancolli E. The paralysed hand. Edinburgh (United Kingdom): Churchill Livingstone; 1987.

77. Boyer MI, Gelberman RH. Operative correction of swan-neck and boutonniere deformities in the rheumatoid hand. J Am Acad Orthop Surg 1999;7: 92–100.

78. Nalebuff EA, Millender LH. Surgical treatment of the swan-neck deformity in rheumatoid arthritis. Orthop Clin North Am 1975;6:733–52.

79. Heywood AW. Correction of the rheumatoid boutonniere deformity. J Bone Joint Surg Am 1969;51: 1309–14.

80. Harrison SH. Rheumatoid deformities of the proximal interphalangeal joints of the hand. Ann Rheum Dis 1969;28(Suppl):20–2.

81. Harrison SH. The proximal interphalangeal joint in rheumatoid arthritis. Hand 1971;3:125–30.

82. Zancolli E. Structural and dynamic bases of hand surgery. Philadelphia: JB Lippincott Company; 1968.

83. Nalebuff EA. Diagnosis, classification and management of rheumatoid thumb deformities. Bull Hosp Joint Dis 1968;29:119–37.

84. Rozental TD. Reconstruction of the rheumatoid thumb. J Am Acad Orthop Surg 2007;15:118–25.

85. Saffar P. Flexor tendon synovectomy in rheumatoid arthritis. Amsterdam: Elsevier; 2006.

86. Ertel AN, Millender LH, Nalebuff E, et al. Flexor tendon ruptures in patients with rheumatoid arthritis. J Hand Surg Am 1988;13:860–6.

Intrinsic Flaps in the Hand

Günter Germann, MD, PhD[a],*, Nina Biedermann, MD[b],
Scott L. Levin, MD, PhD[c]

KEYWORDS

• Intrinsic flaps • Hand • Reconstruction

Advances in anatomical knowledge, progress in surgical instrumentation, and innovative surgical techniques have significantly changed soft tissue reconstruction of the hand. Continual improvements in design and harvesting techniques have led to flap refinements, resulting in improved aesthetic and functional results following soft tissue reconstruction. This holds true for microsurgical free flaps, as well as for regional flaps, such as the intrinsic flaps in the hand.

Soft tissue defects of the fingers resulting in exposed tendons, bones, or joints are frequently encountered in hand surgery. Reconstruction can be challenging if the principle of replacing like with like is followed. Extensive literature is available concerning the variety of local and regional flaps that may be used for coverage of these defects.

Intrinsic flaps in the hand can be classified by

> Vascular anatomy (axial/random pattern)
> Donor site location
> Perfusion pattern
> Tissue components included.

Following descriptions by Littler[1] and Bunnell,[2] soft tissue reconstruction in the hand was limited to a small variety of flaps, often resulting in unsatisfactory results, due to considerable donor site morbidity and long rehabilitation times.

This changed with the first descriptions of dorsal metacarpal flaps by Earley and Milner[3] as early as 1980. Their work was based on anatomical dissections performed by Manchot,[4] Salmon[5] and Spalteholz,[6] who described the vascular architecture of the hand. Although, this knowledge was available, it was not applied in reconstructive surgery until the authors' excellent results were reported. These publications also ignited a new wave of research in the vascular anatomy of the hand.

Much of the research was focused on the interconnections between the palmar arterial system and its perforating vessels into the vascular network of the dorsum of the hand.

In the last 20 years, many new flaps have been developed. These are based on small perforating vessels supplying defined skin areas mostly on the dorsal, but also on the palmar side of the hand. Due to the delicate nature of the feeding vessels, harvesting techniques have relied on microsurgical techniques. The authors have coined the term microsurgery without anastomosis for these dissection techniques. Since these flaps are raised within the territory of the hand and based on intrinsic vessels, they have been named intrinsic flaps.

This article will provide an overview of the most commonly used intrinsic flaps of the hand, covering the well-known dorsal metacarpal flaps, as well as some more exotic flaps that can be used for particular indications under suitable anatomical conditions. This article includes the anatomical base for the intrinsic flaps, harvesting techniques, indications, and the important tricks and pitfalls that should be considered to achieve the optimal results. With these flaps the majority of small-to-moderate-sized defects in the hand can be reconstructed with minimal donor site morbidity and excellent functional results.

[a] ETHIANUM – Clinic for Plastic & Reconstructive Surgery, Aesthetic and Preventive Medicine at Heidelberg University Hospital, Vosstrasse, Heidelberg 69115, Germany
[b] ETHIANUM – Clinic for Plastic & Reconstructive Surgery, Aesthetic and Preventive Medicine at Heidelberg University Hospital, Heidelberg 69115, Germany
[c] Department of Orthopedic Surgery, University of Pennsylvania, Philadelphia, PA, USA
* Corresponding author.
E-mail address: guenter.germann@urz.uni-heidelberg.de

Clin Plastic Surg 38 (2011) 729–738
doi:10.1016/j.cps.2011.07.007

ANATOMY

Anatomical knowledge is the basis for successful flap surgery. Understanding the location of tiny perforating vessels, the angiosomes supplied by them, and their connective network to vascular system is essential in order to raise a well-perfused flap that can be reliably rotated or transferred into a defect.

The vasculature of the hand is based on 2 major feeding vessels, the radial and the ulnar artery. Although they are constant, their contribution to the perfusion of the hand varies significantly. Together with both interosseus arteries (posterior and anterial), they feed the carpal network of the wrist by forming a system of palmar and dorsal transverse arches.

The common digital arteries and their cutaneous perforators provide the blood supply of the palm. Two palmar arches (the superficial and deep palmar arch) are formed by the terminal divisions of the ulnar and radial artery and many communications in the palm. The main tributary of the deep palmar arch is the radial artery, while the ulnar artery mainly supplies the superficial palmar arch.

The common digital arteries arise from the superficial palmar arch and run distally until they reach the web space, where they divide into a pair of proper digital arteries. Proximal to their division, the common digital artery usually gives off a branch that runs dorsally to connect with the dorsal metacarpal arterial system.

The palmar metacarpal arteries originate from the deep palmar arch and run distally along each metacarpal. At the metacarpophalangeal (MP) joint they divide into 2 arches, which connect the palmar with the dorsal metacarpal network and form an anastomosis between the deep, superficial palmar arch, the palmar and dorsal metacarpal arteries, and the common digital artery. This network provides the blood supply to the synovial sheaths and intrinsic muscles of the hand. At the MP and interphalangeal (IP) joints, transverse arches connect the palmar and dorsal arterial arches. Vincular vessels arise from the transverse arches to the flexor tendons and palmar structures. Similar to this arrangement, at the distal phalanx the 2 digital arteries connect through a terminal transverse arch and provide nutrient branches to the nail germinal matrix.

FREQUENTLY USED FLAPS
Homodigital Island Flaps

Homodigital island flaps are designed on the digital arteries as well as their concomitant veins. Grayson ligaments on the palmar side and Cleland ligaments on the dorsal side protect these vessels. From the digital arteries at the proximal interphalangeal joint (PIP) or distal interphalangeal joint (DIP) runs a palmar arch to provide retrograde blood flow, on which a retrograde pedicle can be harvested.

Due to the rich vascularization of the hand, flaps can be harvested on a proximal or distal pedicle. Proximally based flaps are called antegrade flaps. Flaps that are nourished by distal inflow are called retrograde flaps.[7] Retrograde flaps can be used to cover distal defects over the DIP or the PIP. These are usually insensate flaps, but can be reinnervated when defects of the fingertips are reconstructed. The proper digital nerve is then included and reconnected to the distal stump of the contralateral proper digital nerve at the defect site. Antegrade flaps usually do not reach further than the PIP, but can also be employed to reconstruct defects over the MP joints or the distal metacarpals.

Antegrade flaps are ideally centered over the feeding vessels and should not exceed an arc of rotation of 90° to 120°, whereas reverse pedicle flaps may have up to 180° rotation arc, with an increased risk of kinking of the pedicle. Adding 10% to 15% more length to the pedicle, avoiding the use of narrow tunnels for the pedicle, and using a loose closure of the wound should avoid these complications.[8] The size of the flap should be slightly bigger than the size of the defect, due to shrinking of the harvested flap.

The donor site can be closed primarily in many cases. A full-thickness skin graft should be employed, when primary closure is not possible, to achieve an inconspicuous donor site (**Figs. 1** and **2**).

Dorsal Metacarpal Artery Flaps

The dorsal metacarpal artery (DMCA) flap (and its modifications) is one of the most frequently used flaps for soft tissue reconstruction in the hand. Detailed knowledge of the anatomical vascular basis is required to achieve reproducible results. Credit has to be given to Paturet,[9] who, for the first time in 1951, distinctively described the anatomy of the first DMCA. "The first DMCA arises from the outer side of the radial artery between the crossing of the extensor pollicis longus and is penetrating into the apex of the first interosseus space. It passes over the interosseus muscle, where it divides into 2 branches: a radial one, the internal dorsal artery of the thumb and an ulnar one, the external dorsal artery of the index finger".[9]

Further research confirmed his findings. The dorsal carpal branch of the radial artery usually originates at the level of the trapezium and runs in an ulnar direction, forming the dorsal carpal

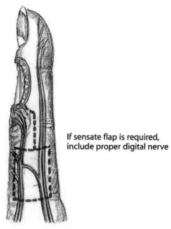

If sensate flap is required, include proper digital nerve

Center flap over neurovascular bundle

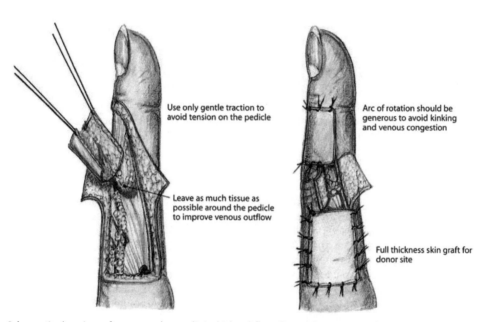

Use only gentle traction to avoid tension on the pedicle

Arc of rotation should be generous to avoid kinking and venous congestion

Leave as much tissue as possible around the pedicle to improve venous outflow

Full thickness skin graft for donor site

Fig. 1. Schematic drawing of a reverse homodigital island flap. (*From* Germann G, Sherman R, Levin LS. Decision making in reconstructive surgery. New York: Springer; 1999; with permission.)

rete after penetrating the radiocarpal ligaments. The dorsal metacarpal arteries run distally between the metacarpal bones in a fascial pocket of the dorsal interosseus muscles, usually giving off six to eight cutaneous perforators.

Not all of the dorsal metacarpal arteries are constant. In 97% of cases, the second dorsal metacarpal artery runs distally as an axial vessel in the fascia, between the 2 heads of the second dorsal interosseus muscle. The third metacarpal artery can be found in 93% of the cases. Distal anastomoses between the dorsal metacarpal branches and branches of the palmar arterial systems are usually located at the level of the deep transverse metacarpal ligament. The fifth dorsal metacarpal artery is absent in 17% to 30% of cases. In 66% of cases, palmar branches provide the vascular supply to the distal skin area.

The dorsal metacarpal arteries bifurcate at the level of the web spaces into the dorsal digital branches, supplying adjacent dorsal areas of the index, middle, ring, and little fingers. Multiple anastomoses with the palmar arterial system can be found at the level of the proximal interphalangeal and the metacarpophalangeal joints. The dorsopalmar anastomoses form the basis for

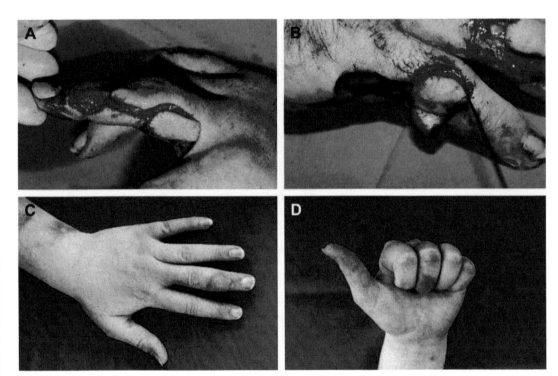

Fig. 2. (*A*) Distal dorsal defect over the DIP. The flap is already raised and centered over the vascular axis. (*B*) Flap rotated into the defect without kinking of the pedicle. (*C, D*) Excellent aesthetic and functional result.

modifications of the dorsal metacarpal artery flaps. The dorsal metacarpal branches are accompanied by venae comitantes, which permit venous drainage of the dorsal metacarpal artery flaps.[10]

There is an ongoing discussion about the correct terminology of these flaps. Earley and Milner first described the proximally based second DMCA flap in 1987.[3] In 1990, Maryuama[11] introduced the reverse DMCA flap, based on the dorsal metacarpal arteries 2 to 4, while Quaba and Davison described the distally based hand flap.[12]- Maryuama's report was supported by the anatomical studies of Dautel and Merle in 1991.[13] Since the initial publications, several modifications of the dorsal metacarpal artery flaps have been developed.

While the proximal DMCA flap first described by Earley and Milner[3] was based on the first and second dorsal metacarpal artery, the distally based flap (distal hand flap) described by Quaba and Davison[12] did not include the dorsal metacarpal arteries, but was based on the main palmar dorsal perforator in the web space. Following the studies of Earley and Milner.[3] the distally based dorsal metacarpal artery island flap was described by Maryuama[11] in 1990 and Dautel and Merle[13] in 1991.

Their modifications of this technique involved the constant anastomoses between the dorsal metacarpal artery and the palmar arterial system in the web space, thereby providing the vascular basis for the flap by securing a sufficient retrograde blood flow.

Thus, the flaps gained a wider arc of rotation and could be safely rotated 180° to reach the palmar and dorsal aspects of the proximal phalanges and also the proximal interphalangeal joint. This type of flap is usually referred to when the term DMCA flap is used. However, based on the author's clinical experience and the scientific exchange with colleagues, it can be stated that in many clinical situations, the flaps are raised without incorporation of the dorsal arterial system. This would support Quaba's[12] hypothesis that the dorsal flaps can be safely raised without inclusion of the dorsal metacarpal arteries (**Fig. 3**).

The first DMCA flap (kite flap) will be described in detail, since it is predominantly used for thumb reconstruction.

The Extended Distally Based DMCA Flap

The extended distally based DMCA flap was introduced by Pelissier and colleagues[14] in 1999. The

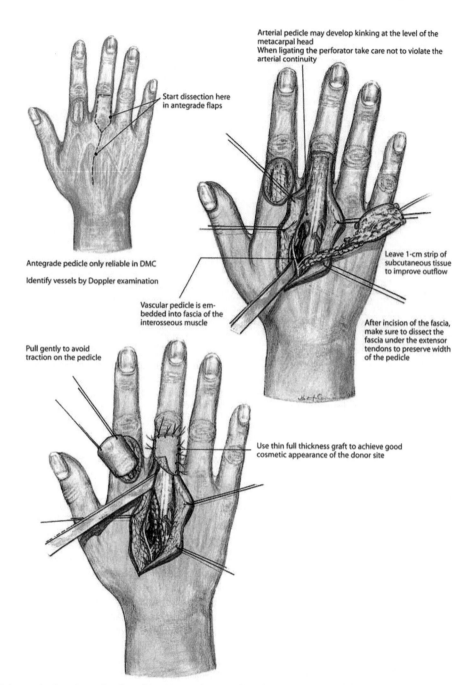

Arterial pedicle may develop kinking at the level of the metacarpal head
When ligating the perforator take care not to violate the arterial continuity

Start dissection here in antegrade flaps

Antegrade pedicle only reliable in DMC

Identify vessels by Doppler examination

Vascular pedicle is embedded into fascia of the interosseous muscle

Pull gently to avoid traction on the pedicle

Leave 1-cm strip of subcutaneous tissue to improve outflow

After incision of the fascia, make sure to dissect the fascia under the extensor tendons to preserve width of the pedicle

Use thin full thickness graft to achieve good cosmetic appearance of the donor site

Fig. 3. Schematic drawing of a dorsal metacarpal artery flap for coverage of a dorsal defect over the PIP. (*From* Germann G, Sherman R, Levin LS. Decision making in reconstructive surgery. New York: Springer; 1999; with permission.)

blood supply of the extended distally based dorsal metacarpal artery flap is based on the first dorso–palmar perforator at the level of the web spaces in the proximal third of the proximal phalanges. Multiple small arterial branches in the web space connect the feeding vessel to the vascular network of the flap. This technique permits a wider arc of rotation of the distally based DMCA flap to reach the dorsal aspect of the distal phalanges, the nail bed, or the lateral aspects of the fingers (**Fig. 4**).

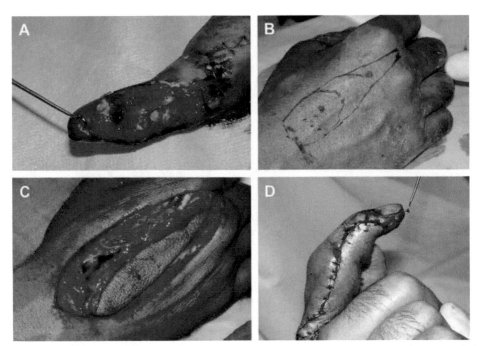

Fig. 4. (*A*) Long distal defect on the mediopalmar aspect of the index finger. (*B*) Design of an extended DMCA flap with a cutaneous tail extension. This extension allows skin/skin closure of the defect with the necessity of tunneling or skin grafting the flap pedicle. (*C*) Flap is raised and ready to be rotated into the defect. (*D*) Flap sutured in place. Note how far distal this type of DMCA flap reaches.

Distally Based DMCA Fascial Flap (Fascial DMCA Flap)

The distally based DMCA fascial flap was developed by Germann.[15] This flap consists solely of the DMCA, a thin subcutaneous layer without adipose tissue and the fascia of the corresponding interosseus muscle. The dissection of the flap follows the same principle as the distally based metacarpal artery flaps. After rotating the flap into the defect, the fascia is covered with a split-thickness skin graft. Primary indications for this type of flap are burns of the hand with defects over the PIP joints or in situations where a skin flap is considered to be too bulky. To date, the authors have used this procedure in 5 cases of burned hands and 1 case of trauma. The results have been very satisfactory; no fascial flap was lost, and the exposed PIP joints showed stable soft tissue coverage.

Distally Based DMCA Compound Flap (Compound DMCA Flap)

A procedure that allows reconstruction of complex defects with all vascularized components is described by Hori and colleagues[16] and Dautel and Merle.[13] All DMCA flaps may be combined with segments of the extensor tendons or a metacarpal bone segment.

DMCA Flaps in Burned Hands

The incidence of the dorsal metacarpal arteries in burned and grafted hands was systematically investigated in a large patient series. The authors were able to establish that even in burned and grafted hands the DMCA arteries can be detected in approximately the same number of cases as in noninjured hands. After using 2 flaps from a skin-grafted area in burned hands, it was recognized that DMCA flaps from grafted areas could be routinely used for coverage of defects over the PIP joints (**Fig. 5**).[10]

Several technical aspects have to be considered when DMCA flaps are raised. The dorsal metacarpal artery runs deep on the muscle between the extensor tendons. The muscle fascia has to be peeled off the synovial sheath of the extensor tendons to secure the inclusion of the vascular pedicle. Frequently, the tendon conjunctions have to be divided to prevent separation of the skin island from the pedicle, since the connections between the skin island and the pedicle are flimsy.

The palmar perforator should be identified under loop magnification. Small vascular connections to

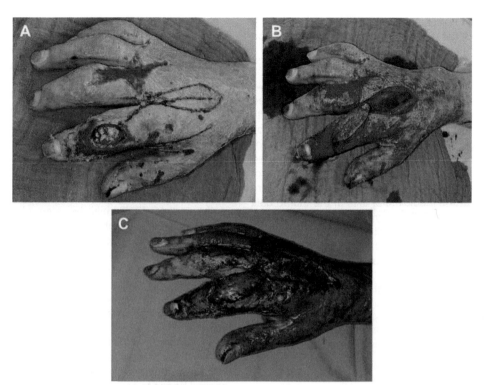

Fig. 5. (*A*) DMCA in burned hands. Typical defect over the PIP in a severely burned hand. (*B*) Although the dorsum of the hand is skin grafted, a flap can be raised. (*C*) The flap is rotated into the defect and shows normal perfusion.

the areolar tissue in the web space should be coagulated to increase flap mobility and extend the arc of rotation. When an extended DMCA flap is planned, the palmar perforator should be temporarily clamped after release of the tourniquet to evaluate retrograde flap perfusion. The perforator can be divided when flap perfusion is secured.

In few cases, there are identifiable veins in the vascular pedicle. Usually venous outflow is provided by a dense network of microveins in the areolar tissue surrounding the pedicle and filling the web space. It is of utmost importance to preserve as much of this tissue as possible to provide sufficient venous outflow.

Kinking of the vascular pedicle can be avoided by adding 10% to 15% to the calculated length of the pedicle.

Closure of the Donor Site

The donor site of the DMCA flaps is closed primarily or grafted with a full-thickness skin graft. The authors prefer full-thickness skin grafts due to the better pliability and the superior aesthetic result that can be achieved.

Cutaneous Tail Modification

The problem of rotating the flap into a distal defect was frequently complicated by tight skin areas around the defect, whereas tunneling always bears the risk of vascular compromise. Applying a skin graft to the pedicle is a possible alternative; however, the result is frequently mechanically unstable and is aesthetically unpleasing. Therefore the authors developed the cutaneous tail modification. This includes a flap extension so that tunneling becomes unnecessary after rotation of the flap, and skin–skin closure is possible with complete coverage of the pedicle. This principle has been extended to other flaps such as sural artery flap, the kite flap, or the radial forearm flap. Since the introduction of this modification, the authors have observed a marked reduction in the failure rate of pedicled flaps.[17]

THUMB RECONSTRUCTION WITH INTRINSIC FLAPS

Extensive thumb defects with exposure of tendons, bone, or joints can be challenging. Immediate closure of the wound has the highest priority to preserve aesthetic and function. A variety of flaps is routinely used for reconstruction of the thumb.

Moberg-Flap

The Moberg-Flap is an advancement flap, based on neurovascular bundles for coverage of defects of the pulp of the thumb. It was first described by Moberg[18] in 1964, and it is considered to be a standard flap for reconstruction of medium-sized defects. Indications are distal palmar defects of the pulp with a size up to 1.5 cm. Incisions are placed at the mediolateral axis of the thumb until short of the MP flexor crease. To raise the flap safely, dissection should start from distal and move in the plain above the flexor tendon sheath. Thus the neurovascular bundles can be preserved under direct vision.

Bilateral Z-plasties at the base of the flap and dividing the subcutaneous septa avoid flexion contracture of the IP joint.[8] Distal procedures such as V-Y extensions,[19] Burrow triangles,[20] or full-thickness skin grafts after division of the proximal skin bridge[21] have been described to increase flap mobility. In large defects, bone amputation must be considered, which may result in a reduced strength in pinch grip. The Moberg flap remains the gold standard in covering distal pulp defects.

Kite Flap (Foucher Flap)

One of the most frequently employed procedures is the kite flap, described by Foucher[22] in 1978 based on the work of Hilgenfeldt[21] in 1950 and Paneva-Holevic (1968).[23] It is based on the first dorsometacarpal artery and usually includes the sensory branch of the radial nerve. The kite flap is suitable for all dorsal defects and is frequently used for restoration of sensibility in case of the

loss of the pulp. Using the kite flap provides immediate sensibility and is therefore especially indicated in older patients. Donor site aesthetics can be markedly improved using a full-thickness skin graft (**Fig. 6**).

Harvest of the kite flap usually starts with a curved linear incision above the second metacarpal, where one of the large dorsal veins is identified. The fascia of the first interosseus muscle is then peeled off the muscle, thereby preserving the vascular bundle that runs deep in a fascial pocket. All the fascia and the connective tissue surrounding one of the veins should be included in the pedicle. To identify the artery at this level is not desirable, since it may lead to a disconnection of the vascular pedicle and the flap.

After the pedicle has been dissected, the flap is incised distally, and dissection starts in the plane above the paratenon. It is of utmost importance to preserve the paratenon to secure healing of the full-thickness skin graft for donor defect closure.

An important step follows at the level of the distal border of the flap at the level of the extensor hood. The authors always include a strip of the sagittal bands to secure the delicate tissue bridge from the pedicle to the skin island. This makes the pedicle more robust against shear forces and allows flap inset without the risk of jeopardizing the vascular supply.[7,15]

Alternatives

Although the kite flap has evolved into the workhorse for thumb reconstruction, alternatives may be needed when the index finger is not available as a donor site. Many anatomical studies have described the constant and predictable anatomy of the dorsoulnar and dorsoradial branch artery of the thumb.[24–28]

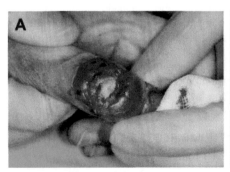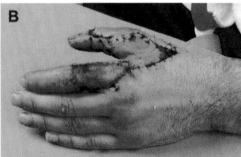

Fig. 6. (*A*) Defect over the dorsal interphalangeal joint in the thumb with exposure of the joint. (*B*) Defect reconstruction with a kite flap with cutaneous tail. This technique results in an excellent contour. Secondary corrections are rarely needed. Donor defects are reconstructed with a full-thickness skin graft.

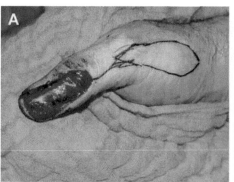
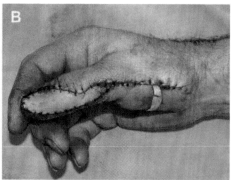

Fig. 7. (A) Moschella flap for distal dorsal defects in the thumb. The defect is already debrided, and the flap is raised on the recurrent dorsal radial artery. (B) Flap is rotated into the defect. Donor site could be closed primarily.

Moschella Flap

Based on detailed description of the dorsal vascularization of the thumb, the reversed flow pedicled flap was first described by Francesco Moschella[29] in 2006. It is raised on the dorsoradial side of the first metacarpal area, and based on the dorsal radial collateral artery, which is constant in course, caliber, and communication with the palmar network.[29]

The dorsoradial artery originates from the radial artery at the level of the snuff box and passes under the extensor pollicis brevis tendon to the central portion of the proximal phalanx, which is the pivot point of the flap. The dorsoradial collateral artery communicates with the palmar network at the level of the middle third of the proximal phalanx.[29]

Flap sizes range from 2 cm × 2 cm to 5 cm × 4 cm. Preoperatively, a Doppler examination helps to identify the course of the vessel and to mark the pivot point. At no point of the surgical procedure must the pedicle be visualized, and a wide strip of subcutaneous tissue should be included to secure venous outflow and avoid kinking of the pedicle. Dissection of the flap should not be extended beyond the middle of the proximal phalanx to protect the anastomosis with the palmar vessels (**Fig. 7**).

Brunelli Flap

A reversed-flow pedicled homodigital flap based on the dorsoulnar collateral artery was first described in 1993 by Brunelli,[30] who used it in 32 cases. The dorsoulnar collateral artery, which originates from the palmar arteries, runs superficially within the subcutaneous tissue; the flap is centered over the dorsoulnar aspect of the the first metacarpal. Flap dissection is similar to the Moschella technique. The Brunelli flap is a suitable flap to cover small-to-medium-sized defects of the dorsal and palmar side of the thumb.[31]

Using these types of flaps, the index finger can be spared as a donor site in many cases of small-to-moderate-sized dorsal defects. Frequently the donor site can be closed primarily, which improves the overall aesthetic appearance of the reconstruction (**Fig. 8**).

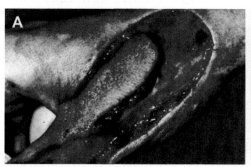
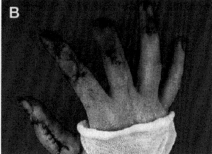

Fig. 8. (A) A Brunelli flap is raised on the dorsoulnar recurrent artery of the thumb to be rotated into a distal dorsal defect. (B) Flap sutured in place.

SUMMARY

Intrinsic flaps offer a wide variety of solutions for the majority of soft tissue reconstructions in the hand. Reconstructive procedures can be individualized to improve aesthetic and functional outcome and decrease donor site morbidity. Profound anatomical knowledge and microsurgical dissection techniques are required to achieve reproducible successful results.

REFERENCES

1. Littler JW. Subtotal reconstruction off the thumb. Plast Reconstr Surg (1946) 1952;10(4):215–26.
2. Bunnell S. Digit transfer by neurovascular pedicle. J Bone Joint Surg Am 1952;34(4):772–4.
3. Early MJ, Milner R. Dorsal metacarpal flaps. Br J Hand Surg 1987;40:333–41.
4. Manchot C. Die Hauptanatomie des menschlichen Körpers (Leipzig 1889). New York: Springer; 1983.
5. Salmon M. Les artéres de la peau. Paris: Masson; 1912.
6. Spateholz W. Die Verteilung der Blutgefässe in der Hand. Arch Anat Med Phys 1893;1–54.
7. Engel H, Germann G. Advanced concepts in vascularised tissue transfer in the hand. Tissue surgery. New Techniques in Surgery 2006;1:23–40.
8. Germann G. Principles of flap design for surgery of the hand. Atlas Hand Clin 1998;3:33–57.
9. Paturet G. Traité d'Ánatomie Humanie. Paris: Masson & Cie; 1951.
10. Germann G, Funk H, Bickert B. The fate of the dorsal metacarpal arterial system following thermal injury to the dorsal hand: a Doppler sonographic study. J Hand Surg Am 2000;25(5):962–8.
11. Maryuma Y. The reverse dorsal metacarpal flap. Br J Hand Surg 1990;43:24–7.
12. Quaba AA, Davison PM. The distally based dorsal metacarpal artery flap. Br J Plast Surg 1990;43:28–32.
13. Dautel G, Merle M. Dorsal metacarpal reverse flaps. Br J Hand Surg 1991;16(4):400–5.
14. Pelissier P, Casoli V, Bakhach J, et al. Reverse dorsal digital and metacarpal flaps: a review of 27 cases. Plast Reconstr Surg 1999;103:159–65.
15. Germann G, Sherman R, Levin LS. Decision-making in reconstructive surgery: upper extremity. Springer; 2000.
16. Hori Y, Tamai S, Okuda H, et al. Blood vessel transplantation to bone. J Hand Surg 1979;4:23–33.
17. Pelzer M, Sauerbier M, Germann G, et al. Free Kite flap: a new FLPA for reconstruction of small hand defects. J Reconstr Microsurg 2004;20(5):367–72.
18. Moberg E. Aspects of sensation in reconstructive surgery of the upper limb. J Bone Joint Surg Am 1964;46A:817–25.
19. Elliot D, Willson Y. V-Y advancement flap with V-Y closure for the thumb tip injuries. J Hand Surg Br 1993;18(3):399–402.
20. Venkatataswami R, Subramanian N. Olique triangular flap: a new method of repair for oblique amputations of the fingertip and thumb. Plast Reconstr Surg 1980;66(2):296–300.
21. Hilgenfeld O. Operativer Daumenersatz. 1st edition. Stuttgart (Germany): Enke Verlag; 1950.
22. Foucher G, Braun JB. A new island flap transfer from the dorsum of the index to the thumb. Plast Reconstr Surg 1979;63:344–9.
23. Paneva-Holevich E. Surgical treatment of congenital malformations of the thumb. Acta Chir Plast 1968;10(3):205–14.
24. Bertelli JA, Pagliei A. Direct and reversed flow proximal phalangeal island flaps. J Hand Surg 1994;19A:671–80.
25. Foucher G. Lambeau cerf-volant. Lambeaux arteriels pedicules du membre superieur. In: Monographies du GEM, editor. ESF; 1990.
26. Kumar VP, Satku K, Liu J. The Brunelli reversed flow pediccled flap from the thumb. Plast Reconstr Surg 1996;98:1298–301.
27. Arria P. Lambeux des arteres interossueses dorsales de la main. In: Monographies du GEM, editor. ESF; 1990.
28. Pistre V, Pelissier P, Martin D, et al. Vascular blood supply of the dorsal side of the thumb, first web and the index finger: anatomical study. J Hand Surg 2001;26B:98–104.
29. Moschella F, Cordowa A. Reverse homodigital dorsal radial flap of the thumb. Plast Reconstr Surg 2006;117:920–6.
30. Pagliei A, Rocchi L, Tulli A. The dorsal flap of the first web. Br J Hand Surg 2003;28B:121–4.
31. Terán P, Carnero S, Miranda R, et al. Refinements in dorsoulnar flap of the thumb: 15 cases. J Hand Surg 2010;35A:1356–9.

Reconstruction of the Ischemic Hand

William C. Pederson, MD[a],*,
Michael W. Neumeister, MD, FRCSC[b]

KEYWORDS

- Hand ischemia • Reconstruction • Arterial perfusion
- Vascular trauma • Raynaud's

Ischemia of the hand remains an uncommon condition, but problems with arterial perfusion of the hand can arise from trauma (open and closed), thrombosis, or as a result of arteriovascular disease. Certain identifiable patterns are seen with hand ischemia, usually discernable according to which one of the major arteries (radial or ulnar) are involved. This article discusses the origin and management of ischemic hand conditions, with an emphasis on recognizing the patterns of ischemia that are commonly seen.

ARTERIAL ANATOMY OF THE HAND

The vascularity of the hand is primarily provided by the radial and ulnar arteries, with secondary contribution through the anterior and posterior interosseous vessels that arborize at the wrist. Although these interosseous vessels do not supply the dominant blood supply to the hand, they may become important in some ischemic conditions involving the major two vessels. The arterial anatomy in the palm has traditionally been considered as having a deep and a superficial arch, whose names describe their positions in the palm. The deep arch is typically fed by the radial artery as it comes around the hand at the base of the thumb in the anatomic snuffbox, and then enters the palm as it pierces the dorsal interosseous muscle in the first web space. This artery then connects with the deep component of the palmar arch. The ulnar artery runs into the palm from the forearm along the radial aspect of the pisiform bone with the ulnar nerve on its ulnar side. This artery continues on to become the superficial arch and supplies the proper digital vessels in the palm. Since the early work of Coleman and Anson[1] on the anatomy of the arch, much discussion has surrounded the potential for ischemia from an incomplete arch if one of the major vessels of the hand becomes occluded. Traditional teaching is that most hand ischemia is caused by this incomplete arch, and the fingers become ischemic from lack of crossover blood flow from the nonthrombosed vessel. In the authors' experience with close to 150 cases of arterial thrombosis of the radial or ulnar arteries, ischemia of the fingers or hand is not generally from a lack of connection between the two portions of the arch, but rather from embolization of clots from the site of original thrombosis (in the radial or ulnar artery) into the downstream digital vessels, leading to ischemia of the fingers fed by these digital arteries (**Fig. 1**). Thus, the authors question the long-held concern about the lack of a complete palmar arch in its contribution to digital ischemia with thrombosis of the radial or ulnar arteries. Some patients unquestionably have an incomplete arch and would experience partial hand ischemia if the radial or ulnar arteries were harvested for a bypass or flap, but in the authors' experience, these patients are significantly few and far between.

Numerous causes of ischemia of the upper extremity have been reported (**Box 1**). The treatment should be individualized depending on the cause and expected outcomes.

[a] The Hand Center of San Antonio and The University of Texas Health Science Center, 21 Spurs Lane, #310, San Antonio, TX 78240, USA
[b] Department of Plastic Surgery, Division of Plastic Surgery, Southern Illinois University School of Medicine, 747 North Rutledge, Third Floor, Springfield, IL 62702, USA
* Corresponding author.
E-mail address: micro1@ix.netcom.com

Clin Plastic Surg 38 (2011) 739–750
doi:10.1016/j.cps.2011.08.007
0094-1298/11/$ – see front matter © 2011 Published by Elsevier Inc

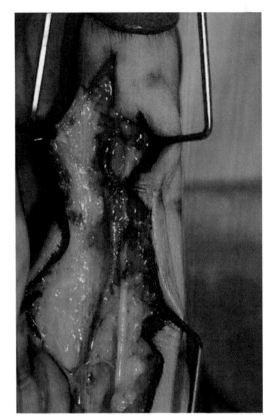

Fig. 1. View of digital vessel with small thrombus from ulnar artery thrombosis.

IATROGENIC HAND ISCHEMIA

Accidental blunt or sharp injury to the radial, ulnar, palmer, or digital vessels may result in vascular insufficiency to the hand or digits. The vascular system could also be disrupted from surgical intervention through flap harvesting. Ischemia from harvesting of the radial artery for coronary artery bypass grafting or flap transfer is fortunately uncommon. Although cases of digital ischemia have been reported after this,[2,3] most studies have shown no significant morbidity from harvest of the radial artery, either for coronary bypass or transfer of a radial forearm flap. Several studies in patients undergoing coronary artery bypass with the radial artery have actually shown improved perfusion of the radial digits after harvest, presumably because of a compensatory mechanism to increase flow to the fingers supplied primarily by the radial artery.[4] Although ischemia of the digits after radial artery harvest has an estimated incidence of 10%,[5] some investigators have found no clinical evidence (hand claudication or ischemic symptoms) after harvest.[6] If the hand is noted to be ischemic after harvest of the radial

> **Box 1**
> **Causes of ischemia of the upper extremity**
>
> *Occlusive arterial disease*
>
> Atherosclerosis
>
> Embolic disorders
>
> Vasculitis
>
> Thromboangiitis obliterans
>
> Thoracic outlet syndrome
>
> Takayasu disease
>
> Traumatic aneurysm
>
> Canalization
>
> Ulnar hammer
>
> Arteriovenous steal/shunt
>
> Arteriovenous malformation
>
> Vasospastic disorders
>
> *Cutaneous small-vessel disease*
>
> Vasculitis
>
> Waldenström's hypergammaglobulinemic purpura
>
> Henoch-Schönlein purpura
>
> Collagen vascular–associated
>
> Acute hemorrhagic edema of infancy
>
> Rheumatoid nodules with vasculitis
>
> Urticarial vasculitis
>
> Hyperimmunoglobulinemia D syndrome
>
> Essential mixed cryoglobulinemia
>
> Familiar Mediterranean fever
>
> Connective tissue disorders
>
> Myeloproliferative disorders

artery for either a flap or coronary bypass, performing a vein bypass graft at that time is probably prudent rather than waiting for symptoms to develop.

Another potential iatrogenic cause of hand ischemia is radial artery catheterization for blood pressure monitoring. Large studies have shown the overall safety of radial artery catheterization, with one study quoting a "permanent ischemic complications" rate of only 0.09%.[7] Nonetheless, other large studies have shown flow abnormalities or thrombosis of the radial artery in approximately 26% of patients who have an arterial line.[8,9] Ischemia significant enough to lead to digital amputation is rare but is certainly reported. In their review of eight patients who experienced ischemia of the fingers after radial artery catheterization,

Valentine and colleagues[10] found that all surviving patients developed some gangrene in the hand and most required some level of digital amputation. This article's authors have had three patients in the past 20 years who required significant amputations after radial artery cannulation: one of the entire hand and two of partial hands. All three of these patients had been taking intravenous vasopressor agents for hypotension, which probably worsened the ischemia of the hand after thrombosis of the radial artery.

Geschwind and colleagues[11] believed that their experience did not support surgical intervention, because their patients all subsequently experienced ongoing ischemic problems. They believed that this was because of embolization of a clot to the digits that could not be removed. Although managing these patients with thrombolytic agents might be theoretically beneficial, this article's authors' experience has been that radiologists consider this treatment to present too much of a systemic risk for most of these patients. Therefore, the authors believe that these patients should be explored and have thrombectomy of the radial artery and repair of the damaged segment of artery performed whenever possible. Even if this is unsuccessful, the authors consider the risk to be justified if amputation of a significant portion of the hand can be prevented (**Fig. 2**).

CLOSED VASCULAR TRAUMA
Ulnar Artery Thrombosis

The most common cause of ischemia of the hand is closed trauma to the vessels of the hand, primarily the ulnar artery. This condition is usually caused by banging of the ulnar side of the hand,

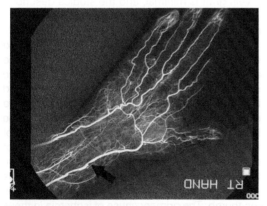

Fig. 2. Arteriogram of patient who experienced ischemia after radial arterial line. Arrow points to intimal flap in radial artery at site of arterial catheter. Note cutoff to flow in index finger and thumb from embolization of clot.

often repetitively, and has been dubbed the *hypothenar hammer syndrome*.[12] It is the result of trauma to the ulnar artery in Guyon's Canal, leading to thrombosis and symptoms of ischemia of the digits. The vascular insufficiency is often found in the ring and little finger and is commonly associated with numbness and tingling in the ulnar nerve–innervated digits. The ulnar nerve may be contused during injury to the ulnar artery, or can simply become involved through its proximity to the inflamed and thrombosed ulnar artery. The thrombosed ulnar artery often becomes tortuous and aneurysmal. Physical examination of these patients will show ischemic digits (and perhaps gangrene or ulceration), and the ulnar artery at the wrist will often still be palpable. An Allen test will usually confirm occlusion of the ulnar artery, but the authors prefer to perform what they call a "dynamic Doppler examination" through listening to the arch with a pencil Doppler and then sequentially occluding the ulnar and radial arteries at the wrist with digital pressure. This technique provides a much better idea of which vessel may be thrombosed. They also prefer to listen to the digital pulps with the pencil Doppler to confirm which fingers have experienced occlusion of the digital arteries from embolization of clot. Patients who have experienced embolization of clot to the digital vessels will usually have recanalization of these vessels after excision and bypass of the injured ulnar artery, and will thus have return of their Doppler pulp signals at some point after bypass.

The natural history of untreated hypothenar hammer syndrome has been somewhat difficult to ascertain. Most surgeons believe that symptomatic patients should probably be managed surgically. A recent study from France, however, analyzed 47 patients who presented to the Department of Internal Medicine at the University of Rouen with hypothenar hammer syndrome[13] (which represented 1.13% of all patients referred for symptoms of Raynaud's disease). They noted that 92% of these patients had "occupational exposure to repetitive palmar trauma." Arteriography showed thrombosis of the ulnar artery in the palm (60%) or ulnar artery aneurysm (40%); 57% were noted to have "embolic multiple occlusions of the digital arteries." Only two of these patients were managed surgically, and these individuals had nonthrombotic ulnar artery aneurysms and continued to be symptomatic on conservative management (probably from recurrent embolization, in the authors' opinion). The remainder of the patients were managed with a variety of conservative measures. All were counseled to change occupational exposure. All received vasodilators (calcium channel blockers and buflo-medil), others also received platelet aggregation inhibitors, and some received hemodilution therapy (intravenous dextran) to lower the hemat-ocrit to 35%. Three patients required a 5-day course of intravenous prostacyclin infusion to manage digital necrosis. Ulcers took an average of 1.6 months to heal on this varied regimen, and, significantly, 28% of patients treated conser-vatively exhibited recurrent symptoms at an average of 11 months after the initial episode. Among these patients, two had undergone thoracic sympathectomy, but none had under-gone surgical bypass of the lesion in the ulnar artery. This study is certainly the only large one examining patients with traumatic ulnar artery thrombosis managed conservatively, and although the results may look encouraging, these patients were managed very aggressively from the nonsurgical standpoint. Approximately 50% of patients required a several-day hospitalization for administration of intravenous dextran or pros-tacyclin. Each of these drugs has its own inherent potential side effects.[14,15] With a recurrence rate near 30% in patients treated nonsurgically, the authors believe that bypass should be strongly considered in patients who remain symptomatic on straightforward management with calcium channel blockers and aspirin. This approach seems to be supported by the literature.

In a follow-up of 14 patients with hypothenar hammer syndrome, Zimmerman and colleagues[16] performed digital blood pressure measurements on each patient to calculate the digital brachial index, which is the digital blood pressure divided by the ipsilateral arm brachial artery blood pres-sure. Patients with a value greater than 0.7 were managed with simple ligation of the artery and excision, whereas those with a value less than 0.7 were managed with excision and bypass. Through excising the ulnar artery, a Leriche's sympathectomy was being performed[17] in the patients who did not have severe diminution of flow. All patients experienced improvement after bypass, but no statistical difference was seen in long-term results between these groups. However, the investigators did not manage any patients without surgery.

More recently, Lifchez and Higgins[18] reported similar findings in an evaluation of 14 patients who underwent surgery for ulnar artery throm-bosis. Two patients had primary excision of the involved segment and direct repair, and the other 12 had the ulnar artery reconstructed with a reversed vein graft. Eight of 12 grafts (67%) were patent at an average of 52 months' follow-up. All patients experienced improvement in their

digital brachial index and subjective symptoms, with those who had experienced thrombosis showing the best improvement in the digital brachial index. Based on the results, the investiga-tors suggest performing reconstruction on patients in whom medical management fails to relieve symptoms, those whose digital soft tissue ulcers fail to heal with conservative management, and those with a reconstructible lesion.[18] Ko-man's[19] group found similar results in their review of 13 hands in 12 patients with ulnar artery throm-bosis. None of the patients had collagen vascular disease, and they found a 77% patency rate of bypass grafts at 24 months' follow-up. Of the three patients who had thrombosis of their grafts, two were symptomatic and one was not. The investi-gators concluded that patients with posttraumatic ulnar artery thrombosis managed with bypass grafting had decreased symptoms and improved function, and experienced a positive effect on health-related quality of life, which confirmed the findings of an earlier study by this group.[20]

Based on these studies and the authors' personal experience, the authors believe that most patients who experience thrombosis of the ulnar artery from external trauma will benefit from either excision and repair of the damaged segment or vein graft bypass. The authors usually manage patients conservatively for a short period with aspirin and calcium channel blockers but, if the patients have or develop gangrene or ulcerations, or the ischemic symptoms do not improve, will proceed with surgical management. With the current widespread training in microvascular surgical techniques and the ease of performing a vein graft, the authors also believe that bypass, rather than simple excision, should be performed in almost all patients. The morbidity of harvesting a vein graft is minimal, and the studies described earlier confirm that increasing inflow will improve symptoms.

In a review of roughly 100 patients who had experienced thrombosis of the ulnar artery, the authors found that 44% presented with ischemic symptoms in the ring finger, whereas 33% had ischemia of the middle finger, 24% had ischemia of the little finger, and 23% had ischemia of the index, but only 2% of patients had evidence of thumb ischemia (most patients had ischemia of more than one finger, thus the results tally more than 100%). Thus, the pattern of digital ischemia seen with ulnar artery thrombosis rarely involves the thumb. The primary cause of ischemia in these individuals is embolization of clot from the original site of injury to the common and proper digital arteries, which leads to the digital ischemia of the involved fingers. The pattern of thrombosis in patients with hypothenar hammer syndrome is typical, because the vessel will usually clot from and to where adequate outflow is present. This process leads to the vessel thrombosing distally to the point at which the superficial arch comes across and anastomoses with the common digital vessel to the fourth web space, and proximally back to either the deep branch in the palm (accompanying the deep motor branch of the ulnar nerve) or, more commonly, the level of the dorsal branch of the ulnar artery (which usually accompanies the dorsal sensory branch of the ulnar nerve). This pattern is commonly seen on arteriograms of the hands in patients with hypothenar hammer syndrome (**Fig. 3**). Patients in a hypercoagulable state or those with collagen vascular disease who experience thrombosis of the ulnar artery may have more extensive occlusion, depending on the severity of their disease.

This pattern of thrombosis leads to fairly straightforward management. If the patient is seen early and little propagation of thrombus has occurred, excision of the damaged segment and primary anastomosis may be possible. Although this finding is uncommon in the authors' practice, it certainly can be seen early after thrombosis of the ulnar artery. The patient usually has a significant area of damage to the intima and media of the vessel, which must be excised (**Fig. 4**). If the thrombus has propagated proximally and distally, a vein graft can be used from where the ulnar artery is open (usually at a level approximately 2 cm proximal to the wrist where the dorsal branch arises) to the bifurcation between the superficial

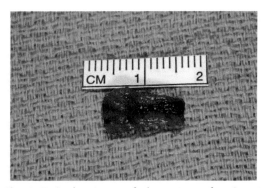

Fig. 4. Excised segment of ulnar artery of patient 1 week after injury to ulnar artery in football game. Note severe disruption of intima and muscular layer.

arch and the branch to the fourth web space. The authors use the basilic vein from the ulnar side of the forearm almost exclusively now for bypass of the ulnar artery, and have not seen any problems with aneurysmal dilatation of the vein over time. Many investigators prefer the saphenous vein, but this article's authors prefer to avoid the donor site on the leg, and also find that the thick wall of the saphenous often makes anastomosis somewhat difficult (particularly to the distal vessel). Some investigators have advocated the use of arterial grafts in the palm,[21] and although these have the potential advantage of a better size match proximally and distally, coupled with the theoretical advantage of a thicker wall, the authors have only used arterial grafts in a few patients who required revision of their original vein graft. Technically, the authors prefer to perform the proximal anastomosis first, which allows the vein graft to unwind and also set the appropriate length for the graft. Once this is accomplished, the graft is flushed with heparinized saline and clamped. Once the graft is trimmed distally to the appropriate length, the distal anastomosis can be performed. Although two anastomoses (to the superficial palmar arch and to the common digital artery to the fourth web space) may need to be performed, this can almost always be accomplished with a single anastomosis at the level of the bifurcation of this vessel. With careful trimming of the distal ulnar artery, a point can usually be reached at which a connection is still intact between the palmar arch and the digital artery to the fourth web space (**Fig. 5**). This structure may look like the end of a double-barreled shotgun, but with care, a single anastomosis can be performed between the vein graft and this bifurcation.

Postoperatively, patients are usually placed in a bulky dressing and the hand is kept elevated.

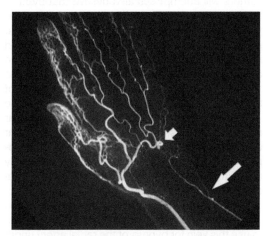

Fig. 3. Typical arteriogram of patient with hypothenar hammer syndrome. Short arrow shows branch at arch connecting to common digital artery to fourth web space. Longer arrow shows takeoff of dorsal branch of ulnar artery. Note small amount of flow through ulnar artery to deep branch in palm.

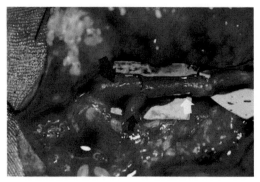

Fig. 5. Reversed basilica vein bypass to branch between superficial palmar arch and common digital vessel to fourth web space. White arrow points to bypass graft, small dark arrow to digital artery to fourth web space, and large dark arrow to superficial arch.

The authors prefer to manage patients with hypothenar hammer syndrome with oral aspirin only (325 mg/d), and will occasionally leave the patients on calcium channel blockers for several months until all symptoms resolve. An early thrombosis of the graft is unusual if reinjury does not occur. Small areas of necrosis and ulcers will generally heal within 6 weeks, and the authors usually find that Doppler ultrasound arterial signals will return to ischemic fingers (in which it was absent preoperatively) by 6 to 8 weeks. In the authors' series of approximately 100 patients with ulnar artery thrombosis, those with hypothenar hammer syndrome have a 2-year patency rate of 88%. Most patients remain asymptomatic (as noted by Higgins[18]) even if the graft thromboses.

Patients with collagen vascular disease and ulnar artery thrombosis present a different set of problems from those of patients with hypothenar hammer syndrome. These patients will often have disease in the arch and digital vessels, which will not be altered through bypassing the occluded segment of ulnar artery. Although they will benefit from bypass if the ulnar artery is occluded, the long-term results are not as good as in patients with traumatic thrombosis.[22] Excision of the ulnar artery will provide an excellent sympathectomy effect and, coupled with periarterial sympathectomy of the palmar arch and digital vessels, may be adequate to improve flow and heal ulcerations in these individuals. Although the authors will perform bypass in patients with collagen vascular disease, they do this on a case-by-case basis. Patients with long segments of thrombosis confirmed on arteriogram or those with severe digital vascular disease may not benefit as much from bypass as from simple ligation and excision of the thrombosed segment. If bypass grafting is performed, the authors will use much the same technique as described earlier.

Radial Artery Thrombosis

Radial artery thrombosis is much less common than thrombosis of the ulnar artery, but when this occurs it is generally in the anatomic snuff-box under the extensor pollicis longus tendon (retrocarpal radial artery thrombosis).[23–25] The origin of this is not entirely clear, but it seems to be caused by compression of the artery under the extensor pollicis longus (EPL) tendon where it crosses over the trapezium.[23] This problem is more common in women than in men, and patients will usually present with ischemia primarily of the index finger or thumb. In review of 40 patients with this entity treated by the authors, 79% had ischemic symptoms in the index finger, with only 42% and 39% having symptoms in the thumb and middle finger, respectively. Only 6% of patients with thrombosis of the radial artery in the snuff-box had ischemic symptoms in the little finger. The authors believe that patients who present with an ischemic index finger have retrocarpal radial artery thrombosis unless proven otherwise. Arteriogram will show either absence of the dorsal branch of the radial artery (caused by propagation of thrombus) or occasionally a single thrombosis in the lumen of the artery at the point of compression (**Fig. 6**).

The issues requiring surgical management mirror those of ulnar artery thrombosis (in patients without collagen vascular disease), and the authors will attempt conservative management of these individuals for a while. However, these patients will frequently have recurrent symptoms, primarily from ongoing compression of the radial artery by the EPL tendon. These patients will often complain of pain in the thenar muscles, which the authors believe is probably from claudication of these muscles caused by ischemia.

Operative management is similar to that for ulnar artery thrombosis, in that the damaged segment can occasionally be excised and the artery repaired primarily; however, this segment usually needs to be grafted after excision. This procedure can usually be performed with a short segment of graft, and the cephalic vein is in the same area and will have surgical exposure, so the authors prefer to use this vein for bypass of the radial artery under these circumstances. The EPL tendon must be moved off of the radial artery or graft to prevent recurrent compression, and this can be accomplished through either making a sling for the EPL out of a portion of the extensor carpi radialis

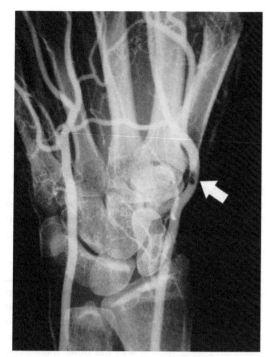

Fig. 6. Arteriogram of patient with ischemic index finger and thrombosis of radial artery in snuff-box. Arrow points to discrete thrombus in radial artery as it passes under extensor pollicis longus tendon.

longus coming off of the base of the second metacarpal[23] or, more simply, releasing the EPL off of the Lister tubercle. Postoperative management is similar to that for hypothenar hammer syndrome, and long-term patency in the authors' series approaches 95%. Only two patients rethrombosed early in the authors' series, but the EPL was not moved in either patient. Both patients re-presented with thumb claudication rather than digital ischemia. Both underwent successful rebypass with vein graft and relocation of the EPL and have remained asymptomatic.

Nontraumatic Ischemia of the Hand

Patients with nontraumatic ischemia of the hand include those with arterial thrombosis from collagen vascular disease and those with arteriosclerotic vascular disease. Management of these patients is different, and although the former is reasonably common, severe vascular disease in the distal upper extremity is fairly uncommon. Many patients with severe arteriosclerotic disease of the vessels of the forearm and hand have diabetes and renal failure, and often have undergone transplantation. Although one-half of patients with Buerger disease are believed to have involvement of the upper extremity,[26] this cause of ischemia of

the hand is increasingly rare in the authors' practice, so much so that this diagnosis is questioned in referred patients. These two problems are discussed in the following sections.

Collagen Vascular Disease

The two primary issues with patients with collagen vascular disease are vasospasm (Raynaud's disease) and vascular occlusion. The vasospastic component of Raynaud's disease can be managed medically or surgically, but most investigators would agree that when ulceration occurs or tissue loss is possible, surgery is the preferred treatment. The mainstay of surgery for patients with Raynaud's disease of the hand is periarterial sympathectomy. Numerous studies have shown that this technique decreases symptoms and heals ulcerations in patients with this condition.[27–29] The work of Koman and colleagues[29] has shown that although periarterial sympathectomy does not increase total flow to the digits, it nonetheless increases nutritional flow through decreasing the amount of blood flow lost from abnormal arteriovenous shunting. Others have shown clinical improvement with periarterial sympathectomy; however, the longevity of this procedure is still uncertain.

The authors perform the operation as per Ruch and colleagues,[27] which involves stripping the adventitia from the ulnar artery from the wrist to the palm, the radial artery in the distal forearm, and the radial artery in the anatomic snuff-box. These patients continue their medical management in the postoperative period, and healing of ulcers is usually seen by 6 to 8 weeks. If the patient has significant gangrene of any individual finger that will require amputation, the authors prefer to wait until this 6- to 8-week postoperative period to maximize arterial flow to the digits and perhaps allow a more distal level of amputation. Occasionally fingers that look like they will require formal amputation will simply slough the eschar and heal. This approach must be tempered by the patient's level and tolerance of pain. If the pain is severe and control with narcotics has been difficult, then the authors will amputate the involved digits during sympathectomy. The short-term results are good, measured in months to years, but occasionally patients will continue to have problems with a particular finger or fingers. In this instance, the authors will sometimes perform a sympathectomy on the digital vessels out in the finger, but the morbidity from this procedure can be high. After sympathectomy in the fingers, patients have a great deal of trouble with the wound healing, and also often develop stiffness of the involved finger, which is difficult to prevent and subsequently treat. These patients may develop further vascular sclerosis and eventually thrombosis of the ulnar artery, but Merritt[30] believes that periarterial sympathectomy may be somewhat preventive in terms of developing later thrombosis.

Some early experience suggests that botulinum A toxin (Botox), when injected around the digital vessels, may be a treatment option in patients with vasospastic disorders, such as Raynaud's disease.[31–33] Typically, Botox is used for conditions that require muscle paralysis. The toxin is taken up by the nerve terminal and subsequently blocks the release of acetylcholine through the blockade of synaptosomal-associated protein 25 (SNAP-25) on the surface of the neurotransmitter vesicles. This process takes 2 to 4 days to occur and 2 to 4 months to resolve. Hence, the natural time frame for the paralytic effects of the toxin. The effects of Botox in patients with Raynaud's disease or syndrome are almost immediate and have so far lasted for years in most people.[33,34] The mechanism of action of the botulinum toxin may be related to paralysis of the smooth muscle fibers in the muscularis layer of the digital arteries; however, other pharmacologic pathways also may be affected.[33] That is, the botulinum toxin may not have a direct action on the vessels but rather may work through modulating the innervation of the vessels or blocking the chronic neuropathic pain pathways. Neurotransmitters, such as substance-P, glutamate, or calcitonin gene–related peptide, have been implicated in the transmission of ischemic pain. Injecting Botox seems to improve perfusion and diminish pain. Botox may also block ectopic sodium channels that are inherently upregulated in patients with chronic pain in conditions such as Raynaud's disease.[34] The pathways of the imbalance of vascular tone and chronic neuropathic pain are complex and multimodal.[33] Neumeister[34] reported greater than 80% success rates with injections of 50 to 100 units into the hand divided equally around each neurovascular bundle (**Fig. 7**). Most patients have experienced an immediate improvement in perfusion and an associated reduction in pain with one injection. The duration of action is unknown, but follow-ups showing no recurrence have lasted longer than 6 years.[34] The case series to date are small, however, and no long-term data are available, but preliminary work is encouraging. The high cost of this drug and issues regarding reimbursement by insurance companies and Medicare remain a challenge for this application. Botox injections for vasospastic disorders remain an off-label use, although clinical trials are underway to verify the benefits.

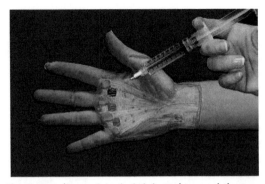

Fig. 7. Botulinum A toxin is injected around the neurovascular bundles around the volar aspect of the metacarpal phalangeal joint. The botulinum A toxin should be injected with preservative free saline.

Arteriosclerotic Disease

Arteriosclerotic disease affecting the smaller arteries of the forearm and hand was unusual 20 to 30 years ago, but with improvements in managing the root causes of vascular disease (diabetes and renal failure) and the other manifestations of it (cardiovascular disease and other large vessel disease), patients with systemic vascular disease are surviving longer. With this longevity, however, an increase in vascular problems in the distal upper extremities has been seen. Another issue that leads to further problems is vascular access procedures for dialysis in the upper extremity. Preexisiting arteriosclerosis is often worsened by arteriovenous shunts placed in the forearm for hemodialysis, which can act to "steal" blood from the hand, leading to ischemia.[35] When evaluating a patient with ischemic disease of the hand from arteriosclerosis, the quality of arterial flow from the shoulder to the hand should be examined. Arterial occlusive disease can exist from the subclavian system to the hand; however, most patients in the authors' practice have severe multivessel disease of the vessels in the forearm, from both arteriosclerosis and vascular access procedures.

Workup of these patients proceeds with a thorough physical examination, with special attention given to the pulses in the upper extremity and the presence or absence of prior vascular access procedures. The presence or absence of gangrene or ulcerations should be noted. The authors perform a complete Doppler ultrasound examination of all the major vessels of the forearm and hand, including the radial, ulnar, and posterior interosseous, to ascertain what is still patent and feeding the hand. The presence of a Doppler signal in a vessel does not mean that vessel has adequate nutritive flow, however. The authors also perform a dynamic Doppler examination of the hand; they believe the gold standard for evaluating these patients remains arteriography. Although other modalities, such as MR angiography and CT angiography, are slowly supplanting direct arterial studies, the authors do not find that these modalities provide enough detail to really evaluate the distal circulation. The authors believe that the primary prerequisite for revascularizing the hand is the presence of some portion or all of the palmar arch. This feature is often not clearly visible in MR or CT studies. Therefore, the authors prefer arteriography. If the arteriogram shows that some portion of the arch is present, they believe that attempting revascularization of the hand is reasonable (**Fig. 8**).

In patients who experience arterial steal syndrome after placement of an arteriovenous shunt, the vascular surgeon and nephrologists rarely want to tie off the shunt. In this instance, if steal can be shown on arteriogram, a reasonable solution is the distal revascularization–interval ligation procedure.[36,37] In this scenario, the shunt is left in situ, but a vein graft is used to jump around the shunt end-to-side from the proximal artery. The artery is ligated just distal to the shunt and the vein graft is then anastomosed into the distal end of the artery going to the hand. In this way the shunt is left open, but now the vein graft actually "steals" from the shunt so that the first branch off the artery (the vein graft) goes to the hand rather than the shunt. The authors have found this procedure to be effective in restoring flow to the hand in the presence of the steal phenomenon.

In the case of occlusive vascular disease of the forearm with an ischemic hand, the authors prefer to perform a bypass from the brachial artery to the wrist or hand level. If a forearm vein is available,

the authors believe that the best option is an in situ bypass, using the forearm vein in a nonreversed fashion through rendering the valves in the vein incompetent (**Fig. 9**).[38,39] The primary reason that this is preferable in the authors' opinion is that the size match is much better than a reversed segment of vein; the in situ vein is large proximally (allowing a large end-to-side anastomosis to the brachial artery) and small distally (allowing end-to-end anastomosis to one of the smaller vessels of the hand). The authors remove the valves with a Leather-Mills reverse-cutting valvulotome, which is passed distally to proximally from either the end of the vein graft or a side branch. All side branches are ligated under direct vision to prevent the formation of arteriovenous fistulae. Once the side branches have been ligated and the valves removed, a large end-to-side anastomosis is performed to the brachial artery, usually just proximal to its bifurcation in the antecubital fossa. Once this is completed, flow is allowed down the graft and is evaluated to ensure all valves are gone. If brisk flow from the end of the graft is absent, an intact or partially intact valve must be sought in the vein graft. Once good flow is established out the end of the graft, it is irrigated with heparinized saline and clamped. After adjusting the length, the distal anastomosis is performed to the chosen distal artery in the hand. The authors have found that the radial artery in the anatomic snuff-box is often patent just proximal to its bifurcation into the princeps pollicis artery and deep palmar arch. Likewise, in patients with severe calcific disease of the forearm arteries, the radial artery in this position is often soft enough to allow passage of the needle on a vascular suture. A standard anastomosis to a calcified radial artery

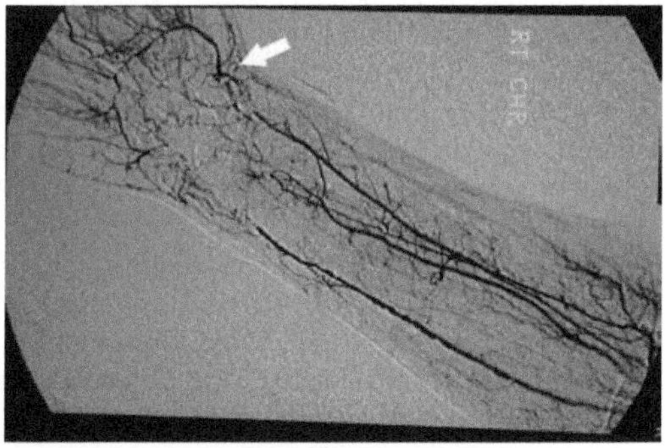

Fig. 8. Arteriogram of patient with diabetes, renal failure, and severe arteriosclerosis. Note multiple levels of narrowing of forearm arteries and no native flow into hand. Arrow points to radial artery in snuff-box, which communicates with patent arch.

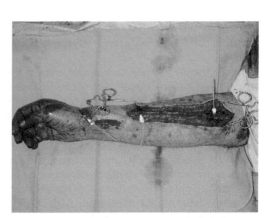

Fig. 9. Intraoperative view of patient undergoing in situ bypass from brachial artery to radial artery in snuff-box for end-stage ischemia. Spears point to proximal, mid-portion, and distal ends of in situ bypass graft with cephalic vein.

is often not possible, and in these instances the authors will usually perform a sleeve anastomosis, feeding the vein graft into the radial artery using 6-0 or 7-0 vascular polypropylene mattress sutures. More discussion of the technique involved in this type of bypass can be found in a previous article.[38] In the postoperative period, the digital ulcers and gangrene are managed conservatively for 6 to 8 weeks. At that time, if the graft is patent, the involved digits can be safely amputated with a reasonable healing rate.

In a review of 26 hands in 21 patients in whom the authors performed a long bypass for chronic ischemia, 23 of 26 grafts remained patent for the follow-up period, which averaged 29 months (range, 1–118 months). Not unexpectedly, however, 52% of patients died during follow-up. Three graft thromboses occurred in the first 3 months, all of which led to major amputation (metacarpal hand or proximal).

Several salvage procedures are available for these patients if bypass is not an option; however, these procedures require that the risks of surgery not outweigh the benefits. If no arch is apparent on the arteriographic study, arterialization of the venous system can be performed. This procedure has been shown to improve capillary bed perfusion through allowing retrograde inflow into the capillary system. The authors' results and those of others have been encouraging, especially in the presence of severe end-stage ischemic disease without any available outflow.[40–42] An increased perfusion and an actual decrease in ischemic symptoms and healing of ulcers can be seen after this procedure. Arterialization of the venous system is to be avoided in patients with active infection; however, the authors have seen two patients in whom the hand became severely edematous, and the infection progressed rapidly after this procedure in the presence of active infection. Both of these patients required amputation of the hand.

The technique is similar to in situ bypass of the hand, because the local arm vein is used. However, the primary difference is that the distal end of the vein is not disconnected nor are the venous branches at the level of the hand and wrist ligated.[38] The valves are removed as discussed earlier via a side branch, and proximal anastomosis is performed to whatever patent vessel is closest. Attempting to remove the valves from the dorsal hand is not necessary, because this can damage these thin-walled veins. The authors have found that the pressure of arterial flow is enough to render the valves in these small dorsal veins incompetent. Patients undergoing this procedure will experience a decrease in symptoms and healing of superficial ulcerations of the digits. The authors do not believe, however, that this procedure is a substitute for revascularization of the arterial system if this can be accomplished.

A final option in patients with end-stage ischemia is to perform microvascular transfer of the omentum to the forearm or hand. This procedure has been used in the lower and upper extremities to augment limb salvage,[43,44] particularly in patients with Buerger disease. In this approach, the omentum is harvested on its gastroepiploic vessels and transferred as a free flap to proximal open vessels (usually in the antecubital fossa for the forearm and hand). It is placed in pockets under the skin of the forearm and hand if possible. However, it may require coverage with a skin graft if the skin is too tight. The authors have seen a return of signals in the native vessels of the hand 3 months after omental transfer, with relief of symptoms and healing of ulcers on the hand. The authors have used this procedure primarily in patients who have ischemic problems posttransplant, because they often will have occlusion of the distal vasculature without any evidence of available outflow via the arch. Again, this complex procedure should not be used instead of revascularization of the arterial system if this procedure is possible. The authors have used it in a few patients in whom bypass or venous arterialization has failed, and it should be considered a backup procedure to these.

REFERENCES

1. Coleman SS, Anson BJ. Arterial patterns in the hand based upon a study of 650 specimens. Surg Gynecol Obstet 1961;113:409–24.
2. Heller F, Wei W, Wei FC. Chronic arterial insufficiency of the hand with fingertip necrosis 1 year after harvesting a radial forearm free flap. Plast Reconstr Surg 2004;114:728–31.
3. Liava'a M, Theodore S, Wagner T, et al. Late presentation digital ischemia after radial artery harvest for coronary artery bypass. Ann Thorac Surg 2009;87: e21–2.
4. Lee HS, Chang BC, Heo YJ. Digital blood flow after radial artery harvest for coronary artery bypass grafting. Ann Thorac Surg 2004;77:2071–4.
5. Manabe S, Tabuchi N, Tanaka H, et al. Hand circulation after radial artery harvest for coronary artery bypass grafting. J Med Dent Sci 2005;52:101–7.
6. Allen RH, Szabo RM, Chen JL. Outcome assessment of hand function after radial artery harvesting for coronary artery bypass. J Hand Surg Am 2004; 29:628–37.

7. Brzezinski M, Luisetti T, London MJ. Radial artery cannulation: a comprehensive review of recent anatomic and physiologic investigations. Anesth Analg 2009;109:1763–81.

8. Sfeir R, Khoury S, Khoury G, et al. Ischaemia of the hand after radial artery monitoring. Cardiovasc Surg 1996;4:456–8.

9. Slogoff S, Keats AS, Arlund C. On the safety of radial artery cannulation. Anesthesiology 1983;59:42–7.

10. Valentine RJ, Modrall JG, Clagett GP. Hand ischemia after radial artery cannulation. J Am Coll Surg 2005;201:18–22.

11. Geschwind JF, Dagli MS, Lambert DL, et al. Thrombolytic therapy in the setting of arterial line-induced ischemia. J Endovasc Ther 2003;10:590–4.

12. Conn J Jr, Bergan JJ, Bell JL. Hypothenar hammer syndrome: posttraumatic digital ischemia. Surgery 1970;68:1122–8.

13. Marie I, Herve F, Primard E, et al. Long-term follow-up of hypothenar hammer syndrome: a series of 47 patients. Medicine (Baltimore) 2007;86:334–43.

14. Hardin CK, Kirk WC, Pederson WC. Osmotic complications of low-molecular-weight dextran therapy in free flap surgery. Microsurgery 1992;13:36–8.

15. Wigley FM, Wise RA, Siebold JR, et al. Intravenous iloprost infusion in patients with Raynaud phenomenon secondary to systemic sclerosis: a multicenter, placebo-controlled, double-blind study. Ann Intern Med 1994;120:199–206.

16. Zimmerman NB, Zimmerman SI, McClinton MA, et al. Long-term recovery following surgical treatment for ulnar artery occlusion. J Hand Surg Am 1994;19:17–21.

17. Leriche R. Surgery of the sympathetic system. Indications and results. Ann Surg 1928;88:449–69.

18. Lifchez SD, Higgins JP. Long-term results of surgical treatment for hypothenar hammer syndrome. Plast Reconstr Surg 2009;124:210–6.

19. Koman LA, Lucas RM, Li Z, et al. Post-traumatic ulnar artery thrombosis: outcome of arterial reconstruction using reverse interpositional vein grafting at 2 years minimum follow-up. J Hand Surg Am 2008;33:932–40.

20. Koman LA, Ruch DS, Aldridge M, et al. Arterial reconstruction in the ischemic hand and wrist: effects on microvascular physiology and health-related quality of life. J Hand Surg Am 1998;23:773–82.

21. Rockwell WB, Hurst CA, Morton DA, et al. The deep inferior epigastric artery: anatomy and applicability as a source of microvascular arterial grafts. Plast Reconstr Surg 2007;120:209–14.

22. Jones NF, Raynor SC, Medsger TA. Microsurgical revascularisation of the hand in scleroderma. Br J Plast Surg 1987;40:264–9.

23. McNamara MG, Butler TE, Sanders WE, et al. Ischaemia of the index finger and thumb secondary to thrombosis of the radial artery in the anatomical snuffbox. J Hand Surg Br 1998;23:28–32.

24. Pomahac B, Hagan R, Blazar P, et al. Spontaneous thrombosis of the radial artery at the wrist level. Plast Reconstr Surg 2004;114:943–6.

25. Richards RR, Urbaniak JR. Spontaneous retrocarpal radial artery thrombosis: a report of two cases. J Hand Surg Am 1984;9:823–7.

26. Piazza G, Creager MA. Thromboangiitis obliterans. Circulation 2010;121:1858–61.

27. Ruch DS, Holden M, Smith BP, et al. Periarterial sympathectomy in scleroderma patients: intermediate-term follow-up. J Hand Surg Am 2002;27:258–64.

28. Tomaino MM, Goitz RJ, Medsger TA. Surgery for ischemic pain and Raynaud's' phenomenon in scleroderma: a description of treatment protocol and evaluation of results. Microsurgery 2001;21:75–9.

29. Koman LA, Smith BP, Pollock FE Jr, et al. The microcirculatory effects of peripheral sympathectomy. J Hand Surg Am 1995;20:709–17.

30. Merritt WH. Comprehensive management of Raynaud's syndrome. Clin Plast Surg 1997;24:133–59.

31. Sycha T, Graninger M, Auff E, et al. Botulinum toxin in the treatment of Raynaud's phenomenon: a pilot study. Eur J Clin Invest 2004;34:312–3.

32. Fregene A, Ditmars D, Siddiqui A. Botulinum toxin type A: a treatment option for digital ischemia in patients with Raynaud's phenomenon. J Hand Surg Am 2009;34:446–52.

33. Neumeister MW, Chambers CB, Herron MS, et al. Botox therapy for ischemic digits. Plast Reconstr Surg 2009;124:191–201.

34. Neumeister MW. Botulinum toxin type A in the treatment of Raynaud's phenomenon. J Hand Surg Am 2010;35(122):2085–92.

35. Malik J, Tuka V, Kasalova Z, et al. Understanding the dialysis access steal syndrome. A review of the etiologies, diagnosis, prevention and treatment strategies. J Vasc Access 2008;9:155–66.

36. Knox RC, Berman SS, Hughes JD, et al. Distal revascularization-interval ligation: a durable and effective treatment for ischemic steal syndrome after hemodialysis access. J Vasc Surg 2002;36:250–5.

37. Yu SH, Cook PR, Canty TG, et al. Hemodialysis-related steal syndrome: predictive factors and response to treatment with the distal revascularization-interval ligation procedure. Ann Vasc Surg 2008;22:210–4.

38. Pederson WC. Surgical techniques for revascularization in the chronically ischemic hand. Tech Hand Up Extrem Surg 1997;1:103–15.

39. Pederson WC. Revascularization of the chronically ischemic hand. Hand Clin 1999;15:629–42.

40. King TA, Marks J, Berrettoni BA, et al. Arteriovenous reversal for limb salvage in unreconstructible upper extremity arterial occlusive disease. J Vasc Surg 1993;17:924–32.

41. Chloros GD, Li Z, Koman LA. Long-term successful outcome of severe hand ischemia using arterialization

with reversal of venous flow: case report. J Hand Surg Am 2008;33:1048–51.

42. Kind GM. Arterialization of the venous system of the hand. Plast Reconstr Surg 2006;118:421–8.

43. Serletti JM, Hurwitz SR, Jones JA, et al. Extension of limb salvage by combined vascular reconstruction and adjunctive free-tissue transfer. J Vasc Surg 1993;18:972–8.

44. McCarthy WJ III, Matsumura JS, Fine NA, et al. Combined arterial reconstruction and free tissue transfer for limb salvage. J Vasc Surg 1999;29: 814–8.

Small Joint Reconstruction of the Hand

Derek L. Masden, MD, Matthew L. Iorio, MD,
James P. Higgins, MD*

KEYWORDS

- Arthroplasty • Arthrodesis of PIPJ • Arthrodesis of MCPJ
- Posttraumatic osteoarthritis of the PIPJ
- Posttraumatic osteoarthritis of the MCPJ

METACARPOPHALANGEAL JOINT RECONSTRUCTION

Anatomy

The metacarpophalangeal joint (MCPJ) is a diarthrodial joint that is critical for functional hand motion and is based on an articulation of the head of the metacarpal and the proximal phalanx. The joint allows for extension, flexion, abduction, adduction, and rotational motion of the proximal phalanx. Extrinsic musculotendinous units and the intrinsic joint elements of capsule and collateral ligaments serve as joint stabilizers during key pinch and static loading.[1]

The capsule of the joint is based on the composite structure of the flexor tendon sheath and the collateral ligaments. Along the volar capsule of the joint, the fibrous volar plate of the flexor sheath is firmly anchored to the base of the proximal phalanx with relatively weak attachments to the metacarpal head. This plate has an accordion-like or thatched structure that allows it to compress with the joint during motion, whereas its counterpart, the proximal interphalangeal joint (PIPJ) volar plate, is much more rigid. On the dorsal and lateral aspects of the joint exist longitudinal ridges that are in continuity with 2 pairs of stout collateral ligaments. The proper collateral ligaments (PCL) originate from the dorsal metacarpal head tubercle and insert along the volar lateral margin of the proximal phalangeal base. The accessory pair of collateral ligaments has a similar origin along the metacarpal tubercle but is more volarly inclined from its origin and inserts along the lateral margin of the volar plate.[1]

Further differentiation of the collateral ligaments is based on the ulnar or radial basis of the PCL. These eccentrically oriented ligaments are the primary stabilizing force against joint dislocation in all 4 planes of movement.[1] The radial collateral ligament is usually more clinically relevant because it is responsible for stability of the finger during pinch and grasp functions.[2]

Unique to the MCPJ is the so-called cam effect created by the nonspherical shape of the metacarpal head. The distance from the axis of rotation of the metacarpal head to the base of the proximal phalanx is greater for flexion than extension.[2] As the MCPJ is brought out of flexion, the collateral ligaments shorten to maintain joint stability by dynamically changing ligamentous length relative to the fixed joint axis. This intrinsic compensatory ability may explain the pathophysiology of MCPJ stiffness and decreased range of flexion after joint trauma or prolonged immobilization in MCPJ extension. Inflammation and decreased motion may decrease the elastic potential of the collateral ligaments, thereby restricting motion that requires a lengthening of the ligaments, such as during active flexion. For this reason, prolonged immobilization and splinting of the hand with the MCPJs in flexion provide a greater chance of return of motion compared with a posture of extension.

The authors have nothing to disclose.

The Curtis National Hand Center, Union Memorial Hospital, 3333 North Calvert Street, Baltimore, MD 21218, USA

* Corresponding author. The Curtis National Hand Center, 3333 North Calvert Street, #200 Johnston Professional Building, Baltimore, MD 21218.

E-mail address: jameshiggins10@hotmail.com

MCPJ Arthrosis

Although traumatic indications and late sequelae of osteoarthritis (OA) may account for many of the indications for joint reconstruction, systemic arthritides, such as rheumatoid arthritis, also deserve special consideration. Unlike traumatic or idiopathic OA, which is usually asymmetric and joint specific, rheumatoid arthritis is a systemic disease that affects multiple joints of the hand in a diffuse manner.

The pathophysiology of the disorder involves an overgrowth of the joint synovium causing secondary deformities with articular destruction and loss of normal soft tissue architecture. The MCPJ develops a posture of volar subluxation, ulnar deviation, and slight pronation. The extensor tendon migrates ulnarly and volarly in relation to the metacarpal head, and active extension, followed by passive extension, is ultimately lost. This migration in turn creates tendon imbalance in the distal digit and may be seen in conjunction with boutonniere or swan neck deformities.[3]

Rheumatoid disease of the hand is a continuous process. Despite severe disease, the hand may still be quite functional for the patient. The residual function is dependent on a delicate balance of the musculotendinous units. As a result, a cosmetic deformity may be a poor indication for intervention and may incur the risk of only worsening function. The alleviation of pain and functional stability should be the primary indicators for surgery in the rheumatoid hand. The perioperative considerations of impaired immune function, wound healing, and the tendency for disease recurrence must always be considered. Because reconstructive options, including arthroplasty and arthrodesis, are frequently dependent on adequate bone stock and healing, the rates of fracture, nonunion, and malunion may be significantly increased, and both the patient and the provider should be prepared for such outcomes.

MCPJ Arthrodesis

Frequently, hand and finger function is not simply limited by a lack of range of motion or strength but by debilitating pain. In the patient in whom active or passive range of motion is limited, arthrodesis may offer the practitioner and the patient an opportunity to markedly reduce the symptoms of a painful joint.

Fusion of the MCPJ can also be applied in other clinical settings. In the laborer with traumatic arthritis, fusion may create a functional grip. By determining the angle that best provides a powerful or stable grip, such as during grasp of a specific tool or instrument, the patient may enjoy a functional reconstruction with a short recovery period.[4] Index finger MCPJ arthrodeses are generally recommended to be performed in approximately 25° flexion. Fusion angles of other digits are planned with a slight cascade of increasing flexion moving ulnarward, which is typically at an increase of about 5° flexion in each successive ulnar adjacent digit.

Consideration is given to arthrodesis if the benefits of pain relief and stability outweigh the cost of loss of motion. The selection between motion-sparing and motion-eliminating salvage procedures is different for each digit. In digits 2 through 5, the MCPJ contributes significantly to total arch of motion (TAM) of the digit. A loss of this motion changes the function of the hand dramatically from baseline. Alternatively, the thumb MCPJ often provides little contribution to the thumb TAM, and arthrodesis at this site is well tolerated. Furthermore, because the hand is a dynamic construct with different needs at the MCPJ between the small to index finger, the fusion of a joint that has increased coronal forces or a tendency toward subluxation, such as the index MCPJ during key or pinch grasp, may be a more stable alternative.

The techniques commonly used for arthrodesis of the MCPJ include plate fixation, Kirschner wire (K-wire) fixation, tension band wiring, and screw fixation.

MCPJ Silicone Implant Arthroplasty

Silicone implant arthroplasty uses a 1-part constrained device for MCPJ reconstruction. The constrained nature of the device allows it to be used in settings of severe ligamentous and articular surface destruction. The rheumatoid joint is an excellent example of the type of pathologic condition in which a constrained device may provide benefit because the surrounding capsular structures may be lax or may require reconstruction, and soft tissues are often inadequate or unable to provide joint stability independently. The 1-piece flexible-hinge design of the device was originally created and popularized by Swanson[5] and is under maximal stress during flexion. His initial results held promise of the use of this implant to serve as a spacer for the development of stability through encapsulation. Multiple studies have continued to show favorable early results but with a possible decline in outcomes after long-term review.

Olsen and colleagues[6] (1994) provided 7-year follow-up data on 60 silicone implant arthroplasties performed in 16 patients with rheumatoid arthritis. The investigators noted continued improvement of passive motion years after surgery but limited active motion (30°) despite longer follow-up. They also noted a high incidence of continued pain (8/16 patients) multiple years after arthroplasty, and only 9 of 16 patients reported satisfaction with their reconstruction.

Kirschenbaum and colleagues[7] provided 8.5-year follow-up data on 27 patients with rheumatoid arthritis with 144 MCPJ silicone implant arthroplasties. The investigators reported stable improvement of ulnar deviation and extension deficit. Although fracturing of 15 of the implants was noted, no patients reported pain at long-term follow-up, and all patients were satisfied with their arthroplasties. Alternatively, Blair and colleagues[8] reported limited improvement in the flexion-extension arc of motion in a longer-term follow-up (54 months average) as compared with preoperative motion (17° increase overall). The investigators also noted a frequent decline of ulnar deviation to preoperative values.

Bieber and colleagues[9] compared the initial postoperative motion of MCPJ silicone implant arthroplasties with a follow-up average longer than 5 years. Their study demonstrated that the ulnar deviation, extension deficit, and total arc of motion again deteriorated at long-term follow-up.

An even longer-term retrospective review of 1336 implants in 381 patients undergoing metacarpophalangeal silicone joint arthroplasty for rheumatoid arthritis was performed by Trail and colleagues.[10] The investigators sought to assess the rate of implant failure and need for revision surgery. Using Kaplan-Meier survival curves based on the terminal events of implant loosening or revision, a total of 1336 implants were identified with 83% survival of the implant at 10 years, and 63% at 17 years. Although the revision rate was very low, the rates of fracture or displacement of the implants was significantly higher (42% at 10 years, 66% at 17 years). This finding indicated that implant failure did not prohibit the construct from serving as a good long-term functional reconstruction. Although the scar tissue surrounding the implant is believed to impart some stability, the study by Trail and colleagues[10] noted that additional soft tissue rebalancing procedures correlated with increased survivorship of the implant.

Less enthusiastic results were reported by Goldfarb and Stern,[11] who reviewed their long-term outcomes of 208 MCPJ silicone arthroplasties at an average follow-up period of 14 years. The investigator's early results demonstrated an improvement in extension and ulnar drift, but they noted an overall decline in function and position over time. The average initial arc of motion improved from 30° to 46° postoperatively but

returned to 36° at the time of follow-up. Extension deficit and ulnar drift also improved postoperatively but diminished at long-term follow-up. In terms of implant survival, 63% were broken and another 22% were deformed at the time of final follow-up. Similarly, pain-free motion was seen in only 27% of the hands, and 38% of patients expressed satisfaction with their hand function.

The use of silicone arthroplasty in the MCPJ has been most widely studied in the rheumatoid population. The initial encouraging results observed with its use have been demonstrated to diminish with longer-term follow-up. Because the enthusiasm for MCPJ arthroplasty in this population has waned, the need for surgical reconstruction has also diminished with the advent of increasingly effective methods of medical management for rheumatoid arthritis. Although much less frequently performed than decades past, silicone implant arthroplasty has remained the standard offering for surgical reconstruction when required.

MCPJ Pyrolytic Carbon Arthroplasty

In an effort to overcome some of the problems associated with silicone arthroplasty, such as implant pistoning, bone and/or implant fracture, and recurrent deformity, efforts have been directed at the creation of a device that might better mimic normal joint kinematics.[12] The pyrolytic carbon arthroplasty device attempts to mimic the normal motion seen in the joint, but its nonconstrained 2-part design must rely on surrounding soft tissue constraints to provide joint stability.

The implant is a synthetic construct engineered from the pyrolysis of hydrocarbon gas, and it achieves an elastic modulus similar to that of cortical bone. This property may allow it to better share loading forces with the proximal and distal cortical bone for implant-bone stress transfer and decrease implant failure, fracture, or wear. In a retrospective review performed by Cook and colleagues,[13] long-term follow-up and functional status of 151 metacarpophalangeal pyrolytic carbon arthroplasties were assessed. Most of these implants were performed for rheumatoid arthritis. At an average follow-up of 11.7 years, the investigators identified a statistically significant increase in the arc of motion from 39° preoperatively to 52° after arthroplasty. In addition, the arc of motion achieved was in a more extended posture (an average of 16° greater extension), resulting in an increasingly functional and extended finger. Survivorship analysis identified an annual failure rate of approximately 2.1% and a 10-year survival rate of 81.4%. Also, radiographic changes indicative of periprosthetic bone lucency and bone erosion were approximately 23% for pyrolytic carbon implants compared with 87% for silicone constrained implants, as reported by Derkash and colleagues.[14] About 82% of implants maintained their original postoperative reduced position. Of 151 implants, 18 necessitated revision due to various reasons, including stiffness, malpositioning of the components, loosening, implant fracture, subluxation, and dislocation.

In a similar analysis, Parker and colleagues[12] reviewed their experience with 142 consecutive arthroplasties using a newer-generation pyrolytic carbon implant in the MCPJ for both OA and rheumatoid arthritis with an average follow-up of only 17 months. Early gains in the arc of motion after implant placement were seen in both groups of patients. Preoperative arc of motion in the OA group improved from 44° to 58° at 1 year, and the rheumatoid arthritis group experienced gains from 32° to 45° in total motion. However, although radiographs demonstrated stable implants in all patients with OA, the rheumatoid arthritis group had a markedly increased rate of axial subsidence and periprosthetic erosions, at 10.5% and 16.4% of joints, respectively. In addition, in those patients with rheumatoid arthritis with more than a year of follow-up, the rate of axial subsidence continued to increase to 55%, and 45% of implants demonstrated periprosthetic erosions.

The pyrolytic carbon joint arthroplasty may offer a durable and biomechanically stable option for joint reconstruction in the patient with modest deformity, whereby joint stability and soft tissue constraints are not markedly compromised.[13] However, given the recent data on short-term follow-up of the newer-generation design, with increasing rates of subsidence, periprosthetic fracture, and joint instability, the pyrolytic carbon implant may suffer from similar long-term deforming sequelae as the silicone implant, especially in the patient with rheumatoid arthritis.

Vascularized Joint Transfer MCPJ Reconstruction

The loss of joint congruity and cartilage integrity after acute injury or chronic attrition of the MCPJ can lead to a painful and stiff finger. Arthrodesis offers reliable pain relief at the cost of motion. Implant arthroplasty offers pain relief with motion preservation with a risk of instability and limited longevity. The concept of autologous vascularized joint transfer could theoretically provide pain relief with lasting stability and motion preservation. Vascularized joint transfer may also provide a ligamentous and tendon/soft tissue reconstruction alternative in addition to the arthroplasty component.

Initially described as a nonmicrosurgical procedure, the PIPJ or metatarsophalangeal joint (MTPJ) of the toe was harvested as an avascular graft and used in the total joint arthroplasty of the MCPJ. The nonvascularized nature of these grafts resulted in cancellous and cartilaginous resorption during the early phase of healing and ultimately the collapse of the construct.[15,16]

Later described by Bunke and colleagues[17] in 1967, vascularized joint transfer may avoid the issues of chronic avascular collapse and synovial degeneration. Modified by Foucher[18] and others, the vascularized joint transfer is usually obtained from either the PIPJ or the MTPJ of the toe. The donor toe joint defect is usually arthrodesed with a bone graft.

Although the procedure has demonstrated a reliable means of providing stabile reconstruction and pain relief, the results in motion preservation have been disappointing. Regardless of use of the MTPJ or PIPJ of the toe as a donor site, the resultant range of motion for digital MCPJ reconstruction in the hand is limited to approximately 30°. The greatest advantage of vascularized joint transfer may exist in treatment of the pediatric trauma patient. The MTPJ, as in the analogous hand joint, has an epiphyseal growth plate at the proximal and distal borders of the joint. These growth plates are in the metatarsal and proximal phalangeal bones, respectively. If the joint is harvested with these growth plates, some continuation of bony growth may be demonstrated in the graft after the joint transfer.[19] Therefore, in pediatric patients with joint damage, including those with epiphyseal damage, joint transfer may offer a reconstructive option that maintains some joint motion and stability and an appropriate anatomic growth potential.

In addition, using the concept of "spare parts" surgery in the setting of multiple digital amputations or crush injuries, the reconstruction of the most functional finger and MCPJ may be aided by using a heterodigital transfer of a vascularized joint from a digit that would otherwise not be saved.[18]

PROXIMAL INTERPHALANGEAL JOINT RECONSTRUCTION
PIPJ Pathology

As with any hand injury, trauma can result in a wide variety of injuries that can affect the PIPJ. Specifically, bony and soft tissue destruction can cause the joint to become unstable, while extended immobilization can contribute to joint stiffness. Bony destruction can range from simple fracture dislocation to total bone loss, whereas soft tissue destruction includes joint capsule disruption or volar plate avulsion leading to instability. The effects of trauma may require immediate joint reconstruction techniques if the fracture is not amenable to conventional reduction and fixation procedures, or delayed reconstruction may be required to address posttraumatic OA.

In addition to these mechanical derangements, chronic joint pain can be the predisposing factor to joint reconstruction. Chronic pain can be a result of idiopathic OA or inflammatory arthritis. As with most treatments, the cause of joint destruction guides the modality of reconstruction.

PIPJ Anatomy

The PIPJ is configured to permit a large range of flexion and extension with limited radial or ulnar deviation. The stability of this joint is achieved via a combination of the bony architecture and the joint capsule. Because of this configuration, approximately 100° motion is capable at the joint. Despite the similarities in function of the 2 joints, the anatomy of the PIPJ differs from that of the MCPJ in distinct ways.[20–22]

Unlike the MCPJ, in which the metacarpal has a cam shape with a volar flare, the proximal phalanx has a bicondylar circular head. The lack of volar flare permits a uniform tension on the collateral ligaments throughout joint motion. However, similar to the MCPJ, the collateral ligaments are composed of both PCL and accessory collateral ligaments (ACLs). Both originate from the condylar recess of the proximal phalanx, with the larger PCL inserting into the volar third of the middle phalanx and the volar plate. The more proximally located ACLs run in a more volar direction and insert onto the volar plate only.

The volar plate of the PIPJ differs from that of the MCPJ. The distal insertion is the strongest, particularly at the lateral margins where the ACLs insert. Paired extensions, called checkreins, extend proximally and insert onto the proximal phalanx at the level of the A2 pulley. These structures limit hyperextension of the PIPJ and provide a strong volar stabilizing force. The PIPJ volar plate does not contract with flexion as the metacarpophalangeal volar plate does but instead slides with finger movement for increased stability during axial loading.

PIPJ Implant Arthroplasty

The primary indication for PIPJ implant arthroplasty is pain from idiopathic and posttraumatic arthritis or inflammatory arthritis. Although this condition provides a motion-sparing option for joint reconstruction, patients primarily seeking improvement in range of motion should be cautioned. Patients with active infection or poor soft tissue coverage or those who have lost the use of the extensor or flexor function are also poor candidates.

Implant composition has undergone numerous changes and evolved since the first description 70 years ago. Currently, 2 frequently used options for PIPJ implant arthroplasty are constrained flexible silicone implants and nonconstrained surface replacement arthroplasty (SRA) options.

Flexible silicone elastomer implants, unlike their hinged predecessors, are implanted as a single spacer. The implant has flexible tapered intramedullary stems that provide stability and a fulcrum for flexion and extension. Lin and colleagues[23] reviewed 69 silicone arthroplasties at an average of 3.4 years of follow-up. The cohort included a heterogeneous group of patients with OA and inflammatory arthritis. The investigators found no significant improvement in motion, but pain relief was achieved in 66 of 69 joints. Ashworth and colleagues[24] followed up 99 proximal interphalangeal (PIP) silicone implant arthroplasties in rheumatoid arthritis cases for an average of 5.8 years. The investigators noted very good pain relief but a loss in average range of motion from 38° preoperatively to 29° postoperatively. These findings were echoed by Takigawa and colleagues[25] in a 2004 study of 70 silicone PIP arthroplasties for an average follow-up period of 6.5 years. This cohort also included a variety of patients with OA and inflammatory arthritis. Although pain relief was very good, there was no significant change for range of motion in postoperative compared with preoperative examinations.

SRA is an alternative to silicone spacers. Similar to other joints, including the MCPJ of the hand, PIP SRA attempts to re-create the normal anatomic geometry of the joint. This arthroplasty uses 2 implants, one that replaces the proximal joint surface and another distal component that allows the implants to articulate. These 2-piece nonhinged implants rely on collateral ligament integrity to maintain PIPJ stability. The first PIPJ SRA was described in the 1990s and includes a chromium-cobalt alloy proximal component and an ultra-high–molecular weight polyethylene distal component.[26] A second type of SRA, made of pyrolytic carbon, is also available. When compared with silicone arthroplasty, SRA has been shown to have analogous results. Particularly with the metal on polyethylene SRA, multiple studies have shown improvement in arc of motion and pain relief.[26,27]

Regardless of implant type, the surgical technique is similar. Volar, dorsal, or lateral approaches may be used, although it has been suggested that better results may be achievable with dorsal access.[26] Osteotomies are made to remove the subchondral base of the middle phalanx and head of the proximal phalanx, taking care to preserve the attachments of the collateral ligaments, particularly with SRA. Implants are chosen after appropriate trials have been selected and inserted in place, confirming adequate motion of the joint.

Regardless of technique or implant material, the range of motion of the PIPJ after arthroplasty is considerably less than an unaffected joint. In 2008, Squitieri and Chung[28] reported the outcomes of their systematic review of finger joint replacement. The investigators found that the mean arc of PIPJ motion for silicone and pyrocarbon (pyrolytic carbon) implants was 44° ± 11° and 43° ± 11°, respectively, with the pyrocarbon group having a considerably higher complication rate. Overall the outcomes for pyrolytic carbon SRA have been varied. Most of the literature indicates that although pyrocarbon arthroplasty may be helpful in reducing pain, there is minimal, if any, improvement in the range of motion of the joint. Nunley and colleagues[29] studied posttraumatic OA PIPJs treated with pyrocarbon implant arthroplasty. At 1-year follow-up, the investigators noted no significant pain relief and loss of motion averaging 10°. These results led the investigators to abandon the implant use and the study protocol. Tuttle and Stern[30] studied 18 pyrocarbon implant arthroplasties in OA joints followed up for 13 months. The investigators noted good pain relief but no improvement in range of motion and a high complication rate. Bravo and colleagues[31] examined 50 PIP pyrocarbon implants at an average of 27-month follow-up in a heterogeneous group of patients with inflammatory, idiopathic, and posttraumatic OA. Pain relief was satisfactory; however, range of motion improved only 7° and the rate of secondary operations was 28%, with 8% patients requiring revision arthroplasty because of complications. Sweets and Stern[32] reported very disappointing results in a 5-year follow-up study of 31 pyrocarbon PIP implant arthroplasties in patients with OA, noting an eventual loss of motion from 56° preoperatively to 28° at longer-term follow-up. Complications were frequent, and patient satisfaction was variable.

It seems that PIP pyrocarbon implant arthroplasty excels greatest for pain relief. This arthroplasty does not provide improvement in range of motion and may be accompanied by a high rate of complications.[28,32] Complications include joint squeaking, subsidence, dislocation, and need for revision.[29,30] Given these limitations, as well as the technical demands of the procedure and relative material cost, the role of these implants may be limited.

PIP Arthrodesis

Indications for PIP arthrodesis are the same as for other reconstructions, with pain and joint instability being the most pertinent. This indication includes severe arthritic pain that limits function at sites where arthroplasty is not an option or has failed or is precluded by joint instability. Arthrodesis can be very successful at relieving pain while still providing the patient with a finger that maintains length and can be functional. For the ulnar digits, fusion may be more unfavorable because it can negatively affect grip strength, and the finger frequently gets caught up in pockets or tight spaces. However, for the more radial digits, particularly the index finger, fusion may provide the patient with a stable digit with effective key pinch.

As arthrodesis is often the last option before amputation, a significant discussion with the patient must take place before surgery. It can be helpful to temporarily splint the joint or immobilize it with a K-wire before surgery so that patients can experience how their hand will function with a stable motionless joint. As with the MCPJ, the amount of flexion for each finger may vary, and this should be adjusted to fit with the patient's needs. Typically the amount of flexion increases from the radial to the ulnar digits, with the index finger being placed in 40° of flexion, 45° for the middle finger, 50° for the ring finger, and 55° for the small finger.

Although there are several techniques for PIP arthrodesis, there are basic components that each must accomplish. Key points may include a dorsal approach that preserves the extensor mechanism and joint capsule to close over hardware. To achieve bony fusion, the articular cartilage must be removed from the proximal and middle phalanx before hardware fixation. This removal can be done in either a cup and cone manner to allow adjustments of the fusion before hardware fixation or an angled resection. Once accomplished, the joint is immobilized until bony fusion occurs (about 6–8 weeks). Frequently used techniques include

K-wire fixation

A combination of multiple crossing K-wires are used to obtain stability at the desired angle and rotation. This type of arthrodesis is the simplest in technique, with comparable rates of nonunion and malunion but higher complication rates.[33]

90–90 interosseous wiring

This technique uses 2 perpendicular steel wire loops.

Tension band wiring

Tension band wiring includes 2 parallel K-wires across the arthrodesis site with a transversely placed interosseous wire through the base of the middle phalanx progressing proximally in a figure-of-eight model along the dorsal cortex of the proximal phalanx. This wiring works to counteract the forces of the flexor tendons and causes compression at the volar surface of the arthrodesis.[34]

Plate fixation

This technique uses a single plate along the dorsal cortex and bent to the desired angle.

Compression screws

In this method, a lag or headless screw is fixed in an axial orientation. This technique is shown to have favorable success compared with other methods of fixation, with the main drawback being the palpability of the screw head; however, this is reduced with the headless screws.[35] This technique is more difficult in arthrodeses performed in significant flexion and is often reserved for extended interphalangeal fusions (ie, distal interphalangeal [DIP] joint arthrodesis).

Volar Plate Arthroplasty

Fracture dislocations of the PIPJ can be unstable if the osseous support of the volar lip of the base of the proximal phalanx is significantly compromised. This instability is directly proportional to the percentage of volar base of the middle phalanx fractured. If less than 20% of the articular surface of the middle phalanx is involved, the joint is typically stable. If 30% to 50% is involved, the joint is tenuous, and greater than 50% is unstable. If the fragments are large enough to permit restoration of architecture through bony fixation, fracture management options are used. If the fragments are highly comminuted and affected and preclude joint restoration, salvage options are considered to achieve joint congruity and stability.

Volar plate arthroplasty (VPA) uses the volar plate to reconstruct the volar joint surface of the middle phalanx and restore joint congruity in these larger nonreconstructible comminuted fractures. This technique can be performed acutely or in a delayed manner.

For exploration and repair, the joint is exposed via a volar approach and hyperextended after release of the collateral ligaments. After removal of comminuted fragments, the volar plate is released from the collateral ligaments and mobilized distally into the defect in the middle phalanx. The plate is then secured with a suture anchor or pullout wire or suture through the middle phalanx. The joint is temporarily stabilized in slight flexion with K-wire fixation for approximately 3 weeks.

Reported outcomes for VPA are satisfactory with better results obtained when surgery is performed in the acute period. In a review of patients with at least 10 years of follow-up after VPA, the average range of motion was 95° when performed within 6 weeks, compared with 78° when performed after 6 weeks.[36] The same senior investigator reviewed results from patients with an average of 11.5 years of follow-up and found that those patients treated within 4 weeks attained a range of motion of 85°, whereas those receiving arthroplasty after 4 weeks achieved a motion of 61°.[37]

In addition, there have been reports of VPA to treat OA of the PIPJ. Although the investigators did not show a difference in range of motion or grip strength, all patients had significant reduction in pain symptoms.[38]

Osteochondral Autografting

Hemihamate arthroplasty provides a reconstructive option for PIP dorsal fracture dislocations in which 50% or more of the articular surface is involved and cannot be restored. This technique involves using a hemihamate osteochondral autograft to reconstruct the base for the middle phalanx and was first described in 1999. The technique can be used acutely or as a salvage procedure. Use of the hamate fragment with articular cartilage attempts to re-create the joint surface of the middle phalanx to restore joint function. This re-creation is possible because of the similarity between the distal dorsal aspect of the hamate and the proximal volar portion of the middle phalanx. The sagittal ridge of the articular surface of the hamate that divides the cartilage contacting the fourth and fifth metacarpals is used to mimic the interfossal ridge of the proximal phalangeal base, which divides the ulnar and radial fossae, respectively.[39]

To determine the amount of hamate required for reconstruction, the PIPJ must first be examined. This examination is done through a volar approach, hyperextending the joint to expose the volar surface of the middle phalanx. Once it is confirmed that the base of the middle phalanx is not suitable for internal fixation, the size of hamate required for reconstruction can be estimated in 3 dimensions. The hamate autograft is harvested via a dorsal approach exposing the distal articular surface with the central ridge between the ring and small finger. Two sagittal (longitudinal) cuts determine the length, whereas the axial (transverse) cut determines the width. The coronal cut through the distal surface of the hamate, which is the most difficult, corresponds to the volar-dorsal dimensions of the fragment. The graft is fixed into place with interfragmentary screws and contoured appropriately. The joint is then reduced, stability is confirmed, and the volar plate and soft tissues are repaired.

Retrospective studies evaluating this technique have shown positive outcomes in both acute and chronic PIP fracture dislocations. After hemihamate reconstruction, active PIP motion ranges from 70° to 85° with low pain and Disabilities of the Arm, Shoulder, and Hand scores and comparable grip strength to the contralateral hand.[40,41]

Other donor sites for osteochondral autografting have been described for reconstruction of small joints of the hand, including the opposing surfaces of the second and third carpometacarpal joints,[42] MTPJ,[43] and osteochondral segments of ribs.[44] The hemihamate reconstruction has become the most widely used and studied technique for replacement of the base of the proximal phalanx.

For injuries related to the condyles of the proximal phalanx, perhaps the most promising innovation was recently described by Cavadas and colleagues.[45] This team performed cadaveric evaluation of the similarities of the ulnar base of the small finger metacarpal with the proximal phalangeal condyles. The investigators demonstrated a similar shape but a greater arc of curvature of 40% to 50% of the donor surface than the PIP condyles. Despite this anatomic discrepancy, the team reported on a clinical series of 16 unicondylar osteochondral reconstructions using this technique with a 4.8-year average follow-up. An average of 49° active motion was achieved in these difficult cases. This finding suggests that this technique may serve as a useful tool in the setting of unicondylar bone loss of the PIPJ.

Vascularized Joint Transfer for PIPJ Reconstruction

Vascularized PIPJ reconstruction involves the transfer of an autologous joint, either from a toe or another finger to reconstruct the PIPJ. The

indications mentioned earlier for joint transfer reconstruction of the MCPJ are also applicable to the PIPJ. The pertinent clinical difference in consideration of vascularized joint transfer for PIPJs is the important contribution of the PIPJ to the digits' total active motion. Achieving minimal motion with such a transfer may be functionally more acceptable at the MCPJ than the PIPJ. Although the studies are limited, it seems that the average range of motion achieved in PIPJ reconstruction (24°) is even less than is achieved in MCPJ reconstruction (32°–34°) using toe joints as donors.[19]

After multiple digital amputations or trauma, a finger joint can be used for transfer from a nonsalvaged digit. In this case, a double osteotomy is performed to isolate the donor joint, with care taken to preserve the volar plate and digital vessels. The recipient site is prepared with extensor tendon preparation and bone cuts, ideally preserving the flexor sheath. The donor joint is inset with bone stabilization via K-wires or interosseous wiring. The flexor tendon sheath is reattached to the donor volar plate, and the extensor tendons are secured by separating into 2 slips, one secured to the central slip and the other to a lateral band.

Heterodigital joint transfers can be performed in the setting of multidigital trauma. Joints from otherwise nonsalvageable digits may be used as pedicled or free microvascular transfers.

If the donor joint is from the same finger, the transfer is termed homodigital DIP to PIP transfer. In this instance, the DIP joint is transferred proximally on its digital pedicle to reconstruct the PIPJ. The finger becomes a 2-joint system but gains motion as the PIP contributes more to the arc of the finger than the DIP.

Reports on outcomes for vascularized joint transfers are few. One study compared the different types of joint transfer performed in 26 patients. These included heterodigital island, homodigital island, free heterodigital, and second toe transfers. The mean active range of motion was 56° for heterodigital island, 52° in the homodigital island, greater than 65° in the free heterodigital island, and only 33° in the second toe transfers. All had significant extension lag ranging from a mean of 21° to 39°.[46] In a series of 11 second toe to PIPJ transfers, the investigators found an average range of motion of 47°, with 41° extensor lag at a mean follow-up of 15 years.[47]

Restoration of stability, resolution of pain, and preservation of motion are ideal goals in the setting of secondary small joint reconstruction of the hand. The surgeon must be familiar with the relative benefits of each of these options and the specific demands of the diseased joint to maximize results and function.

REFERENCES

1. Rubin LE, Miki RA, Taksali S, et al. Metacarpophalangeal collateral ligament reconstruction after band saw amputation: case report with review of MCP anatomy and injury. Iowa Orthop J 2008;28:53–7.

2. Tosun B, Kocaturk M. Chronic posttraumatic rupture of bilateral collateral ligaments of the fourth metacarpophalangeal joint: a new method of reconstruction using a palmaris longus tendon graft. Curr Orthop Pract 2009;20:209–12.

3. Feldon P, Belsky MR. Degenerative diseases of the metacarpophalangeal joints. Hand Clin 1987;3: 429–47.

4. Boulas HJ. Autograft replacement of small joint defects in the hand. Clin Orthop Relat Res 1996;327:63–71.

5. Swanson AB. Flexible implant arthroplasty for arthritic finger joints: rationale, technique, and results of treatment. J Bone Joint Surg Am 1972;54: 435–55.

6. Olsen I, Gebuhr P, Sonne-Holm S. Silastic arthroplasty in rheumatoid MCP-joints. 60 joints followed for 7 years. Acta Orthop Scand 1994;65:430–1.

7. Kirschenbaum D, Schneider LH, Adams DC, et al. Arthroplasty of the metacarpophalangeal joints with use of silicone-rubber implants in patients who have rheumatoid arthritis. Long-term results. J Bone Joint Surg Am 1993;75:3–12.

8. Blair WF, Shurr DG, Buckwalter JA. Metacarpophalangeal joint implant arthroplasty with a Silastic spacer. J Bone Joint Surg Am 1984;66:365–70.

9. Bieber EJ, Weiland AJ, Volenec-Dowling S. Silicone-rubber implant arthroplasty of the metacarpophalangeal joints for rheumatoid arthritis. J Bone Joint Surg Am 1986;68:206–9.

10. Trail IA, Martin JA, Nuttall D, et al. Seventeen-year survivorship analysis of silastic metacarpophalangeal joint replacement. J Bone Joint Surg Br 2004; 86:1002–6.

11. Goldfarb CA, Stern PJ. Metacarpophalangeal joint arthroplasty in rheumatoid arthritis. A long-term assessment. J Bone Joint Surg Am 2003;85: 1869–78.

12. Parker WL, Rizzo M, Moran SL, et al. Preliminary results of nonconstrained pyrolytic carbon arthroplasty for metacarpophalangeal joint arthritis. J Hand Surg Am 2007;32:1496–505.

13. Cook SD, Beckenbaugh RD, Redondo J, et al. Long-term follow-up of pyrolytic carbon metacarpophalangeal implants. J Bone Joint Surg Am 1999;81: 635–48.

14. Derkash RS, Niebauer JJ Jr, Lane CS. Long-term follow-up of metacarpal phalangeal arthroplasty with silicone Dacron prostheses. J Hand Surg Am 1986;11:553–8.

15. Entin MA, Alger JA, Baird RM. Experimental and clinical transplantation of autogenous whole joints. J Bone Joint Surg Am 1962;44:1518–652.

16. Yablon IG, Brandt KD, Delellis R, et al. Destruction of joint homografts. An experimental study. Arthritis Rheum 1977;20:1526–37.

17. Buncke HJ Jr, Daniller AI, Schulz WP, et al. The fate of autogenous whole joints transplanted by microvascular anastomoses. Plast Reconstr Surg 1967; 39:333–41.

18. Foucher G. Vascularized joint transfers. In: Green DP, editor. Operative hand surgery. 3rd edition. New York: Churchill Livingstone; 1993. p. 1201–21.

19. Chen SH, Wei FC, Chen HC, et al. Vascularized toe joint transfer to the hand. Plast Reconstr Surg 1996; 98:1275–84.

20. Kuczynski K. The proximal interphalangeal joint. Anatomy and causes of stiffness in the fingers. J Bone Joint Surg Br 1968;50:656–63.

21. Holguin PH, Rico AA, Gomez LP, et al. The coordinate movement of the interphalangeal joints. A cinematic study. Clin Orthop Relat Res 1999;362: 117–24.

22. Dumont C, Albus G, Kubein-Meesenburg D, et al. Morphology of the interphalangeal joint surface and its functional relevance. J Hand Surg Am 2008;33:9–18.

23. Lin HH, Wyrick JD, Stern PJ. Proximal interphalangeal joint silicone replacement arthroplasty: clinical results using an anterior approach. J Hand Surg Am 1995;20:123–32.

24. Ashworth CR, Hansraj KK, Todd AO, et al. Swanson proximal interphalangeal joint arthroplasty in patients with rheumatoid arthritis. Clin Orthop Relat Res 1997;342:34–7.

25. Takigawa S, Meletiou S, Sauerbier M, et al. Long-term assessment of Swanson implant arthroplasty in the proximal interphalangeal joint of the hand. J Hand Surg Am 2004;29:785–95.

26. Linscheid RL, Murray PM, Vidal MA, et al. Development of a surface replacement arthroplasty for proximal interphalangeal joints. J Hand Surg Am 1997; 22:286–98.

27. Jennings CD, Livingstone DP. Surface replacement arthroplasty of the proximal interphalangeal joint using the PIP-SRA implant: results, complications, and revisions. J Hand Surg Am 2008;33:1565. e1–11.

28. Squitieri L, Chung KC. A systematic review of outcomes and complications of vascularized toe joint transfer, silicone arthroplasty, and PyroCarbon arthroplasty for posttraumatic joint reconstruction of the finger. Plast Reconstr Surg 2008;121:1697–707.

29. Nunley RM, Boyer MI, Goldfarb CA. Pyrolytic carbon arthroplasty for posttraumatic arthritis of the

proximal interphalangeal joint. J Hand Surg Am 2006;31:1468–74.

30. Tuttle HG, Stern PJ. Pyrolytic carbon proximal interphalangeal joint resurfacing arthroplasty. J Hand Surg Am 2006;31:930–9.

31. Bravo CJ, Rizzo M, Hormel KB, et al. Pyrolytic carbon proximal interphalangeal joint arthroplasty: results with minimum two-year follow-up evaluation. J Hand Surg Am 2007;32:1–11.

32. Sweets TM, Stern PJ. Proximal interphalangeal joint prosthetic arthroplasty. J Hand Surg Am 2010;35:1190–3.

33. IJsselstein CB, van Egmond DB, Hovius SE, et al. Results of small-joint arthrodesis: comparison of Kirschner wire fixation with tension band wire technique. J Hand Surg Am 1992;17:952–6.

34. Uhl RL. Proximal interphalangeal joint arthrodesis using the tension band technique. J Hand Surg Am 2007;32:914–7.

35. Leibovic SJ, Strickland JW. Arthrodesis of the proximal interphalangeal joint of the finger: comparison of the use of the Herbert screw with other fixation methods. J Hand Surg Am 1994;19:181–8.

36. Eaton RG, Malerich MM. Volar plate arthroplasty of the proximal interphalangeal joint: a review of ten years' experience. J Hand Surg Am 1980;5:260–8.

37. Dionysian E, Eaton RG. The long-term outcome of volar plate arthroplasty of the proximal interphalangeal joint. J Hand Surg Am 2000;25:429–37.

38. Burton RI, Campolattaro RM, Ronchetti PJ. Volar plate arthroplasty for osteoarthritis of the proximal interphalangeal joint: a preliminary report. J Hand Surg Am 2002;27:1065–72.

39. McAuliffe JA. Hemi-hamate autograft for the treatment of unstable dorsal fracture dislocation of the proximal interphalangeal joint. J Hand Surg Am 2009;34:1890–4.

40. Williams RM, Kiefhaber TR, Sommerkamp TG, et al. Treatment of unstable dorsal proximal interphalangeal fracture/dislocations using a hemi-hamate autograft. J Hand Surg Am 2003;28:856–65.

41. Calfee RP, Kiefhaber TR, Sommerkamp TG, et al. Hemi-hamate arthroplasty provides functional reconstruction of acute and chronic proximal interphalangeal fracture-dislocations. J Hand Surg Am 2009;34:1232–41.

42. Ishida O, Ikuta Y, Kuroki H. Ipsilateral osteochondral grafting for finger joint repair. J Hand Surg Am 1994;19:372–7.

43. Boulas HJ, Herren A, Buchler U. Osteochondral metatarsophalangeal autografts for traumatic articular metacarpophalangeal defects: a preliminary report. J Hand Surg Am 1993;18:1086–92.

44. Sato K, Sasaki T, Nakamura T, et al. Clinical outcome and histologic findings of costal osteochondral grafts for cartilage defects in finger joints. J Hand Surg Am 2008;33:511–5.

45. Cavadas PC, Landin L, Thione A. Reconstruction of the condyles of the proximal phalanx with osteochondral grafts from the ulnar base of the little finger metacarpal. J Hand Surg Am 2010;35:1275–81.

46. Foucher G, Lenoble E, Smith D. Free and island vascularized joint transfer for proximal interphalangeal reconstruction: a series of 27 cases. J Hand Surg Am 1994;19:8–16.

47. Tsubokawa N, Yoshizu T, Maki Y. Long-term results of free vascularized second toe joint transfers to finger proximal interphalangeal joints. J Hand Surg Am 2003;28:443–7.

Reconstruction of the Hand with Wide Awake Surgery

Donald H. Lalonde, MD, MSc, FRCSC

KEYWORDS

- Wide awake hand surgery • Epinephrine finger
- Tourniquet-free hand surgery • Sedation-free hand surgery
- Hole-in-one local anesthesia • Wide awake tendon repair

HOW DO MOST PATIENTS REACT TO BEING AWAKE DURING THE SURGERY?

Most people prefer wide awake hand surgery to having work done on their teeth. The pain is similar if not less with the hand surgery, there is no one working in their mouth, and they do not have to look or listen if they do not want to. Those who want nothing to do with the surgery can look away, listen to music with earphones, or watch movies. As there is no tourniquet used, the patients are totally comfortable. Many patients, if not the majority, are interested in seeing what is happening, and those who are interested are allowed to wear a mask and observe.

Surgeons who have never used the technique often remark, "My patients need sedation." Although some patients are better off asleep or sedated, most prefer the wide awake alternative if it is offered to them in a positive light and if they understand it. After all, most dental procedures are now performed using the wide awake approach, and that is with the surgeon working inside their mouth in which there are airway and communication issues that are not present in hand surgery. Despite these problems, most patients do not want sedation or general anesthesia to have a tooth filled. Patients who have had a wide awake carpal tunnel release feel the same way about their hand surgery.

If patients really need sedation or general anesthesia, it is provided to them. This is in the minority of hand surgery patients, as it is in dental surgery.

WHY DO MOST PATIENTS PREFER WIDE AWAKE HAND SURGERY ONCE THEY HAVE BEEN EXPOSED TO IT?

Most patients prefer wide awake hand surgery for the same reasons they prefer being wide awake when they have a tooth filled. It reduces surgeries like carpal tunnel, trigger finger, operative reduction of fractures, and tendon repairs to the simplicity of going to the dentist. After the surgery, they simply sit up, elevate their totally comfortable hand, and walk out to go home. They never get nausea or vomiting. They get no urinary retention or sedation-induced dizziness. They do not need to get anyone to stay with them or look after them or their children the night of the surgery. They do not have to be admitted to hospital overnight.

They have only 1 visit to the hospital because they do not need to have a second preoperative testing visit. This means that they only need to leave work or get a babysitter one time, the day of the surgery.

They do not need to endure or pay for blood tests, electrocardiography, chest radiography, preoperative medical consultations, anesthesiology fees, or postoperative admissions for the interaction of their medical problems with sedation or general anesthesia.

Many patients do not like to leave control of their faculties to sedation or general anesthesia they do not need to have.

They get to speak to their surgeon during the surgery. The surgeon can answer their questions

Department of Plastic Surgery, Dalhousie University, Hilyard Place, Suite C204, 600 Main Street, Saint John, New Brunswick, Canada E2K 1J5
E-mail address: drdonlalonde@nb.aibn.com

Clin Plastic Surg 38 (2011) 761–769
doi:10.1016/j.cps.2011.07.005

and educate them on good postoperative care and activity as well as return-to-work instructions. They can establish a verbal relationship with the surgeon outside the preoperative consultation.

WHY DO SURGEONS WHO HAVE USED THIS APPROACH LIKE IT?

The surgeons no longer have to wait for an anesthesiologist to do a hand surgery case. The surgery no longer has to be done in the main operating room because all the monitoring required for sedation or general anesthesia is not required. The only 2 medications that are given to the patient are lidocaine and epinephrine, which have now been given to millions of patients in dental offices without monitoring with ultimate safety for more than 60 years. Hand surgery in the office or clinic is more efficient and convenient for the surgeon. Efficiency is increased because of minimal turnover time. Surgeons no longer have to admit and look after patients who underwent hand surgery with medical problems aggravated by sedation or general anesthesia postoperatively.

The initial impetus for the widespread use of wide awake hand surgery in Canada was the difficulty surgeons had in getting hand surgery into the main operating room with an anesthesiologist. The approach is now preferred in many surgeries because watching patients actively move reconstructed parts during the surgery has improved outcomes.[1]

EPINEPHRINE IN THE FINGER FOR HEMOSTASIS DELETES THE TOURNIQUET REQUIREMENT

There was a myth that epinephrine should never be injected into the fingers, nose, ears, and toes. It was based on the theoretical risk that epinephrine caused infarction in body parts with end arteries. The myth originated between 1920 and 1945 and was cemented with the writing of the first American textbook on hand surgery by Stirling Bunnell in 1945. This myth has been clearly shown to be not valid by the following 4 seminal papers and several others.[2–9]

The first of the 4 papers was published in 2007 and traces the root of the epinephrine myth to its true source, procaine.[10] There are 48 cases of finger infarction with local anesthetics in the world literature; almost all of them were before 1950. Twenty-one of those were with epinephrine mixed almost exclusively with procaine. Twenty-seven of those were with procaine without epinephrine. More fingers died with procaine *without* epinephrine than with procaine *with* epinephrine. Procaine

was the first synthetic local anesthetic and replaced injected cocaine in 1903. It was the new caine, hence the term Novocaine. It was the only widely used local anesthetic agent until lidocaine became available in 1948. Procaine was quite acidic with a maximum stability pH of 3.6, less than the physiologic pH of 7.4. It became more acidic as it sat on the shelf.[11] Yellowish procaine that had been on the shelf for some time was injected into patients in the 1940s,[12] as the first law requiring expiration dates was passed in 1979 by the US Food and Drug Administration (FDA).[13] In 1948, the US FDA issued a warning about toxic batches of acidic procaine (Novocaine) that had induced tissue necrosis. One batch had a pH as low as 1, which is extremely acidic.[14] Clearly, aged acidic procaine was responsible for tissue death before 1950 and likely was the cause of the death of the fingers attributed to epinephrine. There is not 1 case of finger death caused by lidocaine with epinephrine in the world literature.[15]

The second paper that ended the epinephrine myth was written in 2003.[16] This paper showed that epinephrine-induced vasoconstriction could be reliably reversed in the human finger with the injection of the α-antagonist phentolamine (available since 1957[17]). This study was performed by the Dalhousie University alumni plastic hand surgeon volunteers. If 1 mg of phentolamine in 1 cc of saline is injected wherever epinephrine is injected, the vasoconstrictive effect of 1:100,000 epinephrine is reliably reversed in the human finger in an average of 85 minutes.

The third paper was a 2-year prospective consecutive clinical series of 3110 surgeries in the fingers and hand with elective epinephrine injection published in 2005.[18] In this 6-city, 9-surgeon study, there were no cases of digital infarction and phentolamine rescue was never required.

The fourth paper was a review of all 59 cases of accidental high-dose (1:1000) epinephrine injection in the finger in the world literature.[19] There was not 1 case of finger death even though only 13 patients were treated with phentolamine. If 1:1000 epinephrine has yet to be reported to kill a finger, it is unlikely that 1:100,000 ever will, especially with the availability of the phentolamine antidote.

Epinephrine in the fingers and hand deletes the need for tourniquet, which deletes the need for sedation, Bier block, brachial plexus block, or general anesthesia. Patients with sedation, general anesthesia, or motor nerve block are mostly unable to cooperatively, comfortably, and reliably move the reconstructed hand and finger structures during the surgery in most cases.

CONTRAINDICATIONS TO EPINEPHRINE IN THE FINGER

If a fingertip is nice and pink before a surgery, it will be nice and pink after the surgery unless the surgeon damages the blood supply to the skin during the surgery. However, if a finger is dusky or blue before the surgery, it may be wise not to use epinephrine.

A surgeon probably should not inject epinephrine in the finger if he does not know about phentolamine, the antidote to epinephrine-induced vasoconstriction. This would be similar to a surgeon who injects morphine when he does not know about naloxone. All that the surgeon needs to know about phentolamine is that 1 mg of the antidote in 1 cc of saline will reliably reverse epinephrine-induced vasoconstriction, as described previously.

HOW TO INJECT LIDOCAINE AND EPINEPHRINE FOR THE HAND AND FINGER SURGERY

The tumescent concept is used. The goal is to get the lidocaine and epinephrine molecules wherever there is likely to be any incision or dissection. Injection of low concentration with large volume is preferred to high concentration of anesthetic agents in nerve blocks. To stay less than 7 mg/kg of lidocaine with epinephrine, the dosage shown in **Table 1** is used.

The local anesthesia can be injected rapidly (painfully) with a 25-gauge needle, as the author did in the first 22 years of his practice, or slowly with a 27-gauge needle and bicarbonate to provide an almost pain-free experience as described in the hole-in-one local anesthetic technique, which means that all that the patient feels for pain is the first poke of the first injection.[20,21] The last 2 references clearly explain with text and film

how to inject a local anesthetic in an almost pain-free fashion.

A large volume is injected in the most proximal location that any dissection is likely to take place to block the nerves distally. For example, for a zone 1 flexor tendon repair in the hand in which the dissection may reach into the palm, 10 cc would be injected at the most proximal of likely incisions as shown in **Fig. 1** to block the distal nerves (see **Fig. 1**). After waiting 15 to 30 minutes to allow for distal anesthesia to set in, the distal parts of the palm and finger are injected for the epinephrine-induced vasoconstriction effect in a pain-free fashion as described in **Fig. 2**. The same technique would be used for the Dupuytren palmar fasciectomy.

The technique of injection for carpal tunnel surgery has been recently described in detail in text and film.[21] **Figs. 3** and **4** summarize the technique; 10 cc is injected between the median and ulnar nerves, and then 7 to 10 cc is injected under the skin down into the palm to tumesce at least 5 mm of skin on either side of the incision.

For tendon transfer such as extensor indicis to extensor pollicis longus, normally 30 to 40 cc of local anesthesia is now injected in the area shown in **Fig. 5**. For trapeziectomy, the radial side of the hand is injected volarly and dorsally as well as in the joint with a total of 40 cc of local anesthesia as in **Fig. 6**. For spaghetti wrist, 100 to 150 cc of 1/4% lidocaine with 1:400,000 epinephrine is

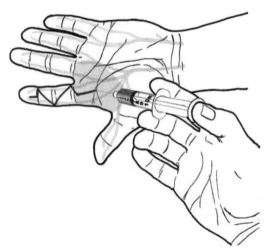

Fig. 1. For flexor tendon repair or the Dupuytren palmar fasciectomy, 10 cc of 1% lidocaine with 1:100,000 epinephrine plus 1 cc of 8.4% bicarbonate is injected into the hand in the most proximal part of the likely dissection to block the distal nerves. (*Reproduced from* Lalonde DH. Wide-awake flexor tendon repair. Plast Reconstr Surg 2009;123(2):623; with permission.)

Table 1	
Dosage and concentration of lidocaine with epinephrine tumescent fluid to be injected in the forearm, hand, and finger	
Volume Required to Tumesce the Area of Dissection	**Concentration of Lidocaine and Epinephrine**
Less than 50 cc	1% lidocaine with 1:100,000 epinephrine
Between 50 and 100 cc	1/2% lidocaine with 1:200,000 epinephrine
Between 100 and 200 cc	1/4% lidocaine with 1:400,000 epinephrine

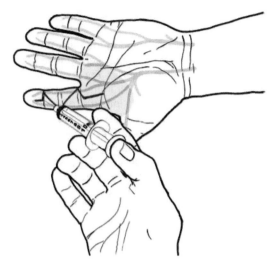

Fig. 2. Secondary injections in flexor tendon repair or the Dupuytren palmar fasciectomy. Another 4 cc is injected between the first injection and the proximal phalanx, 2 cc into the center of each of the proximal and distal phalanges, and 1 cc into the middle of the distal phalanx. (*Reproduced from* Lalonde DH. Wide-awake flexor tendon repair. Plast Reconstr Surg 2009;123(2):623; with permission.)

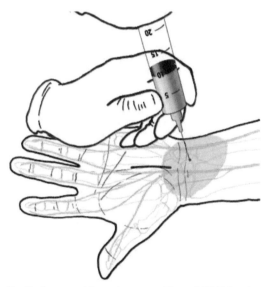

Fig. 3. For carpal tunnel surgery, 10 cc of 1% lidocaine with 1:100,000 epinephrine plus 1 cc of 8.4% bicarbonate is injected very slowly under the skin and under the forearm fascia to bathe the space between the median and ulnar nerves. The needle is moved very little as shown in the film in Lalonde (2010).[21] The tumescent effect of a slowly injected large volume and a nonmoving needle permits the patient to feel the pain of only the first poke of the 27-gauge needle going into the skin (hole in one). (*Reproduced from* Lalonde DH. "Hole-in-one" local anesthesia for wide-awake carpal tunnel surgery. Plast Reconstr Surg 2010;126(5):1642–4; with permission.)

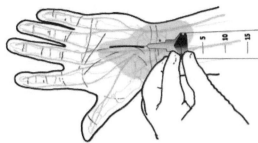

Fig. 4. The final 7 to 10 cc is injected underneath the incision by advancing the needle very slowly without jerking forward and never letting the needle get ahead of 3 to 4 mm of firm, white, tumescent subcutaneous tissue so that the needle never contacts unanesthetized nerves. The goal is to get at least 4 to 5 mm of firm, white, tumescent subcutaneous tissue on either side of the incision. (*Reproduced from* Lalonde DH. "Hole-in-one" local anesthesia for wide-awake carpal tunnel surgery. Plast Reconstr Surg 2010;126(5):1642–4; with permission.)

injected wherever dissection and incisions will take place as shown in **Fig. 7**. For ulnar nerve decompression or transposition at the elbow, 60 cc of 1/2% lidocaine with 1:200,000 is injected wherever incisions and dissection are to be performed (**Fig. 8**), beginning proximally and working distally as in all surgeries.

WIDE AWAKE FLEXOR TENDON REPAIR

The wide awake approach has 4 major advantages to conventional tourniquet methods.

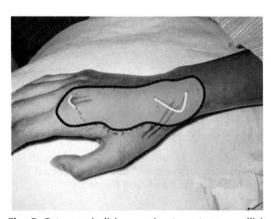

Fig. 5. Extensor indicis proprius to extensor pollicis longus tendon transfer. The blue area is injected with 20 mL of 1% lidocaine with 1:100,000 epinephrine 30 minutes before the operative procedure. Yellow lines indicate incisions. (*Reproduced from* Bezuhly M, Sparkes GL, Higgins A, et al. Immediate thumb extension following extensor indicis proprius to extensor pollicis longus tendon transfer using the wide awake approach. Plast Reconstr Surg 2007; 119(5):1507; with permission.)

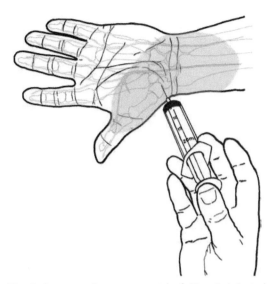

Fig. 6. For trapeziectomy, a total of 40 cc is injected volarly and dorsally as well as in the joint to totally anesthetize the radial side of the hand. (*Reproduced from* video 4 in Mustoe TA, Buck II DW, Lalonde DH. The safe management of anesthesia, sedation and pain in plastic surgery. Plast Reconstr Surg 2010; 126(4):165–76e; with permission.)

1. Intraoperative testing of the flexor repair by the pain-free cooperative unsedated patient ensures that there is no gapping of the flexor repair. After each core suture is inserted and tied, the wide awake patient is asked to flex and extend the finger through a full range of motion. Occasionally, the tendon will be seen to bunch up in the suture with active movement because the suture was not pulled tightly enough and a gap in the repair is identified (**Fig. 9**). Tendon gap is the most common cause of flexor tendon repair rupture. Any gaps revealed in the repair with active movement testing can be repaired before the skin is closed. This intraoperative testing has been documented to result in very low rupture rates in patients with compliants.[1] After seeing no gap with active movement intraoperatively, the surgeon can be confident that postoperative gapping will not likely occur unless accidental excessive forces are applied to the repair and he can be more comfortable about initiating early active movement as opposed to passive movement of flexor tendons such as in the Kleinert or Duran regimes. Bier or axillary blocks paralyze forearm muscles, and the patient cannot actively flex finger tendons during surgery.
2. Intraoperative active movement lets the surgeon see that the repair fits through the pulleys.

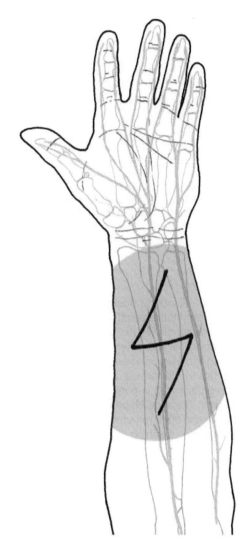

Fig. 7. For spaghetti wrist, 100 to 150 cc of 1/4% lidocaine with 1:400,000 epinephrine is injected wherever dissection and incisions will take place. (*From* Lalonde DH, Kozin S. Tendon disorders of the hand. Plast Reconstr Surg 2011;128(1):1e–14e; with permission.)

If it does not, additional sutures, repair trimming, or pulley division is performed so that there is a full range of movement before the skin is closed. This helps to avoid postoperative tenolysis.
3. Sheath and pulley destructions are minimized, and good 1-cm bites of tendon are permitted because flexor tendons can be repaired through small transverse sheathotomy incisions through which the sutures for intra-sheath/intra-pulley tendon suturing are inserted (**Fig. 10**).
4. The surgeon gets more than a full hour to talk to the patient during the surgery and gets a feeling

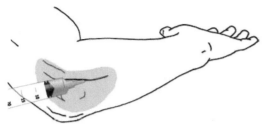

Fig. 8. For ulnar nerve decompression or transposition at the elbow, 60 cc of 1/2% lidocaine with 1:200,000 is injected wherever incisions and dissection are to be performed, beginning proximally and working distally as in all surgeries. (*Reproduced from* video 4 in Mustoe TA, Buck II DW, Lalonde DH. The safe management of anesthesia, sedation and pain in plastic surgery. Plast Reconstr Surg 2010;126(4):165–76e; with permission.)

for the likelihood of postoperative compliance. In addition, intraoperative patient teaching by the surgeon allows the patient to practice the postoperative movement regime in a pain-free comfortable environment. In the author's hospital, this is performed by the hand therapist who participates in patient teaching during the surgery. The sedated patient may not be cooperative and often remembers very little about intraoperative teaching.

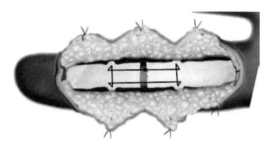

Fig. 9. This tendon has also just been repaired with a core suture that is too loose. This too loosely repaired tendon has been tested with intraoperative full range of active movement of the freshly repaired flexor tendon during wide awake flexor tendon repair. Tendon bunching in the suture has occurred, and a gap has revealed itself. The gap can now be corrected before the skin is closed, and repeated active movement testing will verify that the suture is snug enough to withstand the forces of active flexion. It is better to discover that a core suture is too loose during the surgery when it can be redone than after the surgery when a postoperative rupture occurs. (*Reproduced from* Higgins A, Lalonde DH, Bell M, et al. Avoiding flexor tendon repair rupture with intraoperative total active movement examination. Plast Reconstr Surg 2010;126(3):941; with permission.)

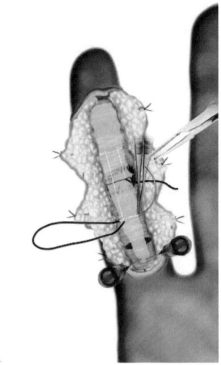

Fig. 10. The needle and thread are passed through proximal and distal sheathotomies to purchase 1 cm of tendon bite without destroying sheath and pulleys. The sheathotomy incisions can be closed with a fine absorbable suture. This type of repair can only be performed in awake patients who can actively test the repair to verify that the suture is only in the tendon and has not been caught inside the sheath. (*From* Lalonde DH, Kozin S. Tendon disorders of the hand. Plast Reconstr Surg 2011;128(1):1e–14e; with permission.)

TENDON TRANSFERS

In tendon transfers such as extensor indicis proprius to extensor pollicis longus or flexor digitorum superficialis to flexor pollicis longus, the tension of the transfer can be tested by the patient with active movement during the surgery to be sure that the transfer is not too loose or too tight.[22] The tension of the transfer can be adjusted by the surgeon to be sure it is just right before the skin is closed.

TENOLYSIS

With tenolysis, the tourniquet-free, comfortable, unsedated, and therefore cooperative patient can use his own muscles to assist the surgeon in performing tenolysis during the surgery by pulling hard on the tendon to rupture adhesions in between bouts of surgical lysis of adhesions by the surgeon. In addition, these patients get to see their final range of active motion in a totally pain-free state at the end of the surgery so that they know where they will end up if they are faithful to their therapy after surgery. As there is no tourniquet, there is no rush for the surgeon to perform this often difficult surgery.

FINGER FRACTURES

In open or closed operative reduction of finger fractures with Kirschner (K) wires, the patient can comfortably actively move the fingers after fixation under fluoroscopy to see if there is enough stability in the fixation to support early protected movement or if further K wires or other forms of fixation will be necessary before the end of the procedure.

JOINT FUSION

In fusions such as of the thumb metacarpal phalangeal joint, the unsedated patient can help to choose the final angle of the joint during the surgery. The patient and surgeon can watch the thumb actively move in all directions after temporary K-wire fixation of the joint during the surgery to verify if the angles are ideal. Permanent angles can then be fixed as desired before closing the skin.

PROXIMAL INTERPHALANGEAL JOINT ARTHROPLASTY AND FINGER EXTENSOR TENDON SURGERY

In proximal interphalangeal joint arthroplasty and finger extensor tendon surgery, such as sagittal band reconstruction or boutonniere surgery, the surgeon reconstructs the extensor mechanism and then sees that he has placed the sutures in such a way that they will support the active range of motion performed by the patient during the surgery. Sometimes the surgeon sees the sutures let go or restrict movement as they have not been placed in an ideal location. He gets the opportunity to replace the sutures in a more favorable location before closing the skin.

TRAPEZIECTOMY FOR BASAL JOINT ARTHRITIS

In trapeziectomy with or without ligament reconstruction, the surgeon can see the patient actively move the thumb during the surgery to see if the metacarpal base is grinding on anything after the trapeziectomy so that adjustments can be made before the skin is closed, if necessary. Many of these patients are older with medical comorbidities. They just get up and go home like after they have been to the dentist as there has been no sedation.

THE DUPUYTREN CONTRACTURE

This surgery is one of the more difficult ones to perform using the wide awake approach because of the close proximity of the digital vessels to the cords. This may not be the best surgery for a tourniquet hand surgeon to start with. Even though the digital arteries are bathed in epinephrine, they continue to pump and their little branches can produce troublesome bleeding during the surgery. Surgeons who love a totally dry field may be a little troubled by this at the beginning. However, the patient gets to see the whole range of motion obtained with his active pain-free movement during the surgery and understands the goal that he can reach with therapy after the surgery.

With needle aponeurotomy, the patients are wide awake in any case. Some prefer to just anesthetize the skin and leave the digital nerves live so that the surgeon is unlikely to cut the nerves with the needle. Others simply anesthetize the whole area as in other wide awake surgeries so that the patient feels no pain during the surgery, the risk being perhaps a higher incidence of nerve injury.

TRIGGER FINGER OR THE DE QUERVAIN RELEASE

In trigger finger, 4 cc of lidocaine with epinephrine is injected in the fat just below the center of the skin incision as the A1 pulley itself does not seem to be tender and does not need to be injected. The A1 pulley is released just enough to allow full nontriggering active movement during the surgery by the patient. This approach is particularly helpful when the swelling in the tendon has prevented full flexion preoperatively. The patient gets to see his finger fully flex and extend during the surgery and knows what is possible after surgery.

In the De Quervain release, 10 cc of lidocaine with epinephrine is injected starting proximally and local injection into the tender tendon sheath is included. Active movement during the surgery by the patient helps the surgeon distinguish the 2 different tendons in the canal and aids with identification and deroofing of separate tunnels within the De Quervain canal.

CARPAL TUNNEL RELEASE

In Canada, more than 70% of carpal tunnel surgeries are now being performed with the wide awake approach.[23] Many of these surgeries have moved outside the main operating room to minor procedure rooms, in which twice as many procedures can be performed in the same time at one-quarter the cost.[23] In the hospitals in Canada, 3 carpal tunnel procedures are regularly performed per hour with just the surgeon and a nurse assistant who also circulates and turns the room over in a minor procedure room. The surgeon gets a full uninterrupted 15 minutes to speak with the totally sober patient to answer questions and discuss postoperative management, how to avoid problems, and return-to-work issues. Patients appreciate this opportunity. The technique of injection and other details of wide awake carpal tunnel release have been described in detail in text and film.[21]

ULNAR NERVE DECOMPRESSION AT THE ELBOW

After decompression or transposition, the patient can take the elbow through an active range of motion so that the surgeon can see that the nerve does not subluxate. The nerve can be supported with sutures, or the operative plan can be changed if subluxation is seen. In addition, patient positioning is unencumbered by the tourniquet or anesthesia apparatus. Now, this surgery is usually performed with the shoulder flexed and the elbow lying comfortably at the level of the patient's face. The hand can be behind the patient's head if this is comfortable for the patient's shoulder. Many patients do have shoulder position discomfort problems, and these problems can easily be accommodated for in the wide awake patient.

COMPLEX SURGERIES SUCH AS TENDON GRAFTING, SECONDARY SURGERY

The opportunity to watch the comfortable unsedated patient move the structures being analyzed adds a new dimension to the surgery. This helps greatly in complex surgeries in which the surgeon is not sure what he will find to reconstruct. An example is a complex maneuver such as tendon grafting. In secondary surgery, this approach has often resulted in changes in intraoperative strategy for the patients for the better. The more complicated the case, the better the patient be wide awake.

CAUTERY, LET DOWN BLEEDING AND HEMATOMA

Cautery is rarely used any more for hand surgery. The skin always bleeds during the initial incisions. However, the field gets the time to dry up and clot before the skin is closed in any lengthy surgery. Larger veins can be tied or clipped. Hematoma

has not been a problem despite no cautery for the past 15 years in brief procedures such as trigger finger and carpal tunnel release.

REFERENCES

1. Higgins A, Lalonde DH, Bell M, et al. Avoiding flexor tendon repair rupture with intraoperative total active movement examination. Plast Reconstr Surg 2010;126(3):941.
2. Wilhelmi BJ, Blackwell SJ, Miller J, et al. Epinephrine in digital blocks: revisited. Ann Plast Surg 1998;41:410.
3. Wilhelmi BJ, Blackwell SJ, Miller JH, et al. Do not use epinephrine in digital blocks: myth or truth? Plast Reconstr Surg 2001;107:393.
4. Andrades PR, Olguin FA, Calderon W. Digital blocks with or without epinephrine. Plast Reconstr Surg 2003;111:1769.
5. Wilhelmi BJ, Blackwell SJ. Epinephrine in the finger. Plast Reconstr Surg 2002;110:999.
6. Johnson H. Infiltration with epinephrine and local anesthetic mixture in the hand. JAMA 1967;200:990.
7. Sylaidis P, Logan A. Digital blocks with adrenaline. An old dogma refuted. J Hand Surg Br 1998;23:17.
8. Steinberg M, Block P. The use and abuse of epinephrine in local anesthetic. J Am Pod Assoc 1971;61:341.
9. Burnham PJ. Regional block anesthesia for surgery of fingers and thumb. Ind Med Surg 1958;27:67.
10. Thomson CJ, Lalonde DH, Denkler KA. A critical look at the evidence for and against elective epinephrine use in the finger. Plast Reconstr Surg 2007;119(1):260.
11. Terp P. Hydrolysis of procaine in aqueous buffer solutions. Acta Pharmacol 1949;5:353.
12. Uri J, Adler P. The disintegration of procaine solutions. Curr Res Anesth Analg 1950;29:229.
13. Available at: http://www.livestrong.com/article/105520-expired-medication-vitamins/. Accessed November 29, 2010.
14. Food and Drug Administration. Warning-procaine solution. JAMA 1948;138:599.
15. Denkler KA. Comprehensive review of epinephrine in the finger: to do or not to do. Plast Reconstr Surg 2001;108:114.
16. Nodwell T, Lalonde DH. How long does it take phentolamine to reverse adrenaline-induced vasoconstriction in the finger and hand? A prospective randomized blinded study: the Dalhousie project experimental phase. Can J Plast Surg 2003;11(4):187.
17. Zucker G. Use of phentolamine to prevent necrosis due to levarterenol. JAMA 1957;163:1477.
18. Lalonde DH, Bell M, Benoit P, et al. A multicenter prospective study of 3110 consecutive cases of elective epinephrine use in the fingers and hand: the Dalhousie Project clinical phase. J Hand Surg Am 2005;30:1061.

19. Fitzcharles-Bowe C, Denkler KA, Lalonde DH. Finger injection with high-dose (1:1000) epinephrine: does it cause finger necrosis and should it be treated? Hand 2007;2(1):5.

20. Mustoe TA, Buck DW II, Lalonde DH. The safe management of anesthesia, sedation and pain in plastic surgery. Plast Reconstr Surg 2010;126(4):165e–76e.

21. Lalonde DH. "Hole-in-one" local anesthesia for wide-awake carpal tunnel surgery. Plast Reconstr Surg 2010;126(5):1642–4.

22. Bezuhly M, Sparkes GL, Higgins A, et al. Immediate thumb extension following extensor indicis proprius to extensor pollicis longus tendon transfer using the wide awake approach. Plast Reconstr Surg 2007;119(5):1507.

23. Leblanc MR, Lalonde J, Lalonde DH. A detailed cost and efficiency analysis of performing carpal tunnel surgery in the main operating room versus the ambulatory setting in Canada. Hand 2007; 2(4):173.

Index

Note: Page numbers of article titles are in **boldface** type.

Moving?

Make sure your subscription moves with you!

To notify us of your new address, find your **Clinics Account Number** (located on your mailing label above your name), and contact customer service at:

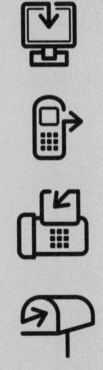

Email: journalscustomerservice-usa@elsevier.com

800-654-2452 (subscribers in the U.S. & Canada)
314-447-8871 (subscribers outside of the U.S. & Canada)

Fax number: 314-447-8029

Elsevier Health Sciences Division
Subscription Customer Service
3251 Riverport Lane
Maryland Heights, MO 63043

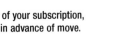

Printed and bound by CPI Group (UK) Ltd, Croydon, CR0 4YY

03/10/2024

01040359-0004